An Inflammation Nation

An Inflammation Nation

**THE DEFINITIVE 10-STEP GUIDE TO PREVENTING AND
TREATING ALL DISEASES THROUGH DIET, LIFESTYLE, AND
THE USE OF NATURAL ANTI-INFLAMMATORIES**

Sunil Pai MD

RocDoc Publications
ISBN-13: 9780692514870 (Custom Universal)
ISBN-10: 0692514872
Library of Congress Control Number: 2015949549
RocDoc Publications, Albuquerque, NM

A Note To The Reader

The information contained in this book is for educational purposes and is not intended to replace individualized, direct medical advice or care by your current health-care professional. If you are taking medications or have health concerns, please consult with your health-care provider prior to making any lifestyle changes or implementing any recommendations in this book. However, if you feel that your current physician will not respond favorably to your request for assistance in implementing any of the lifestyle changes contained within this book, you may wish to seek out a physician trained in integrative medicine who will. Although the information presented herein will place you on a healthier path, your individual needs and specific requirements may vary; thus, a team approach with a qualified medical professional is highly recommended. Throughout the book, dietary recommendations, products, and therapeutic modalities have not been approved by the FDA are denoted by an asterisk (*). The Food and Drug Administration has not evaluated these statements, and "these products are not intended to diagnose, treat, cure, or prevent disease." However, since the products discussed in the book are foods, natural dietary supplements, and traditional cultural medicines, thousands of years of historical use, current scientific evidence, and positive clinical outcomes support our continued use of these natural medicines and integrative treatment modalities.

Sunil Pai, MD, is an internationally recognized medical doctor, expert, health influencer, and specialist in integrative medicine as well as a sought-out motivational lecturer on integrative medicine and holistic health. In addition, he conducts training programs for other integrative-medicine doctors and clinics. Dr. Pai is also a deacon of Priory of Santa Fe, Native Health Service Providers. The information herein is given as health and life-style educational information only and is provided by his position as deacon. This teaching is constitutionally protected through our freedom of religious practices, including practices that *incorporate all-natural health and healing modalities*—both historical and current—to provide these options for health to all people worldwide. The purpose of the Priory of Santa Fe is to provide safe haven and a sacred space in which Holistic/Integrative health-care, as instruments of the Creator, can gather together and share their gifts, vision, faith, in fellowship as well as their experiences. It is the belief of the Priory of Santa Fe that Indigenous Medicine Principles known and unknown as well as all forms of Religious Healing Principles known and unknown, are ordained by the Creator.

House of Sanjevani is an Integrated Auxiliary of the Priory of Santa Fe, a Title 26 Section 508 (c)(1)(a) church, a Special Ministry, Medical Diocese. Therefore, proceeds from our services, sales of this book, and sales of products from our website and lifestyle center recommended herein help continue our mission to protect indigenous medicines and other healing modalities and to promote the right of all people to choose natural healing as part of their overall health care.

In addition to being an integrative MD and deacon of the House of Sanjevani, Dr. Pai enjoys hobbies that include playing guitar and drums. Since the book contains over seven hundred references and scientific data, musical quotes have been used within each chapter to evoke thought, emotion, or ideas. These quotes are for entertainment purposes only and do not reflect the views of the artist, the content of the section that they accompany, or imply endorsement. They are provided to enhance learning, since music is an educational tool that we all can relate to and a fun way to remember new information.

Asatoma Ma Sadgamaya

Asato ma sadgamaya
tamaso ma jyotirgamaya
mrtyor ma amrtam gamaya
Om shantih shantih shantih

Brihadaranyaka Upanishad 1.3.28

Translation of "Asatoma Ma Sadgamaya"

Lead me from death to life,
from falsehood to truth.
Lead me from despair to hope,
from fear to trust.
Lead me from hate to love,
from war to peace.
Let peace fill our heart, our world, our universe.
Peace, peace, peace.

—Adapted from the Hindu Upanishads by Satish Kumar

Native American Prayer

Great Spirit,
Give us hearts to understand
Never to take from creation's beauty more than we give,
Never to destroy wantonly for the furtherance of greed,
Never to deny to give our hands for the building of earth's beauty,
Never to take from her what we cannot use.

Give us hearts to understand
That to destroy earth's music is to create confusion,
That to wreck her appearance is to blind us to beauty,
That to callously pollute her fragrance is to make a house of stench,
That as we care for her she will care for us.

Give us hearts to understand
We have forgotten who we are.
We have sought only our own security.
We have exploited simply for our own ends.
We have distorted our knowledge.
We have abused our power.
Great Spirit,
Whose dry lands thirst,
Help us to find the way to refresh your lands.

Great Spirit,
Whose waters are choked with debris and pollution,
Help us to find the way to cleanse your waters.

Great Spirit,
Whose beautiful earth grows ugly with misuse,
Help us to find the way to restore beauty to your handiwork.

Great Spirit,
Whose creatures are being destroyed,
Help us to find a way to replenish them

Great Spirit,
Whose gifts to us are being lost in selfishness and corruption,
Help us to find the way to restore our humanity.

Christian Prayer

Lord, please walk beside me through this day.
Clear the heavy air with the lightness of Your Presence.
Guide my hands and steady my heart that I may give comfort
When I cannot give hope, that I may give relief when I do not have a cure,
And that I may radiate Your healing peace when the limits of science, time,
and the human body overwhelm us all.
Amen.

Table of Contents

Acknowledgments xvii
Forward xix
Introduction xxi

Chapter 1 1
Inflammation— The Common Link To All Diseases 1
What Is Inflammation? 2
Types of Inflammation 3
Conventional Medicine vs. Integrative Medicine 6
The Integrative-Medicine Approach 9
Inflammation 101: The Triggering Mechanism
That Makes Any Disease Worse 10

Chapter 2 14
An Introduction: Ten Steps to Optimum Health And Longevity 14
Point of Entry: The GI Tract 15
Point of Entry: Screening in the GI Tract 16
Probiotics: The GI "Foot Soldier" Cells 23
GI Tract: The Command Center Where 80 Percent of
Your Immune System Resides 25
The Genetic Misunderstanding 30
Food and Nutrition: The Foundation of Health 34
Not Eating Enough Vegetables and Fruits—Eating Too Much Refined
Wheat, Refined Sugar, and Animal Proteins, Fats, and Oils 35

Chapter 3. 37
    The Ten-Step Approach to Optimum Health and Longevity. 37
    STEP 1: Eating an Organic, Non-GMO, Plant-Based,
    Anti-inflammatory Diet. 37
    The GMO Myth: Are GMOs Really That Bad for
    You and the Environment? 37
    Top GMO Foods to Avoid and What You Must Eat Organic. 43
    Tips for Healthier Shopping Choices. 45
    What Are We Eating? 47
    Pro-inflammatory (Animal Proteins) vs.
    Anti-inflammatory (Plant-Based Proteins) 51
    Anti-inflammatory Proteins = Plant-Based Proteins
    (Have No Cholesterol and Contain Protein, Fiber,
    Antioxidants, and Phytonutrients) 52
    Pro-inflammatory Proteins = Animal Proteins
    (Contain Cholesterol, Cause Inflammation, Have
    No Fiber, Have Few Antioxidants, and Have No Phytonutrients). 54
    Omega-6s: The Pro-inflammatory Cascade .55
    Omega-3s: The Anti-inflammatory Cascade .58
    Omega-3s: What about Fish?. 61
    Wild Caught vs. Farmed. 63
    What about the Mediterranean Diet?. 64
    Omega-3s: What about Fish-Oil Supplements?. 66
        Fish-Oil Processing. 67
        Fish-Oil Potency 68
        Fish-Oil Purity and Safety 69
        Ethyl Esters vs. Natural Triglycerides 72
        What about Salmon Oil?. 73
        Krill Oil vs. Fish Oil. 75
        Fishy Labeling. 78
    Omega-3 Supplements: What to Avoid. 79
    What about Omega-3s for Vegetarians or Vegans?. 79
    So what are the best sources of plant-based EPA and DHA? 80
    SAD = Inflammation Overload 81
    Cheap Food: The Common Denominator for
    Expensive Health Care 83

Farm Raised vs. Factory Farmed 87
The Grass Is Not Greener on the GMO Side. 92
"Where's the Beef?" Not in Your Burgers!. 93
Keep Your Eyes on the Fries 94
"When Pigs Fly"—Is Your Pork from China? 95
Ditto Foods. 98
Colorless, Odorless, Tasteless 99
Winner, Winner, Chicken Dinner?. 100
Chicken of the Sea: Is Seafood a Healthier Option? 102
Moo Gloo 103
Factory Farms: A Clear and Present Danger 105
Foodborne Illness: More Common Than You Think. 106
Dietary Protein and Cancer 109

Chapter 4. 118
STEP 2: Testing What Is Triggering Inflammatory
Responses in Your Body. 118
1) Contact Allergies: The Inflammation That We Touch 118
2) Inhalant Allergies: The Inflammation That We Breathe. 123
Allergy-Drops Therapy: Safer, More Accurate, and More
Convenient. 125
Skin-Prick Testing vs. Blood Testing. 126
SAAT (Soliman Auricular Acupuncture Treatment) 129
3) Food Allergies: The Most Important Triggers of
Systemic Inflammation. 131
    My Personal Experience with Food Allergies 133
    The Factors That Contribute to Inflammation from Foods . . . 135
Inflammation's Four Favorite Targets 138
The Levee Point. 150
The Wheat Misunderstanding: Not the Root of All Illness 151
    Gluten Sensitivity and Celiac Disease 155
The Paleo Myth: Caveman Thinking Sold to the Masses. 160
What Do I Do with the Results of Laboratory
Testing for Sensitivities? 165
ADHD/Behavior Problems in Children and
Psychiatric Problems in Adults 166

Chapter 5. 170
     STEP 3: Detoxification—Clearing the Toxins 170

Chapter 6. 174
     STEP 4: Avoid Smoking. 174

Chapter 7. 178
     STEP 5: Avoid NSAIDs—The Unknown Dangers. 178
     What Are the Side Effects of NSAIDs?. 181
         Common Reactions (Side Effects) of NSAIDs 182
         Serious Reactions (Side Effects) of NSAIDs. 183
     The Black-Box Warning—Your Worst Nightmare. 184
     The Black-Box Warning—The Unknown,
     Unconsented Agreement 188

Chapter 8. 195
     STEP 6: Decrease Inflammation through
     the Use of Bosmeric-SR. 195
     What Is Bosmeric-SR? 195
     What Are the Benefits of Bosmeric-SR? 196
     How Does Bosmeric-SR Work?. 196
     What Makes Bosmeric-SR So Effective and Different from
     Other Natural Anti-inflammatories?. 199
     Curcumin C3 Complex. 201
     Curcumin—A Vital Component of Turmeric. 202
     Curcumin: Activities and Actions. 203
     Curcumin: A Natural Pharmaceutical without
     Side Effects? 205
     Conditions Helped by Curcumin 208
     What Form of Curcumin Is Best for Me? 208
     What about Generic Curcumin Extract Standardized to
     95 Percent Curcuminoids?. 210
     All That Glitters Is Not Gold: All That Is Yellow Is
     Not Curcumin C3 Complex 211
     What about the Newer Forms of Curcumin
     That Claim to Be Better Absorbed?. 213

Bioavailability: A Path and Not a Destination 213
Turmeric Cultivation and Processing: What Is Best? 217
How Much Curcumin C3 Complex Should One Take?............. 222
What about Taking Curcumin Products during Chemotherapy,
Radiation, or Imaging Such as CT and PET Scans? 223
Boswellia: Activities and Actions 226
Which Boswellia Extract Is Best for Me?.......................... 228
Boswellia serrata—Boswellin PS: The New Gold Standard 229
How Much Boswellin PS Should I Take?........................... 230
Ginger and Gingerols.. 230
Ginger: Activities and Actions.................................... 231
What about Ginger Supplements—Which Is Best for Me?......... 233
Black Pepper—Not Just the Other Shaker on the Table............ 234
BioPerine: Activities and Actions 236
How Much BioPerine Should I Take in a Supplement?............. 237
Can Black Pepper Be Dangerous? 237
What Is the Recommended Dosage of Bosmeric-SR? 238
Why Is the Price So Different from Other
Products with Similar Ingredients?............................... 239
What about Other Similar Turmeric and
Boswellia Combinations?... 240

Chapter 9.. 243
STEP 7: Increase Immune-System Functioning 243
Vitamin D3 244
Beta Glucans 248
Physical Vascular Therapy—BEMER 250

Chapter 10... 254
STEP 8: Maintain Healthy Glucose Levels and Avoid
Excess Sugar and Salt.. 254
Sugar and Health-Care Costs 255
Sugar and Addiction 258
Sugar and Aging 259
Sugar and Appetite Suppression.................................. 259
Sugar and Heart Disease 260

Sugar-Sweetened Beverage Consumption Increases the Risk
for Both Diabetes and Heart Disease 261
Sugar and Childhood Learning 262
Sugar and Childhood Behavior (or, More Accurately,
Misbehavior) 264
Sugar and Childhood Obesity 265
Sugar and Dental Cavities 266
Sugar, the Immune System, and Inflammation 266
The Unsweet History of Sugar 267
Disparities in Sugar-Sweetened-Beverage Consumption 268
Keeping Healthy Blood-Glucose Levels 269
Sugar and Cancer 273
What about Natural Sugars? 276
Artificial Sweeteners—Are They Effective and Safe? 279
The Question of Salt 281
Is All Salt the Same? 283

Chapter 11 286
STEP 9: Stress Reduction through Meditation and Yoga 286
Sympathetic vs. Parasympathetic Response 287
The Benefits of Yoga 291
The Benefits of Meditation 294
Sanjevani REST Pod 296
BIO-WELL and BIOCOR 301

Chapter 12 304
STEP 10: Love, Happiness, Social Relationships, Faith, and
Spiritual Practices 304

Chapter 13 310
Summary: Moving Forward and Taking Action 310
Side Notes 313
Functional Medicine 313
Acid Blockers 313
Sanjevani Acid-Blocker Support 316
Dr. Pai's Recommended Laboratory Testing 317

Manufacturing of Probiotics 318
Natural Antimicrobial Support............................... 323
Sanjevani Immune Support Protocols 324
Books and Movies 328
Growing an Inexpensive Garden and Growing Boosters 330
Safer Alternatives for Weed and Bug Control 330
Omega-3 Recommendations................................. 331
Water Filtration.. 334
Structured Water 334
Humic and Fulvic Acids 335
Cosmetics and Body-Care Products 338
Sinus Polyps and Surgery.................................... 340
Exelon Patch... 341
Absolute Risk Versus Relative Risk with Statins and Other
Medications 343
Preemptive Protocols for Food Allergies 344
Plant-based Health Shakes 345
Detoxification Support Protocols............................. 346
Therapies to Help with Anxiety, Depression, and Insomnia 348
Curcumin C3 Complex* In Bosmeric-SR 350
Boswellin PS in Bosmeric-SR................................. 356
Ginger Elixir Recipe 357
Ginger in Bosmeric-SR...................................... 358
BioPerine in Bosmeric-SR.................................... 358
BEMER Physical Vascular Therapy Device..................... 359
Neuro-acupuncture... 360
Peripheral Neuropathy Protocols............................. 361
Sanjevani Intensive Support Pack............................. 361
Sole Protocol 362
Bio-Well and Biocor... 362

References... 367
About the Author 423

Acknowledgments

would like to thank the following: My mentors, Dr. Deepak Chopra and Dr. Andrew Weil who pioneered the field of integrative medicine. Dr. Chopra inspired me to return to my roots of Ayurveda and mind-body medicine. Dr. Weil created the formal postgraduate training program in integrative medicine which has allowed me to practice medicine with a holistic approach. My grandmother and grandfather for helping to raise me and introducing me to cultural practices, belief systems, and foods that helped shaped the way I live and practice today. My mom and dad for their support and encouragement in helping me pursue my personal interest in integrative medicine. Despite our cultural expectations of "just being a regular doctor," sixteen years ago they allowed me to join the first formal fellowship integrative medicine training program in the United States and become the youngest practitioner in the country. My brother, who is visually impaired taught me that through hard work and perseverance one can overcome all odds, including physical hardship and social stereotypes. Maureen Sutton—who has been my partner (and greatest supporter) in my journey of taking Sanjevani to an international level by providing a gold standard for the future of holistic health care, education, and services—for ensuring that I stick to my core beliefs and preventing me from compromising my values and goals. Princess Winnie, our Sanjevani therapy dog, for teaching me patience and always providing me with unconditional love. All my patients who have placed their trust and belief in Sanjevani and me—I thank them for taking this journey with me, improving their health conditions despite the odds and what the conventional health-care providers told them, and proving that almost all conditions can be improved and even reversed. Finally, the Great Creator, Mother Earth, and Father Sky for providing us this beautiful blue planet that we live on. Hopefully this book directly and indirectly will provide guidance for everyone to help conserve, preserve, and be thankful for all that we have received and to always work together toward the preservation of health, community, and our environment.

Forward

have known Dr. Sunil Pai since he was a medical student at the University of Arizona doing a rotation in the integrative medical clinic I directed. Later, as a family medicine resident, he spent more time with the University of Arizona Center for Integrative Medicine, and on completing his residency, began our intensive fellowship training. From our first meeting he expressed a deep desire to learn and incorporate the integrative approach into his practice.

Over the two-year fellowship, Sunil was an excellent student who was able to apply new ideas and therapies to his patients with ease and skill. He was quick to challenge the conventional medical system, always working to improve outcomes and increase patient satisfaction. Sunil graduated at the top of his class, becoming the youngest integrative medicine fellow in the country. Since then, he has – as I have done – pushed the boundaries of his profession and traveled the world to gain first-hand experience of traditional systems of healing and treatments used in other cultures.

I have been working for more than 40 years to educate the public and my medical colleagues about the need to shift our health care system from disease management to prevention and health promotion. American health care is in crisis and faces total collapse due to increasing and uncontrollable costs of dependence on high-tech interventions (including pharmaceutical drugs) and our inability to curb epidemics of lifestyle-related conditions like obesity, diabetes, and hypertension. Integrative medicine offers safe, effective, and low-cost strategies to solve these problems and create a new kind of health care for the future. I consider Sunil Pai a leader in this transformation.

In *An Inflammation Nation* he draws on the best scientific evidence to demonstrate the causative role of chronic inflammation in many of the diseases that kill and disable people prematurely and absorb most of our health care spending. And he tells us what we can do to contain it, giving practical, evidence-based information about foods, dietary supplements, and natural remedies. He argues for the benefits of a plant-based diet to optimize health and takes us on an investigative journey to dispel common myths and misinformation about both conventional and alternative medicine. The natural solutions he recommends for common health problems are easy to follow and use on a daily basis.

As a mentor of Sunil Pai early in his professional development, I am more than pleased to see the direction his career has followed. I know that the book he has written will be of great help to readers.

Andrew Weil, MD
Tucson, Arizona
January 2016

Introduction

What if all diseases—from Alzheimer's disease to heart disease, colitis, arthritis, and breast, prostate, and colon cancers—all had a common link that could be addressed by one single approach? What if you could easily improve your current health, prevent the onset of disease, and decrease the risk of future health problems? What if you could reduce the number of prescription drugs you take (which only treat symptoms) and actually *fix* the underlying cause of disease, imbalance, or dysfunction with simple lifestyle and dietary choices and the use of natural medicines and supplements?

You can; it's easy, and I'm going to show you how!

Two fundamental truths of medicine are these: you can treat, reverse, and improve almost every single health condition that you have, and you can prevent and decrease the odds of encountering disease throughout your life.

You may ask, "If there is such a simple way to optimum health, why haven't my doctors, health-care institutions, or pharmaceutical and insurance companies told me about it?" By reading this book you will see that all these systems that have been created *"for your health"* were not put in place to give you simple solutions. They are in fact complex systems that lead you away from the simple solutions.

Health is a journey, and the best part of this journey is that you are in charge of your destination. Think of this book as a guide for your journey; it will not only change your health immediately but will change the way you look at health care, insurance, food, pharmaceutical and dietary supplement industries. I want to help provide you with life-changing solutions that will move you into the direction of optimum health and longevity. I congratulate you on taking these important first steps toward health, happiness, and healing!

Sunil Pai, MD

CHAPTER 1

Inflammation— The Common Link To All Diseases

Something is burning, baby, are you aware?
— Bob Dylan

The common link among almost every disease, and the factor that causes the progression of those diseases, is *inflammation*. From allergies to asthma, from fibromyalgia to arthritis, from colitis to cancer, research now suggests and demonstrates that most, if not all, disease begins and worsens with inflammation.

Regardless of where they are localized in the body and the names that we have given them, all diseases lead back to inflammation. All fields of health science—cellular biology, physiology, biochemistry, and immunology—have been pointing to inflammation as *the* common link to disease for over a decade.

However, inflammation is not always the *cause* of disease; it is always the *trigger mechanism* that makes every health condition worse. In fact, if you want to live a long and healthy life, you must keep your inflammation as low as possible. Research now shows that inflammation not only worsens disease but also accelerates aging. Of the lifestyle factors that can help us reach an age of one hundred, it is the easiest to change.

Our chromosomes, the structures that carry our DNA, are typically in a shape of an X. Our telomeres are caps at the ends of our chromosomes that protect our DNA from damage. Over time, through a variety of environmental influences, these telomeres shorten. The more quickly they shorten, the faster we age, and the sooner we die. Therefore, the way to increase our lifespan is to increase our telomeres or, more importantly, to prevent them from shrinking. Think of your chromosomes as your legs and the telomeres as your running shoes. When running a race over time your shoes will wear down. Once you have no more soles on the bottoms of your shoes, you can no longer run, and your race is cut short. By keeping your telomeres longer and stronger, you help slow down the wear and tear of your running shoes, and you can stay in the race for a longer time and cross the finish line. Telomere length has been at the forefront of antiaging research. Recent studies, however, show that inflammation level is an even better predictor of successful health and aging.[1]

When we investigate traditional medicines such as Ayurveda (traditional medicine from India that has been practiced for over five thousand years), these ancient texts describe most of the common diseases that we still see today as inflammatory responses. As an expert in integrative medicine, I incorporate healing modalities from these ancient traditions and integrate them with current scientific research that points to the same conclusion. We are not inventing anything new here; we are rediscovering what people have already known for thousands of years.

What Is Inflammation?

I'm on fire.
— BRUCE SPRINGSTEEN

Inflammation is a fundamental pathologic process. It consists of a dynamic complex of cellular changes that are visible only under a microscope. These changes include cellular infiltration and mediator release, which occurs in the affected blood vessels and adjacent tissues in response to an injury or abnormal stimulation caused by a physical, chemical, or biological agent. Inflammation includes the local reactions and resulting morphologic changes, the destruction or removal of the injurious material, and the responses that lead to repair and healing.

Although that definition sounds very scientific, inflammation is simply a process in which the body responds to a variety of environmental and physical conditions (both good and bad). Through these responses, the body goes on the defensive and either destroys or repairs itself.

As the United States has been engaged in wars over the past decade, and most people watch or read about them on a daily basis, it (unfortunately) is easy to use military analogies to describe complex medical processes in a simplified way.

In our bodies there are certain cells that help our immune systems. I like to call these cells our "soldier cells," made up of the army, navy, air force, marines, and Special Forces. These "soldier cells" exist to protect and defend our bodies against foreign invaders—infections such as viruses, bacteria, yeasts, and parasites. We also have subsets of service people, such as the Army Corps of Engineers, which help build infrastructure (things like walls, levees, and fences) not only to keep the system running but also to keep invaders out.

Our immune system comprises the total strength of all of these "armed forces" working together to protect our bodies from foreign invaders and to help repair any damage that occurs during attack or normal wear and tear.

Two types of inflammation affect our bodies. Our "armed forces" can address both, but if they're under attack for too long, our soldier cells can wear down, causing many of the chronic health issues most of us face today.

Types of Inflammation
Acute = helpful (in most cases)
Chronic = harmful

Let's start with acute inflammation. Acute inflammation is usually helpful. With an acute injury, inflammation protects the body from further injury and aids in repair and healing.

When you sprain your ankle, for example, your immune system immediately releases inflammatory chemicals called cytokines. These cytokines include NF-kB, interleukin-6, TNF-alpha, interleukin-1 beta, and C-reactive protein—to name a few. These inflammatory signals in the body then cause swelling and stimulate particular soldier cells (white blood cells) to help

3

defend and protect the injured area from infection and further injury. These cells also assist in the repair of any damaged tissues. With an acute injury like an ankle sprain, the body uses inflammation to actively and immediately stabilize the situation and start healing it. A fever during a viral or bacterial infection acts in the same way. Viral or bacterial infections are sensitive to temperature; they thrive at normal body temperature and cannot survive higher temperatures. Our soldier cells however are more tolerant of these changes and actually turn up the heat of the blood so they can gain the advantage over the infection. The fever is a *good* response, letting us know that the body is trying to defend and repair itself from the infectious agents.

When inflammation is controlled, it provides enormous benefits for your body. Think of controlled inflammation as if it were your gas stove or fireplace at home. When at the right level, the fire creates the perfect temperature for cooking or keeping the room warm. But if the fire gets out of control—and we all know how quickly that can happen—your entire house can burn down. Like fire, inflammation follows the Goldilocks rule: not too hot, not too cold, but just right. Too much inflammation can become a problem, while the balance of acute and controlled inflammation can be very useful in most situations, like striking the balance of yin and yang.

Let's talk chronic inflammation. This type of long-term inflammation is always harmful. Using the sprained-ankle analogy again, if your ankle continues to have pain and swelling over an unusually long period of time, and your immune system is not able to repair it, this inflammation can lead to chronic damage to the ankle joint. This also goes for chronic fevers. With an uncontrolled fever, there is a constant release of inflammatory chemicals, and the body can no longer repair itself. This chronic inflammation spirals into degenerative changes and worsening disease. Simply put, if inflammation continues and becomes chronic, then the body loses its ability to maintain a normal state of health. This then leads to progressively worsening disease.

The following list contains some of the diseases and conditions associated with chronic inflammation:

- Allergies—to inhalants (environmental), foods, or chemicals such as colorings and preservatives
- Orthopedic—osteoarthritis and autoimmune arthritis such as rheumatoid arthritis

- Cancers—all types
- Cardiovascular—coronary heart disease, myocarditis, hypertension, phlebitis, varicosities
- Dental—gingivitis, periodontal disease
- Endocrine—diabetes, thyroiditis, obesity
- ENT: Eye—conjunctivitis, uveitis; Ear—otitis; Sinus—sinusitis; Throat—pharyngitis
- Gastrointestinal—gastritis, esophagitis, IBS, Crohn's, ulcerative colitis, diverticulitis
- Injuries—tendonitis, bursitis, broken bones
- Infections—flu, colds, Hepatitis C, HIV, EBV
- Pulmonary—bronchitis, asthma, COPD
- Neurological diseases—Alzheimer's, Parkinson's, dementia
- Skin—eczema, acne, psoriasis, dermatitis

The ending *itis* means "inflammation," which is derived from the word *flam* or *flame*. Thus whenever we place a root word before it, the new word just refers to inflammation of that part of the body or system. For example, *tendonitis* means "inflammation of the tendon(s)." As you can see from the above examples, almost every category of disease has inflammation directly involved with its worsening and its progression.

Conventional medical treatment has classified over two hundred different "itis" conditions, with over a dozen different types of medical specializations that treat these individually and symptomatically. For example, if you have red eyes (conjunctivitis), an ophthalmologist will prescribe drops for your allergies or irritation. If you have a runny nose (rhinitis), your ENT will prescribe a steroid nasal spray or oral antihistamine medications. If you have nasal congestion with pain or fever (sinusitis), you will receive antibiotics to treat that infection. If your gums bleed when you brush them (gingivitis), your dentist will recommend oral care products. If you have asthma, which causes congestion and coughing (bronchitis), a pulmonologist will prescribe an inhaler, oral steroid medications, or an antibiotic. If you have GERD, heartburn, or stomach pain (esophagitis and gastritis), your GI doctor will prescribe an acid blocker; if you have diarrhea and painful colon cramps (colitis), you'll receive a stool stopper and steroids; if you have constipation, you'll get a laxative. If you have joint pain (arthritis), your orthopedic doctor will prescribe a pain medication or a steroid injection. If you have a rash (dermatitis), your dermatologist will prescribe a steroid ointment...and the list goes on from head to toe, with a different doctor for each part of your body, treating each area separately and symptomatically.

While specialization in medicine is necessary for acute conditions, we doctors tend to forget the obvious, but most ignored, questions: "What is causing my patient to have these inflammatory problems in the first place?" and "What triggers are causing these symptoms?"

I am glad that we have medications that treat the immediate symptoms so that patients can find relief. But I have to imagine that most people must stop and ask themselves, "Do I have to take these medications forever?"

Most people have been told that their conditions are lifelong and that they have to take their medications indefinitely or they will get worse. So, they continue to take their medications over years and even decades, yet they never truly get better, nor does their disease resolve or improve. Most people are chronically inflamed regardless of the medications they're prescribed. The culprit is a trifecta of our modern lifestyles:

- Too many pro-inflammatory foods in the diet
- Stressful and unhealthy lifestyles with minimal movement or exercise
- Overuse of prescription drugs that treat the symptoms but mask the underlying causes of dysfunction

The combination of these triggers prevents a person from ever healing and becoming normal and healthy again.

In reading this book, you will learn how you can overcome your "itis" conditions through diet, simple lifestyle changes, and natural therapies. This book outlines a path that will help you to reverse and prevent most chronic diseases and feel "normal" again.

Let's begin by talking about the integrative-medicine approach to inflammation.

Conventional Medicine vs. Integrative Medicine

> *Can't get no help. I say again health-care cutback.*
> — PUBLIC ENEMY

Western or conventional medicine stands above the rest of the world when it comes to acute and emergency care. If you are involved in a car accident, wounded by a gunshot, or experience a heart attack, having access to the scientific wonders of conventional medicine could save your life. For those with life-threatening illnesses that would have meant their death even a generation ago, conventional medicine has saved millions of lives.

But the ER only helps for a crisis when no other intervention method is better. For chronic diseases such as heart disease, diabetes, obesity, arthritis, or depression, conventional medicine has, in my opinion, failed us.

Physicians are trained to treat only the symptoms not the underlying causes of the disease, dysfunction, or imbalance. In an acute situation where it is necessary to go to the ER, the health-care workers can help to stabilize the condition. But if someone goes to the ER with a miserable, chronic condition that has given them a poor quality of life, so much so that they feel like they are dying—but they are not actually dying — then the ER health-care workers have very little to nothing to offer them.

For most chronic conditions, the ER sends the patient home with the standard discharge instructions, such as "take these medications and follow up with your primary physician." And with the current state of health care today, it might take a few weeks to several months to get a follow-up appointment.

Health insurance and *affordable health care* are oxymorons. There is no care or affordability with insurance, especially since insurance companies are mainly private and profit-driven by definition. Politically, it sounds good for those who work in government to tout health care for everyone, but the "benefits" of a mandatory, for-profit health-insurance network are not rooted in reality. In my opinion as a physician, we went wrong when we decided to pay private insurance companies rather than create a universal health plan that everyone participates in. Private insurance companies are only looking out for quarterly profits on Wall Street, exorbitant CEO and management salaries, and their bottom line—not your best health outcome. Although it helps to have some coverage if we get into an accident, mandatory insurance will never really prevent us from getting the most common diseases or from getting sick. It simply provides a system where you receive bills monthly and then have to meet high deductibles, in addition to copays. Even with insurance available to everyone, it is still not affordable once someone gets sick because, as of this writing, the Affordable Care Act (ACA) has still not controlled the costs of health care.

So, although the insurance companies cannot deny coverage because of a preexisting condition as they did previously, they will always charge you more just to accept you. Thus, and many people don't realize this, private insurance companies, hospitals, doctors, and pharmaceutical companies can charge whatever they want without any regulation of health-care costs. Just because we all have health insurance does not mean that we will all have improved overall health outcomes (with the possible exception of the very poor who previously had no health care and those with acute emergencies). But the ACA will improve the private insurance companies' profits and please Wall Street and their shareholders.

Unfortunately for the citizens of the United States, this "profits before people" ethos has spread to medical schools. Conventional medical schools train us in "disease management." We learn how to treat and manage symptoms but not how to treat the underlying causes of disease. This is standard practice in the United States, where pharmaceutical companies, which want to maximize profits over health outcomes, primarily dictate the practice of medicine. Managing symptoms via long-term prescriptions and treatment is far more profitable than alleviating the disease through simple, time-tested, science-backed methods.

Fortunately, many people are rejecting this paradigm. Integrative medicine, as used in my practice and as practiced in most other countries in the world, views patient health through the concept of *disease resolution*. With integrative medicine, we are geared toward finding the underlying cause of dysfunction, imbalance, or disease and then removing or rebalancing those factors. This is, logically, what will lead to resolution of disease. However, conventional medicine and integrative medicine are two radically different philosophies and approaches to health and healing.

I, along with many Americans when given the choice, will choose the integrative-medicine approach when offered. That's because, as a medical doctor, I believe in helping my patients get well, not simply managing their symptoms.

The Integrative-Medicine Approach

I want the best of both worlds, and,
baby, I know what it's worth.
— VAN HALEN

When we look at using an integrative-medicine approach to health—reviewing what other countries and cultures currently use for treating the same conditions—we find that in most cases integrative-medical approaches are safer, more successful, and more cost-effective than what we currently offer in conventional medicine. Have we been ignorant of these differences? The answer is yes, and for many reasons that are usually not in the best interests of the patient. Instead, they benefit the person or organization that continues to make money from "managing" disease and ensuring the chronic disease remains chronic: hospitals, specialty clinics, pharmaceutical companies, high-tech diagnostic/surgical-equipment companies, and insurance companies.

Although we have made many advances through the promotion of medical specialists (particularly in the area of diagnostic testing and surgery), very few of these have changed the underlying diseases themselves. Specialists are only helpful for acute care or emergencies that necessitate immediate control of physiology or when rare conditions need to be diagnosed.

As a country that in 2013 spent $3.8 trillion[2] on health care and $329.2 billion[3] on prescription drugs alone, in almost every category when compared to other countries the United States has very low health outcomes. Most Americans, including our politicians and doctors, think that we rank at least in the top three in most health categories. But when looking at each major health-care parameter, the United States ranks far below most countries that spend only a fraction of what we do, and their populations are healthier than ours. The United States is not even in the top ten worldwide, and we spend more on health care than all of our peer democratic countries![4] This translates to about 17.5% of our GDP on healthcare.[5]

Here are the facts: The United States ranks at the *bottom* of the top sixteen high-income democracies in reference to "death from all causes."[6] This means that we die more from infant mortality, homicides, teen pregnancy, HIV and AIDS, drug-related deaths, obesity and diabetes, heart disease, chronic lung disease and disability than most other industrialized countries. For overall life expectancy, we rank thirty-fourth out of the top thirty-five countries,[7] and most recently, the United States ranks forty-sixth (out of forty-eight countries) in overall health-care outcomes.[8] To put this into perspective, you might ask "which countries are ranked just above us at 43rd, 44th and 45th?". The answer is Dominican Republic (43rd), Turkey (44th) and Iran (45th).

Again, we are lucky in the United States to have the best acute-care system in the world. If you get in a car accident, break a leg, or are a victim of gun violence, our emergency and trauma centers are the best places to be, bar none. But most Americans live outside the ER. We suffer from chronic disease, and our health-care system mainly treats our symptoms, not the underlying causes of our chronic illnesses.

I like to talk to my patients about the idea of *disease resolution*. I see numerous patients with chronic conditions such as diabetes, heart disease, and depression. Here's how a typical discussion of their condition will proceed.

I start by asking patients how long they have had these conditions; most patients will tell me they have had them for decades. At this point, I usually ask them why they think they still have these conditions. They usually answer, "I have been told that this is a lifelong disease, and I must take these medications to control it."

At this point, I ask them when they were first diagnosed with the disease or health condition, and I ask them if they started with only one medication for the treatment. They almost universally answer yes. I then ask them why they are now on multiple medications for the same condition. They usually tell me that their condition has worsened or was not managed appropriately. I then ask why these conditions haven't been resolved or reversed, and they always reply, *"I did not know I could get better or reverse my disease."*

If these answers sound familiar, then this book will change your life. It is possible to improve or resolve your health conditions, and I want to give you the tools to take control of your health care, without a monthly premium or deductible!

Inflammation 101: The Triggering Mechanism That Makes Any Disease Worse

> *You can go for the trigger, but only if you have to.*
> —BON JOVI

A variety of potential sources of inflammation can contribute to acute and chronic diseases, including cancer. Here are some of those important sources:

1. **Food Factors:** for example, animal proteins (including dairy), grilled or fried foods
2. **Environmental Pollutants/Toxic Agents:** for example, industrial pollutants, fuels, smog, fracking chemicals, heavy metals, chemotherapy
3. **Bacteria:** for example, H. pylori, E. coli, chlamydia pneumonia, salmonella typhi, streptococcus bovis
4. **Parasites:** for example, giardia, campylobacter
5. **Viruses:** for example, hepatitis, HIV, HSV, EBV
6. **Cigarette Smoke:** for example, tobacco, e-cigs
7. **Alcoholic Beverages:** for example, liquor, beer, wine
8. **Ultraviolet Radiation:** for example, the sun, tanning booths
9. **Stress:** for example, low pH, hypoxia, fear, anger, anxiety
10. **Environmental Allergens:** for example, grasses, weeds, molds, animals

Now that you know the general categories, let's explore how just one of these inflammatory triggers affects our bodies.

Uncontrolled inflammation caused by toxic environmental exposure, poor dietary habits, and lifestyle factors can trigger the onset of chronic diseases, even cancer. Before we get into the amazing and simple ways to start feeling better and moving toward optimum health, let's start with an understanding of how our bodies work. After you have this understanding, you will find it easier to comprehend how the common factor of having too much inflammation in the body links all of your health conditions together.

Almost everyone has experienced inhalant allergies, commonly known as "seasonal allergies" or "hay fever." Allergies like these are a simple yet powerful example of how inflammation works. *Allergy* is synonymous with *inflammation*. Yes, allergies are caused by inflammation of the eyes, ears, nose, and respiratory tract. Allergies can also cause asthma, COPD, and other respiratory conditions. Here is how all that happens:

Allergies can be triggered by various offenders, such as pollens from grasses, weeds, and trees; molds; dust mites; dogs; and cats. Allergic "triggers" are specific to each individual. (Details on testing for these triggers will be discussed later, in chapter 4, "Inhalant Allergies—The Inflammation That We Breathe.") These allergens cause an inflammatory response in the respiratory tract and surrounding mucosal tissues. In effect, foreign invaders (allergens) provoke the immune system's soldier cells in the eyes, ears, nose, throat, and lungs to pull out their weapons and fight. That means sending inflammation signals (there are hundreds of inflammatory signals, but some of the main categories of these messengers are called cytokines and interleukins) that then travel throughout the bloodstream to stimulate certain cells, called mast cells, which release histamines.

These mast cells act like the Army Corps of Engineers, filling sandbags to wall up flooding waterways. In your immune system's case, those "sandbags" are the histamines. Histamines are the chemicals that cause our eyes and ears to become itchy and red, our sinuses to become congested or runny and full of mucous, and our lungs to become tight and constricted. Many people (as well as doctors) forget that histamines perform a protective role, blocking the body from overexposure to allergens. Those Army Corps of Engineers mast cells release histamines that, in essence, act as barriers to halt the entry of allergens into the body. The body releases mucous to try to capture the allergens, and our sinuses and airways can constrict to reduce the penetration of allergens into our bodies.

Now, while our body creates an allergic reaction to protect us from greater harm, we still have to breathe! Even when we realize that our body is allergic to something, we cannot always avoid allergens in our environment (especially those allergens that are airborne). Voilà! Antihistamines were created.

Since allergies are not new, and neither is treating them, mankind has devised dozens of ways to give the body an antihistamine effect through the use of homeopathics, biotherapeutics, herbs, antioxidants, anti-inflammatories, over-the-counter antihistamines, prescription antihistamines, steroids, and other immune modulators. Although I personally prefer to use natural therapies—since they are as effective but have fewer side effects—there is still one major drawback to using the antihistamine approach: antihistamines only treat the symptoms and not the underlying cause (inflammation).

Once you start taking antihistamines, you are stuck using them—be they natural, OTC, or prescription—whenever you have allergic symptoms.

Even though they may be effective, or somewhat effective, they only help treat allergy symptoms temporarily. When the antihistamine medication wears off, allergy symptoms return; therefore, you only manage the disease, or "dis-ease." For most people, allergies are seasonal. In certain areas of the United States, however, allergies can affect people almost year-round, making antihistamines a continual temporary solution.

Allergies are just one powerful example of out-of-control inflammation in the body. Would you like a more permanent solution to inflammation? In the coming chapters, I will teach you how to manage and even resolve the inflammation that's making you sick!

For every patient whom I see at Sanjevani Integrative Medicine Health and Lifestyle Center, I create a simple step-by-step approach that starts the journey toward optimum health and longevity. You'll get to see the basics of my methods as you go through this book, learning how a straightforward approach to managing inflammation applies to all conditions, from allergies to asthma, chronic migraine headaches, arthritis, ulcerative colitis, and even various types of cancers.

Let's begin on your journey into healing and optimum health!

CHAPTER 2

An Introduction: Ten Steps to Optimum Health And Longevity

The following ten steps provide the foundation on which I guide my patients to greater health. They are incredibly simple and, when implemented fully, incredibly effective. They include physical, emotional, and spiritual health, which are inextricable when seeking to heal a whole person.

1. Eat an organic, non-GMO, plant-based anti-inflammatory diet.
2. Test what triggers inflammatory responses in your body.
3. Detoxify: clear the toxins.
4. Avoid smoking.
5. Avoid NSAIDs—the unknown danger.
6. Decrease inflammation through the use of supplements like Bosmeric-SR.
7. Increase immune-system functioning.
8. Maintain healthy glucose levels and decrease sugar in the diet.
9. Reduce stress through meditation and yoga.
10. Increase love, happiness, meaningful social relationships, and faith or spiritual practices.

If you utilize these ten steps to optimum health, all conditions can improve, resolve, and even reverse!

Let's start with the point at which we have the most control: what we eat and drink.

Point of Entry: The GI Tract

The journey to optimum health and longevity begins first with planning the travel itinerary. Before I teach you the Ten Steps to Optimum Health and Longevity, you must first have a deeper understanding of how inflammation affects our bodies and how our bodies become inflamed.

There are three ways inflammatory triggers get into our bodies: through our skin, our respiratory tract, and through the most vulnerable point of entry, our GI tract (stomach and intestines).

Optimum health starts at our GI tract. Using our travel analogy, the GI tract is the Grand Central Station of the body. It is the point at which we receive the overwhelming amount of exposure to inflammation. This understanding is supported by traditional medical practices, like Ayurveda and Chinese medicine (which are both over five thousand years old), and more modern science and medicine, such as functional medicine **(see Side Notes: Functional Medicine)**, which incorporates all of our Western scientific fields into a functional model to explain how our bodies work.

Now, although you may have learned differently from your doctors, on TV, or at school, our GI tract (the internal mucosal tract containing IgA immune cells) functionally starts from our sinus cavities/oral cavity and moves down our esophagus into our stomach, and then into the small intestine, and then to the large intestine and the colon, and then out through the anus. Although a separate tract, the vagina is still part of this internal mucosal system.

Functionally speaking, the entire internal mucosal tract is a tube that, during embryonic development, starts out as a mouth and an anus. As we develop in the womb, the simple tube connecting the mouth and anus differentiates into multiple organs but still has the same entrance and exit. The new system shares similar functions and features to the original starting point.

Modern medicine dissects the individual into a bunch of separate parts—head and neck, stomach/GI tract, urinary/gynecological tract—and suggests a separate doctor for each part! We have forgotten that this simple tube—seen through the eyes of different doctors depending on the location of symptoms—is part of the entire person, and thus we lose the holistic approach to medicine. A patient is no longer viewed as an entire person, and doctors only treat the individual parts as restricted by medical specialty.

For example, some people might have a sinus infection, some heartburn, some irritable bowel, and some vaginitis. Conventionally, those people would see different doctors for each specific health problem. Each doctor or specialist micromanages the symptoms by only treating the area that he or she specializes in (e.g., conjunctivitis through ophthalmology, sinusitis through ENT specialization, bronchitis through pulmonology, dermatitis through dermatology, and arthritis through rheumatology).

Because of specialization, nobody ever addresses the state of the entire individual. How can a doctor ever hope to get to the source of the problem if the body is separated into parts and dissected by a dozen different specialists with completely diverse opinions?

Point of Entry: Screening in the GI Tract

As I wrote in the previous section, the GI tract starts from the sinus/oral cavity and extends on downward. This starting point takes in the air we breathe and the foods we eat. It is the entry point for our immune system, and it is part of an entire, complex system.

Our first line of defense, called the IgA immune response, is located along the entire internal mucosal tract. These mucosal membranes are the first barriers and walls, the borders and ports of entry where checkpoint soldier cells examine travelers (e.g., food, drugs, viruses, bacteria, fungi, parasites, and cancer cells) and either allow them to pass or reject them. Think of these membranes as customs at an airport, screening for suspicious or unwanted people.

The GI tract is an impressive collection of organs that have functions that no machine can duplicate. The average person's GI tract is about thirty-five feet (about 10.7 meters) long.

I like to describe the stomach as a highly efficient blender—like a Vitamix. You place food inside it, and using the necessary stomach acids, it breaks down all the categories of food—proteins, carbohydrates, fats, sugars, macronutrients, micronutrients, water, and fiber—into smaller particles.

The acid in the stomach is a biological necessity. Without stomach acid, we would have many more digestive problems than we normally do; the advent of acid-blocking medicines is, in fact, creating more harm than good. With very few exceptions, stopping or reducing acid in the stomach through medications—whether OTC or prescriptions—should be done with extreme caution. Most people (even most doctors) do not know that the majority of clinical studies on the acid blockers (H2 blockers, such as Zantac and Pepcid, and proton-pump inhibitors, such as Prilosec and Nexium) covered time periods of less than three months. That's right: most antacid medications have not been studied for use longer than *ninety days*, yet we have millions of Americans who have been taking these drugs for over *thirty years*!

Every day I see patients who tell me that their GI doctor told them that they could take antacid medications indefinitely. This is not only bad medicine; it is, in my opinion, malpractice, as antacid use just masks symptoms of unhealthy food habits, hidden food allergies, and other lifestyle factors that simple tests and dietary improvements could address. By letting patients take antacid medications indefinitely, doctors only create bigger problems for patients down the line. Of course, this practice may benefit GI doctors and could be viewed as strategic, as prolonged antacid use creates a need for more GI procedures, such as endoscopies and colonoscopies.

Why do we Americans take so many medications for GI symptoms such as heartburn, acid reflux, and gastritis? Here are a few reasons:

1. We overeat and consume larger portions than we should;
2. The foods we eat are high in fats and animal-based proteins, which make them more difficult to digest;
3. Some of the foods we eat are causing *inflammatory* or allergic reactions (food allergies/sensitivities);
4. The foods we eat are genetically modified (GMO) and not organic; or
5. We take acid-blocking medications to deal with the side effects of NSAIDs (nonsteroidal anti-inflammatory drugs) such as ibuprofen (Motrin, Advil), naproxen (Aleve), celecoxib (Celebrex).

Let's examine some of these reasons more closely. The majority of people who take antacids, H2 blockers (Zantac, Tagamet, etc.), and proton-pump inhibitors (PPIs, such as Prilosec and Nexium) are using them to treat symptoms of GI distress, but they are not designed to treat the underlying causes of that GI distress.

Thanks to high school biology class, most of us are familiar with the basic process of digestion. After food enters the stomach, where it is broken down (like in a blender) into a soup of all the food categories (e.g., proteins, carbohydrates, fats, vitamins, minerals, fiber, and water), it moves to the small intestine and then to the large intestine, or colon. You experience gastrointestinal symptoms because your body is trying to tell you something is wrong with the amount, type, or source of food you're consuming or the speed at which you're consuming it. The problem with taking medications like the ones described above is that they allow you to ignore the problem and continue with the unhealthy behaviors that actually caused it to begin with.

The stereotypical commercial for these acid-blocking products shows an overweight male at a football game. He complains of heartburn when drinking beer and eating cheeseburgers, nachos, popcorn, and peanuts. When he takes his heartburn medications, he feels better and can continue eating and drinking, since he can no longer feel any symptoms.

In a TV endorsement, Larry the Cable Guy states, "You know what I love about this country? I love everything about this country, including Prilosec OTC. Take one Prilosec each morning to treat your frequent heartburn!" The commercial then shows him handing out corn dogs at a carnival, beneath a big sign advertising Colossal Corndogs. "So, if you're one of those people who gets heartburn from what you eat day after day, block the acid with Prilosec OTC, and don't get heartburn in the first place!"

Other acid-blocker commercials show the food such as pizza and chicken wings beating up the individual. They imply that by taking the medications, you can relieve the feeling of being beaten up by the foods and may continue to eat them as you like.

This type of positive reinforcement for the wrong behaviors has now become part of our culture. Wouldn't it be better for us to learn how to control the foods we eat that cause the symptoms in the first place, instead of being beaten up by those foods? Shouldn't foods nourish us and make us feel better versus try to harm us?

With the rare occurrence of an ulcer (for which one may use an acid blocker for six to twelve weeks) or erosions of the esophagus (for the same period of time), the temporary suppression of stomach acid can assist in the healing process of those damaged tissues. However, people hardly ever discontinue these medications once they start them. Now that most acid-blocking medications are OTC, one can continue taking them indefinitely.

Again, why aren't we asking ourselves, "Even if this drug gives me all-day relief, why do I have to take it every day for the rest of my life?"

The problem is that most people do not want to listen to what their body is telling them. If your food is "slapping you and beating you up," you should be paying attention to what is happening instead of blocking and masking the underlying problems. More of us should be asking, "What is causing these symptoms, and why do I have them every day?"

In my medical opinion, the foods that we eat directly cause GI tract issues. Some foods are inflammatory for everyone (pro-inflammatory foods), and some foods cause specific inflammatory responses that are unique to each of us. (Note: If you currently take acid-blocking medication—whether OTC or prescribed—or have in the past, please **see Side Notes: Acid Blockers and Sanjevani Acid-Blocker Support.**)

Most people who have had an upper endoscopy or colonoscopy have gone to the GI doctor and, under light sedation, had a camera placed into their stomach **(see fig. 1)** and also into their colon **(see fig. 2)**. These procedures can be very helpful and are a wonderful example of one of the benefits of the technology that we have in Western medicine—to actually view areas of the body that we can't see with the naked eye. These scoped procedures allow us to actually *see* gross pathology or disease. By that I mean that we can see if anything looks suspicious or broken. For example, in both procedures we can see internal tissues on the monitor. These tissues should look nice and pink, with normal folds and healthy characteristics. In the stomach, we can see if there are any ulcers, bleeds, areas of inflammation (gastritis), or masses. Similarly, in the colon we can see if there are any polyps (fatty, grapelike projections of tissue hanging from the walls of the colon), areas of inflammation (colitis), pouches (diverticula), or masses (tumors, either benign or cancerous). Again, the benefit of such screening and diagnostic procedures is that we can see gross pathology or disease. If the organ looks abnormal, then most likely there is a problem that can be addressed, sometimes before patients even have symptoms. That is where health screening per appropriate guidelines can be lifesaving.

Unfortunately, if they don't see anything unusual on the monitor, conventional doctors will say that there is nothing wrong. Each year this happens to millions of patients who have these tests done and don't have gross pathology (disease severe enough to be observed) yet have GI symptoms such as heartburn, reflux, stomach pains, gas, bloating, diarrhea, and constipation—or what has been commonly described as *irritable bowel syndrome*. When most—if not all—of these patients are scoped, they are considered negative for visible pathology, meaning their symptoms do not correlate with what their doctors can see. This is because these procedures don't detect *functional changes* in the GI tract. Functional changes are changes in how the GI tract works with regard to absorption, assimilation, and excretion—all the factors that make the GI tract work and all the factors that can also make it dysfunctional.

To illustrate for patients in my office how functional changes work, I like to use an example. I tell them that if I take a picture of them sitting in my office and place it on my computer and then show them that picture, they will see that there is no fire or flood occurring in the room. According to the logic of conventional scoping procedures and the specialists that conduct them, that picture indicates that nothing in the room—including them sitting there—is in any immediate danger.

But what the picture misses, of course, is the *functionality* of the patients sitting in the room. The picture does not tell us the climate of the room (hot, cold, humid, or dry); it does not tell us whether there is electricity running in the walls or if any of the outlets are broken; it does not tell us if there is water running to the sink or with what pressure and temperature; it does not tell us if there is mold in the ceiling or cracks in the foundation. Therefore, while on one hand the picture can help rule out immediate problems (gross pathology), on the other hand, it misses any *functional* problems that might be occurring. Those unseen functional problems could be causing daily symptoms such as heartburn, cramping, bloating, diarrhea, or constipation, which are dysfunctions of absorption, assimilation, excretion, and other jobs of the GI tract.

While we can use an endoscopy (upper GI) or colonoscopy (lower GI) to view the stomach and colon, which are fixed with ligaments, we cannot see the middle section—the small intestine **(see fig. 3)**—from these scoping procedures. Although other types of evaluations can show us certain aspects of the small intestine, we cannot visualize it directly like we can the stomach and colon, so we have to ask patients to swallow a camera pill that will take the pictures.

The small intestine contains thousands of folds **(see fig. 4)**, and within these folds are thousands of even tinier folds that have fingerlike projections. Although these projections look smooth to the naked eye, they are actually textured like fine velvet. This is where food particles are filtered, absorbed, and then excreted. Food gets filtered into specific areas of the GI tract based on the size of those food particles. These areas contain intestinal villi, or crypts, where food particles enter into the system. These crypts are specifically structured to fit with a specific group of food particles. For example, a twelve-amino-acid protein molecule from a vegetable goes into a specific area in the small intestine that can absorb that size of amino acid. A fourteen-amino-acid molecule goes into another area, and so on, as do different-sized carbohydrates, fats, sugars, and other particles.

Each of these food particles is helped along the way by a very important aspect of our immune system that resides inside the GI tract: probiotics. When we're looking at the *functionality* of the GI tract, few things are as important as having the ideal probiotics working in harmony with this critical bodily system.

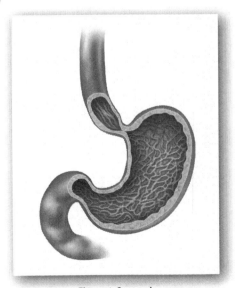

Figure 1: Stomach

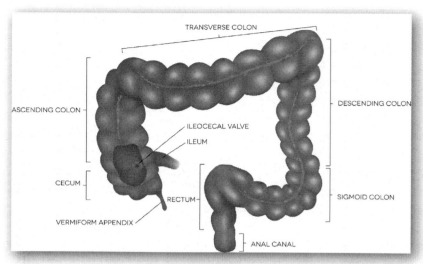

Figure 2: Colon

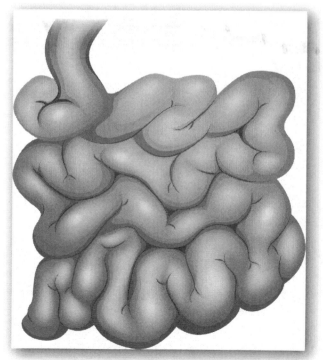

Figure 3: Small intestine

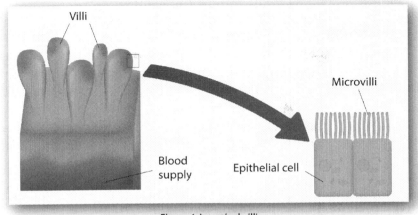

Figure 4: Intestinal villi

Probiotics: The GI "Foot Soldier" Cells

Most of us know about or at least have heard of probiotics, but not everyone understands the critical role that they play in our digestive system, our immune system, and our overall health. This growing area of medicine looks at all the factors that positively and negatively affect what is now called the gut's "microbiome"—that is, all the microorganisms inhabiting the human body in both health and disease—and how lifestyle, diet, pharmaceutical drugs, illness, and stress affect our microbiome.

Probiotics are the helpful inhabitants of our microbiome. The word probiotics is derived from the Latin preposition "pro," which means "for" and the Greek word "biotic" meaning "bios" or "life." They are the healthy bacteria that live in our GI tract and perform a variety of bodily functions. Over 500 species have been identified to date (and there are probably hundreds more to be discovered), and each probiotic plays a specific and communal role. Even more impressive is that the probiotics in our bodies exist in approximately one hundred trillion colony-forming units (yes, trillion with a *t*). *That is more than three times the total number of cells in the entire human body.* So, although we think of them as tiny beneficial microorganisms, probiotics actually exist in much, much larger numbers than we thought. In fact, the total weight of these probiotics is approximately *three to four pounds* (1.3–1.8 kilograms) in the average person.

Each of these probiotic species plays a specific role. Think of the community where you live. Different types of people are doing many different jobs, all of which are necessary for a town to thrive. There are doctors, lawyers, teachers, sanitation workers, police officers, judges, construction workers... you get the idea. Without these important groups doing their specific jobs, your town could not run efficiently. (Think of what your community would look like without sanitation workers!) The same goes for the probiotics in your gut. Even though there are different types and numbers of probiotics in the gut, they all play important roles and have different jobs; without specific species doing their designated jobs, the entire GI system could not run efficiently, either. The probiotics also utilize certain foods to keep healthy themselves called prebiotics (i.e. fiber, inulin).

All probiotics provide protection against bad microbes and toxins and help to move food particles into their specific places. Some probiotics make certain vitamins, excreting heavy metals and toxins; some absorb various nutrients and provide immune protection; some have antimicrobial action against infectious agents and help *reduce inflammatory* reactions. I bet you didn't know how busy your probiotics are!

As mentioned before, the GI tract is about thirty-five feet long in the average person. But when you calculate the entire surface of the GI tract, it is quite amazing how large it really is. If we were to iron out each of those tiny folds in our small and large intestines, the surface area would equal approximately two Wimbledon-sized tennis courts! That is a *huge* amount of surface area to absorb, assimilate, and excrete food particles.

Now you know the average person has about one hundred trillion colony-forming units (CFUs) of probiotics that weigh between three to four pounds. But do they all live uniformly in the GI tract? The answer is no. Many people think that probiotics coat the GI tract in the same way that the old 1980's Pepto-Bismol commercials used to show the pink liquid coat the entire GI tract as it was ingested. This however is not the case.

Probiotics live in their own communities and corresponding "neighborhoods" within the GI tract. This is important because, for example, when people have GI surgeries (e.g., bariatric or weight-loss surgeries) or have trauma from a car accident or gunshot wound or even cancer in their GI tract, standard surgical procedure is to remove the affected sections of the GI tract. However, when sections are removed and the remaining ends placed together, although the overall system still works, the GI tract becomes dysfunctional. GI problems develop over time, along with macronutrient and micronutrient deficiencies, because of the missing probiotics that lived in the section of GI tract that was removed. People who have had these surgeries require daily probiotic supplementation because "homeless" probiotics operate less effectively, leading the patient to become deficient in those probiotic functions. Not only do the probiotics become ineffective, but the surgery also affects the way the body absorbs, assimilates, and excretes food particles—including all vitamins and minerals, proteins, carbs, fats, and sugars. If you have had GI surgery or chronic GI problems, such as diarrhea or other malabsorption issues, go now to **Side Notes: Dr. Pai's Recommended Laboratory Testing.**

GI Tract: The Command Center Where 80 Percent of Your Immune System Resides

How about getting off all these antibiotics?
—ALANIS MORISSETTE

So, what's the big deal about the GI tract size and what it contains—and why am I spending so much time on it? Everything comes back to inflammation, and one of the most important aspects in achieving optimum health is decreasing inflammation through diet. Because over *80 percent* of your immune system resides in your GI tract, decreasing inflammation through diet naturally increases immune-system function. To use the armed-forces analogy again, increasing immune system functioning is like providing more supplies—such as food, training, and weapons—to our troops to keep them strong and always on guard, protecting us from enemy attacks.

The immune system resides in a location collectively called the gut-associated lymphoid tissues (GALT). Think of the GALT as the command centers where the soldier cells are stationed, awaiting their orders. Of these soldier cells, 20 percent circulate and assist in daily bodily protection. For example, the circulating soldier cells (i.e., the Border Patrol or the Coast Guard) are fending off foreign invaders, blocking infections, and protecting and repairing minor damage like a small cut on your finger. However, not all of the military can be on patrol all the time, as that would be inefficient and costly. Instead, they reside at their command centers until they are needed and called into action.

Everything you've consumed—from the breast milk on the day that you were born (hopefully you were breastfed or you plan to breastfeed your children) to the later baby foods and then adult foods, to the most recent meal you ate—has challenged your immune system in positive and negative ways. And your GI tract's border-patrol cells have inspected everything that has ever entered your body.

Again, this GI tract is the point-of-entry area where the border-patrol cells examine travelers (e.g., foods, beverages, medications, supplements, viruses, bacteria, fungi, and parasites) and either allow them to pass through the checkpoints or reject them. These cells allow some food particles to pass through, screen others more stringently, and reject others outright.

At this point you might be asking what happens to the rejected, problem-causing particles once the border-patrol cells turn them back. These rejected food particles cause *inflammatory* reactions like heartburn, reflux, and gastritis in the upper-GI tract and gas, bloating, diarrhea, and constipation in the lower-GI tract. But the problem doesn't end with local GI reactions; once those rejected food particles leak into the gut and are absorbed into the body inflammation will spread systemically (throughout the body). I will soon talk about the effects of systemic inflammation, but let me continue to explain *how* these inflammatory reactions occur because it's not just food that causes them.

Common offenders that disrupt the probiotics in your GI tract include antibiotics, antifungals, infections, stress, drugs, alcohol, and pro-inflammatory foods. Let's take antibiotics as an example, since this is the most common insult to the GI tract's probiotics (in addition, of course, to unhealthy pro-inflammatory foods and stress).

Most Americans have taken antibiotics frequently in their lifetime. Most of us had ear infections and respiratory infections as children and received antibiotics from our pediatricians. Although most clinical data will show that 70 to 80 percent of those infections were viral in nature, we were still given antibiotics. Why? Because our doctors didn't know any better? Or was it because we demanded to be treated with medicines, and doctors prescribed them to show that they were providing treatment? Or was it the influence of pharmaceutical companies taking advantage of both patients and doctors, playing middleman to ensure that both parties got what they wanted—and that pharmaceutical companies got what they wanted: more prescription sales?[9]

As we got older, little changed. Most of us dealt with acne, sinus infections, bronchitis, urinary-tract infections, or gastroenteritis—all of which we treated with antibiotics. On average, most Americans take a few courses of antibiotics every year; some people get antibiotics every few months for one reason or another.

Most people don't understand the risks associated with taking antibiotics. These include reducing the number of probiotics in the GI tract, increasing GI permeability (aka "leaky-gut"), lowering the immune system and increasing overall inflammatory sensitivity to foods (all to be discussed). These risks are especially severe when people do not replenish their gut with probiotics for extended periods of time after taking a course of antibiotics. Most probiotics on the market are not potent enough to provide true benefits, and some are not even viable when you take them. To learn about common probiotic products, **see Side Notes: Manufacturing of Probiotics**.

As an expert in integrative medicine, I restrict prescribing antibiotics to patients with severe infections that have gone untreated. In other instances, most people respond well to natural antimicrobials **(see Side Notes: Natural Antimicrobial Support)**, as well as immune-supportive therapies **(see Side Notes: Sanjevani Immune-Support Protocols)**, which produce none of the harmful side effects that accompany antibiotic use. People should use antibiotics only if absolutely indicated or if no other choice is available.

I would like to emphasize here that although I exercise extreme caution when prescribing antibiotics, I feel it's important to acknowledge that they do play an important role in medicine. Without antibiotics' lifesaving benefits, most of us who have had serious bacterial infections or wounds, or who have needed surgery, would not have survived.

The problem with antibiotics is not the antibiotics themselves but their overuse and the fact that they have been prescribed unnecessarily or for conditions that should have been treated at the source of the disease (e.g., untreated asthma that turned into bronchitis and then required antibiotics).

Antibiotics are very powerful, and many people don't understand or respect that power. Antibiotics are so powerful that when one has an infection, the antibiotic does not just go to the area of infection but travels to all parts of the body, cell by cell. The good news is that the antibiotics kill the bad bacteria that are causing the infection. The bad news is that they kill the good probiotic bacteria as well. To continue with the military analogy, antibiotics are like drones used to attack an enemy. Although the drone drops bombs and kills the enemy proficiently, as we all know, there is collateral damage, where innocent citizens, including women and children, are also harmed. There is no true "smart bomb" that affects only terrorists. The same goes for antibiotics. They successfully kill the bad bacteria, but they also kill many good bacteria along the way.

For example, when you received treatment as a child for an ear infection or as an adult for a sinus infection **(see figs. 5 and 6)**, the antibiotic did not just go to the sinus cavity or the ear. After an antibiotic is absorbed (mainly in the GI tract when taken orally), the antibiotic molecules distribute systemically **(see fig. 6)**. The largest impact begins locally in the GI tract, and then travels through the bloodstream to each cell and organ system in the body—hopefully to eventually arrive at the infected area and then destroy or inhibit the growth of the bacterial organisms. On a Z-Pak (azithromycin pack) prescription, we can't write instructions telling the drug to go to the exact location it needs to address (e.g., "Go to Mrs. Garcia's left sinus cavity"). We just write, "Take one tablet daily for five days," and voilà—after five days, the infection is cleared.

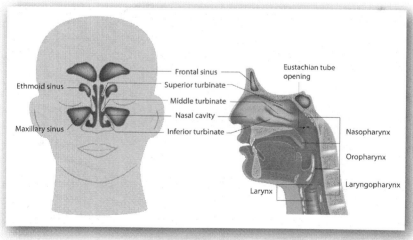

Figure 5: Sinus cavity

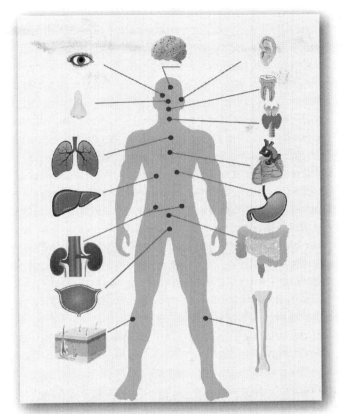

Figure 6: Systemic effects of antibiotics on human organs

The antibiotic does not know where the infection is. Instead, it saturates the entire body and tries to kill all the bacteria it encounters. Most people think that the antibiotic travels only to the site of the infection, but by the time the antibiotic reaches the ears or sinus cavity and penetrates those tissues, it has already penetrated tissues from the bottoms of the toes to the tops of the hair cells—hitting the GI tract the hardest.

So, just how powerful are antibiotics? They are so powerful that one single dose can cause GI dysfunction *up to eighteen months after the exposure.* The reduction of the body's probiotic population—and the consequent damage to the gut's microbiome—causes this dysfunction. Since approximately 80 percent of your immune system is associated with the functioning of the GI tract, antibiotics temporarily weaken, or suppress, the immune system **(see fig. 4)**. Remember, antibiotic use decreases the good probiotic soldier cells and, therefore, their supportive immune function. This is why antibiotic treatments actually put you at risk of a secondary infection.

To illustrate this point, we all know or have heard of someone who has gone to the hospital for a routine procedure, such as a knee, hip, or shoulder operation, and—even though the procedure was successful, without complications—contracted pneumonia or some other infection while in the hospital. Even though surgeons use antibiotics to help protect the surgical area from infections, those antibiotics also affect and decrease the GI-tract probiotics (remember, the GI tract is the entire internal mucosal tract and gastrointestinal system, from the mouth, nose, and lungs to the anus), thus suppressing total immune function. This temporary immune suppression makes anyone undergoing surgery susceptible to secondary infections like pneumonia or even MRSA.

To complicate matters, viruses and bacteria are often transferred to a patient who has just had a surgical procedure from another patient in the hospital (usually via health-care workers who don't wash their hands). These new invaders can cause infections because there are not enough soldier cells on guard. It's a Catch-22 situation: people need antibiotics to prevent infections, but antibiotics often lead to those very infections!

Hospitalized individuals need to be protected from getting secondary infections. Using *probiotics* and helping them get out of the hospital (which I call the Germ Hotel) as soon as possible will decrease their risk of secondary infection. (So will better hygiene from health-care workers, who should make sure they wash their hands between patients.) This is why more people are opting for treatments at outpatient surgical centers.

So now that you have a basic understanding of the gut-immune connection, let's start clarifying some of the myths around *why* we get certain diseases.

The Genetic Misunderstanding

There's something mystical in our genes,
So simplistic it kicks and screams.
—DEPECHE MODE

Over the last fifty years, a persistent belief has wormed its way into our collective consciousness. Most of us have grown up believing that disease runs in our genes and is passed down from our parents. We learned that genes control our biology, and there's nothing we can do to change that fact.

But what if I told you that the gene theory of disease has not actually been proven to be correct?

Here's an interesting fact: over 90 percent of our genome has been shown to be "junk DNA."[10] This means that most of our genome is not functional but is simply carried-over evolutionary material that does nothing. Between 5 and 10 percent of all disease (even cancer) has a direct genetic link,[11] and in fact many researchers are moving this number downward to only 2 to 5 percent. Most of that tiny percentage represents diseases that are metabolic and developmental in nature and that present at birth or at a very young age. This means most chronic diseases—such as heart disease, diabetes, obesity, and even most cancers—are *not* genetically linked. That means that although your genetics may give you an increased tendency toward disease, they are not a direct link to disease.

But why do certain diseases tend to run in the family? One way to think of this phenomenon is to think of a card game where your genes are the cards. For decades, we were told that we had to live with the hand we were dealt. But the truth is that we can change the outcome of the game by *how we play the cards we have been dealt*.

The major causes of disease are environmental, dietary, and lifestyle factors. We are not victims of genes for heart disease or diabetes per se; instead, it's the same dietary habits, lifestyle choices, and stressors that ultimately cause us to experience the same diseases as our parents by affecting how our genetics are expressed. We all tend to teach our children what our parents taught us. Therefore, we pass down the same food habits and environmental stressors, placing us at the same risk of developing the diseases that affected our parents.

There is an emerging field of genetics called epigenetics. Epigenetics emphasizes the understanding that our biology is not *controlled* by our genes, but rather *uses* our genes to make changes to itself.[12] This totally new understanding of genetics suggests that we can exert far more control over our genes than was previously thought possible.

An excellent example of medical hysteria that could have been tempered by a greater understanding of epigenetics came in 2013. In that year the media focused on a set of genes for breast cancer called BRAC1 and BRAC2. A company was encouraging women everywhere to submit to an expensive test to determine the risk of breast cancer in women. This company also tried to get a patent for this test that, fortunately, was blocked by the Supreme Court. I do not have a problem with testing for higher risk of breast cancer; rather, my problem with this test follows:

Only *around 2 percent* of women with breast cancer test positive for BRAC markers. Among those who have these markers, there's only (at most) a 30 percent chance that the gene will express itself. That means that most women (98 percent) would not test positive for BRAC1 or BRAC2, and those who did would have a 70 percent chance that the gene would *never* express.

The media also didn't report the fact that the test was incredibly expensive—sometimes ranging upward of fifteen thousand dollars—and was being pushed as routine screening for all women in the United States. This, of course, would have made the company that owned the test hundreds of millions of dollars very quickly. Thanks to the Supreme Court's blocking of the patent, the test now costs as little as three hundred dollars, but its overall utility to determine breast-cancer risk is still very low.

Unfortunately, through clever marketing to laboratories, doctors, and hospitals, and through sensationalistic news stories directed at the public, this BRAC test remains very popular. Even more unfortunately, many women have opted for bilateral mastectomies to "prevent" breast cancer from occurring, inspired by some famous celebrities who opted for this surgery and were viewed as heroic for it. I don't think it's heroic at all. In fact, I believe it sets a bad example for women to fear disease and try to, misguidedly, lower their risk using drastic measures.

Here is the simple truth of genes and breast-cancer risk. At the last cancer conference that I attended, one of the doctors who specializes in the study of the genetic code—specifically genes that show risk for breast cancer—demonstrated that almost *five hundred* different genes that have been mapped can lead to an increased risk of developing breast cancer. Just one year ago, that number was about four hundred genes. We are learning so much so quickly about the number of genes that can be involved in breast cancer. It is foolish to think that testing only two genes would describe our risk in any significant way. So far we have discovered about 250,000 (500 x 500) possible gene combinations for breast cancer—and that's just what we know as of the writing of this book in 2015!

Genetic testing only indicates risk factors, which isn't a bad thing. But since we are discovering and mapping out more and more factors every year, it will be impossible to avoid them all and impractical to worry about every possible risk. The good news is that genes have switches that can be turned on or off. The even better news is that the major factors that influence those switches are diet, lifestyle, and natural therapies **(see Side Notes: Books and Movies)**—all things within our control. We now have data to show that the right foods and certain easy lifestyle practices can turn down, or even turn off, these risk factors—these genetic switches. For example, we now view cancer as a preventable disease that requires lifestyle changes. The latest data shows that causes and their associated cancer incidences are as follows:

Tobacco—30 percent
Diet—35 percent
Obesity—14–20 percent
Infections—18 percent
Environmental pollution/toxins—7 percent
Genetics—5–10 percent[8]

Thus we should be focusing on the 95 percent of preventable factors that directly cause cancer rather than only the 5 percent.

Many doctors and patients alike depend too much on genetic testing to reduce potential and theoretical risks rather than work on the direct risks. Although genomic testing can help give some guidance to doctors and patients regarding metabolic pathways, sensitivities, and useful information about cellular and immune functioning, this data is not always static, but sometimes dynamic. This is hugely important to understand; most people don't realize that the genetic information that we collect with these tests is not set in stone but actually in flux. Yes, your genes are constantly changing how they function, for better or for worse. How we eat, how we move, how we think, and how we feel can all affect these changes.

Everything we place into our body and into our mind directly affects the expression of our genes. Thus, using genomics to optimize certain drugs or therapies can be helpful, but ultimately limiting lifestyle recommendations to what tests tell you is very shortsighted; doing so can cause problems down the line. Many of my patients repeat genetic tests six months after implementing my lifestyle recommendations. They often see their potentially risky genetic markers change back to normal or their protective genetic markers improve.

Not surprisingly, many people prefer to believe that "removal" of the potential area of worry or risk frees them from the future problem. For example, a recent study showed that double mastectomies given to women with cancer in just one breast did not increase their overall survival when compared to women that treated the cancerous breast alone.[13] The idea of performing surgery before a problem actually appears is the worst kind of reactionary medicine. It encourages an avoidance of responsibility. It comes as a result of not encouraging patients to take personal responsibility for their lifestyle, and of not taking the time to address and understand the underlying, treatable wellness issues.

Food and Nutrition: The Foundation of Health

Building a house on a strong foundation
—SHERYL CROW

Let's start with diet. It's so basic, but it's the most important foundational aspect of health.

We all have heard the saying, "you are what you eat." Now, through science and evidence-based medicine, we can actually demonstrate that concept. It is ridiculous that many doctors—especially GI doctors—and even oncologists say, "Eat whatever you want," or "It doesn't matter what you eat as long as you take your medications."

This way of thinking is not only absurd, it is also completely ignorant, arrogant, and grossly uninformed. All doctors should be well versed in nutrition, since they are authorities who provide you with critical advice about your health. To deny the importance of nutrition is mind-boggling. How do these doctors think the body works? How do they think medicines work? Were they not taught in medical school that most pharmaceutical drugs have been derived from plants and other natural agents? Do they only understand how drugs work, not how the original compounds work in their natural states?

Here is a startling fact: most doctors in the United States do not have any nutrition training—maybe a few hours, if that, out of thousands of hours of medical training. Given this alarming fact, I recommend that you check to see if your health-care practitioner has any formal education in nutrition and ensure that he or she is not using out-of-date information or unscientific recommendations. You can easily verify whether your health-care provider has had formal postgraduate fellowship training in integrative medicine or specific certifications in nutrition (and importantly whether they also look healthy themselves).

Science understands that food fuels our body, giving us the ability to function appropriately. Let me give you an example. If your body were a car, you would be careful to give it the right type of fuel. You wouldn't put kerosene or lighter fluid in your car, nor would you put cheap gas in a Ferrari.

But when it comes to the food we eat, we do just that—choose the cheapest fuel possible. It's easy to understand how kerosene would ruin your car. But when it comes to our bodies, we do not acknowledge the consequences of using the wrong fuel.

So, let's begin by looking at which types of fuels we should be using and which we should be avoiding.

The standard American diet is a paradox—a diet of both deficiency and excess. I will start with a discussion about what we are not eating enough of, and then I will focus on what we are eating too much of.

Not Eating Enough Vegetables and Fruits—Eating Too Much Refined Wheat, Refined Sugar, and Animal Proteins, Fats, and Oils

In 2012, the Union of Concerned Scientists published data showing that Americans are not eating enough vegetables and fruits and are instead eating more refined grains and sugars than recommended. You don't have to be a scientist to agree with their data; just look around you and see what has happened to the average size of the American adult over the past twenty years. Adults and children alike have become "supersized." Is it any wonder we are living in the first period in all of recorded history in which humans are dying of preventable illness at a higher rate than of infectious diseases?

American farmers could easily grow the additional vegetables and fruits our nation desperately needs without any impact on the total acreage of land currently available for crops. In fact, only 2% of U.S. farmland is planted with fruits and vegetables.[14] Without even addressing the larger issue of misguided agricultural subsidies, and instead simply increasing the public support of local farms, we could not only grow the amount of healthy veg-etables and fruits that we need but also boost the prosperity of our local economies. Sadly, there is little community support nationwide for a local food investment—it's a market of about $90 million annually—yet the mas-sive soy and corn (both mostly GMO) subsidies total $5.08 billion annually.[15]

We need to change our focus from industrial farming to local farming, and from unnecessary GMO crops to sustainable agriculture that's good for our health, the environment, and our economy. Estimates show that if we did so, we could create about 189,000 jobs in local food systems and gener-ate $9.5 billion in direct sales of healthy foods.[16]

The good news is that small steps can lead to big change. Therefore, instead of shopping at big-box stores, I recommend supporting local co-ops and community-supported agriculture (CSA), farmers' markets and, if you can, growing as much of your own food as possible by planting a garden **(see Side Notes: Growing an Inexpensive Garden and Growing Boosters)**.

CHAPTER 3

The Ten-Step Approach to Optimum Health and Longevity STEP 1: Eating an Organic, Non-GMO, Plant-Based, Anti-inflammatory Diet

> *Without proper diet, medicine is of no use.*
> *With proper diet, medicine is of no need.*
> —AYURVEDIC PROVERB

Over the past few decades, we have come to understand the importance of eating organic foods. That actually means foods that are grown naturally, without the use of pesticides, herbicides, endocrine (hormone) disruptors, and other carcinogenic (cancer-causing) agents. We have come to understand that the fewer chemicals we consume and are exposed to, the better off we will be. Simply put, we need to eat more organic, non-GMO (genetically modified) foods.

The GMO Myth: Are GMOs Really That Bad for You and the Environment?

> *I want a cup of coffee, but I don't want a GMO.*
> *I like to start my day off without helping Monsanto.*
> —NEIL YOUNG

Organic, Non-GMO Foods = Healthy and safe for us and the environment
GMO and Conventional Foods = Unhealthy and unsafe for us and the environment

GMO foods are neither good for you nor good for the people who grow them or for the environment. Independent data from scientists and consumer organizations (those not paid by the industry and without financial ties to "big agra") have shown this to be true.[17] There is absolutely no health reason to eat GMO foods or to plant GMO crops for the sake of saving the environment—period.

Organic is understood to mean that particular animals and plants are not GMO (genetically modified organisms). This means that organic plants or animals have been grown without certain chemicals and have not been exposed to or created as new organisms. Genetic modification uses biotechnology to introduce the DNA of other animals, plants, insects, bacteria, and so on, to an organic plant or animal. Hence an organic tomato is just a tomato—its DNA is only tomato, nothing else. A GMO tomato, in contrast, can contain the DNA of salmon, pigs, other vegetables, mycobacteria, or insects.

Why, you might be asking yourself, would we want the DNA of vastly different species in our food? The boilerplate reasoning is that these genetic modifications enhance or create certain positive attributes. By creating what are now commonly called "Frankenfoods"—foods that contain a mixture of DNA from other species and categories of life, just like Frankenstein—we have created a monster. The companies that own the technology and produce these types of foods benefit financially, of course, but you and I are the collateral damage. Let's look at the reasoning behind a GMO tomato.

Salmon DNA prevents the GMO tomato from freezing during shipment in the winter; pig DNA makes the skin slightly thicker to prevent bruising; and other genetic modifications allow the tomato to ripen more slowly so it will stay fresh longer during transport, storage, and display. This GMO tomato can be found twenty-four hours a day, seven days a week, year-round in all fifty states; it's ready to eat anytime, anywhere. Until very recently, foods were seasonal, and people ate with the cycles of the harvest and the seasons. Many fruits and vegetables were eaten in the summer, and others were eaten in the winter. Today, we're paying a price for the modern convenience—not in actual costs of food, but in the increased costs of inadequate nutrition making us sick. Through GMO foods, we have created a sophisticated "fix" instead of a sustainable solution.

The problem with GMO is twofold. First, the mixing of DNA of multiple different species into another animal, vegetable, or plant confuses our immune system (remember, this system comprises the soldier cells in our bodies that fight viruses, bacteria, yeast, parasites, and cancers and that repair damaged tissues). When we eat GMOs, our immune system doesn't recognize what food it's consuming. Here's how you can think of it: if you go to the airport for your flight, you will have to show a TSA (Transportation Safety Administration) officer your ID and ticket. These officers not only compare you directly against your picture, they also compare the name on your ticket to your ID, and they place your ID under a black light to make sure the ID and state seals are real. Even if you travel every day and know the TSA officer by name, when you pass through security, that TSA officer will still inspect your ticket and ID.

The same goes for your immune system and food. Even if you eat the same food all the time, each time you eat it, your GI tract's immune "TSA officer" inspects it. Using the GMO tomato example, when you present the food to your immune TSA officer, you're presenting it with an ID that has many faces (through the introduction of other genetic DNA) and a name on the ticket that doesn't match. When the immune TSA officer looks at the ID under the black light one way, it may see a tomato; another way, it may see a salmon or pig. When this confusion occurs, the immune TSA officer interprets the jumbled information to mean that the ID is fake or suspicious and may send you for further screening and holding, and—worst-case scenario—Taser you if it feels threatened.

In essence, your immune system's TSA officer is trying to protect itself and your body. If it cannot recognize the food you're eating, it does what it is supposed to: reject it. Using this fundamental protective mechanism, the body then sends inflammation (like a Taser) to help the TSA officer stop the suspicious passenger.

But the immune system doesn't see the suspicious GMO passenger as an isolated incident. Immune TSA officers instead start to continuously overreact to all suspicious passengers. They fire their Tasers at everything that might be a threat, triggering symptoms of inflammation that worsen all health conditions—especially those starting from the GI tract, like heart-burn, reflux, gastritis, bloating, cramping, diarrhea, and constipation. All of these reactions are just the immune system's response to foods that are offending it, and inflammation is a protective mechanism. Inflammation is an extreme measure, but, like Tasering, it's supposed to function as an effective, *temporary* solution. Inflammation is not a long-term safeguard but a quick way to neutralize a threat. However, if the person does not prevent or reduce exposure to suspicious foods, then inflammation becomes chronic. This leads to worsening disease because inflammation is meant only as a first line of defense—not a permanent strategy.

Another symptom of an overused inflammatory response—this mis-guidance of recognition and overexposure—is food sensitivity or allergic reaction. Like with a "most wanted" list, once the immune system has been challenged, it will be on the lookout for foods that are the same or similar to the suspicious passengers. It will react against such foods with inflammation every time it confronts them.

In addition to confusing the immune system and causing the body to defend itself with inflammation, GMO foods present an additional problem; some of these genetically modified organisms are directly harmful to our bodies.

Most GMO foods are manufactured by or have a relationship with a few companies that control the agricultural industry (e.g., Monsanto, DuPont, Syngenta, and ConAgra Foods). To justify creating a market for GMO foods, these companies promised (more like misled) that farmers would see increased yields, use fewer pesticides and insecticides, and be able to "feed the world" with this new technology. This propaganda is spread not only by these companies but also by lobbyists who influence our representatives in Congress—many of who have financial ties to multibillion-dollar agra-bio-tech companies and their owners.

The problem with GMOs and pro-GMO propaganda is that there is no scientific basis for the claims of increased yields, decreased chemical use, or the suitability of these Frankencrops for worldwide cultivation. The official report by the Union of Concerned Scientists elucidated all this in an article titled, "Failure to Yield: Evaluating the Performance of Genetically Engineered Crops."[18] In addition, the American Academy of Environmental Medicine's position paper on GMO foods states that GMOs pose a "serious health risk in the areas of toxicology, allergy and immune function, reproductive health, and metabolic, physiologic, and genetic health and are without benefit."[19] Most recently, a report by the UN Commission on Trade and Development concluded that small-scale organic farming can create strong local food systems—the only viable, sustainable way to feed the world. Bottom line: GMO foods are not sustainable, not good for the environment, and not good for our health.

Yet again, the United States lags behind the rest of the world in matters of public health. Most of Europe has banned GMO foods since 1999, and most of the world has followed suit. Over sixty other countries, including Russia and China, ban or severely restrict GMO foods. Yes, China, the country in which most of our manufactured items—like our tennis shoes and smartphones—are made with child labor in unhealthy factory conditions. This is not a point of moral superiority, however. China does not permit GMO foods, as the Chinese government doesn't want their laborers to be sickened and to be unable to make our cheap consumer goods!

Why, then, do we in the United States, continue to be exposed to these harmful foods? Let me explain briefly why they have been banned nearly everywhere else.

Mounting scientific data, both in laboratory animals and from the agricultural and farming communities, support the same conclusion about the dangers of GMO foods. Studies have established that GMO foods contain not only other species' DNA but also DNA that performs two main functions that are devastating to our health.

Many GMO plants contain Roundup Ready genes. You may have seen or used Roundup, an herbicide created by Monsanto Company to kill and prevent weeds from growing. Although many people use Roundup on their home lawns and gardens **(see Side Notes: Safer Alternatives for Weed and Bug Control)**, few are aware that companies now alter the genes of plants to help them withstand exposure to Roundup, and that these genetic modifications create a serious danger. Here's how that gene-changing process works.

When the Roundup Ready genes are mixed into the GMO crops, they cause the GMO plant to resist the herbicide in Roundup. Roundup acts as a chelator to prevent weeds from growing in the fields. A chelator is a substance that binds to minerals and removes them. Roundup kills weeds by binding to minerals in the weeds, starving them of nutrition and thus killing them. Studies have shown that these GMO Roundup Ready crops—such as soy and corn fed to cows, pigs, and other live-stock—cause nutritional deficiencies that lead to health problems and even death in the livestock. Studies and data from the Institute for Responsible Technology also show that when humans eat these animals that have consumed GMO foods, we also develop nutritional deficiencies. Terrifyingly, the actions of chelation from GMO foods affect us at the top of the food chain!

The Roundup Ready, resistant genes in crops also kill insects that eat the crops due to the ingredient glyphosate. Even more frightening is that it kills them by cracking open the insects' GI tracts, causing them to die from a leaky gut. Unfortunately, the same effect has also been discovered in animals further up the food chain (cows, pigs, etc.) that eat GMO foods. These animals have much higher incidences of GI distress and related health problems. Dissections of the GI tracts of GMO-fed animals have revealed damage to their digestive linings, similar to what we see in humans with conditions like Crohn's and ulcerative colitis. This damage also causes food particles to leak from the GI tract, creating additional systemic inflammatory conditions.

The introduction of GMO foods in 1999 very strongly correlates with the sharp rise of certain health conditions. Genetic engineers John Fagan and Michael Antoniou and researcher Claire Robinson, authors of GMO Myths and Truths, published an evidence-based examination of the claims made about the safety and efficacy of GMO crops and foods by Big Agra. They discovered that most of the claims about the environmental benefits and safety of GMO foods are simply not true.[20] I strongly encourage you to read this report. In addition, a recent study, titled "Genetically engineered crops, glyphosate and the deterioration of health in the United States of America" and published in the Journal of Organic Systems by Swanson et al., indicates there is a dramatic statistically significant correlation (P value <0.00001) between twenty-two diseases and the consumption of GMO crops and glyphosate use. These include hypertension, stroke, diabetes, obesity, inflammatory bowel diseases, Alzheimer's, Parkinson's, MS, autism, lipoprotein metabolism disorder, and a variety of cancers, such as myeloid leukemia and cancers of the thyroid, pancreas, liver, kidney, and bladder.[21] There is a clear and distinct correlation between the rise of these health problems and the introduction of GMOs into the food supply.

Not only are these chronic diseases now more common, they are also occurring in younger populations. People born after 1999 have lived their entire lives with immune systems that have been fighting these GMOs; they have not been exposed to real foods in any meaningful way. Many of these young people started with fussy eating habits as infants. They had GI problems regardless of the types of formula used. As a population, they experienced more eczemas, behavioral problems, and autoimmune illnesses as children than previous generations.

Older people have experienced a similar increase in incidence of these health issues, reporting symptoms only in the past few years after eating these foods. Remarkably, many of these older people never experienced these symptoms prior to the introduction of GMO into our food supply.

Top GMO Foods to Avoid and What You Must Eat Organic

1. Soy—94 percent of US crops are GMO
2. Corn—88 percent of US crops are GMO including high-fructose corn syrup and corn sugar
3. Canola (Rapeseed)—90 percent of US crops are GMO
4. Sugar Beets (and sugar made from sugar beets instead of cane)—95 percent of US crops are GMO
5. Hawaiian Papaya—95 percent of US crops are GMO
6. Zucchini—11 percent of US crops are GMO
7. Crookneck Squash—11 percent of US crops are GMO
8. Apples—recent approval, data not available at time of publication
9. Potatoes—recent approval, data not available at time of publication

New GMO foods coming soon to a grocery store near you

10. Salmon
11. Wheat
12. Rice
13. Bananas

If you consume any of the foods above, look for specific disclosures that say they are organic and non-GMO.

GMOs affect all of us, even the most careful organic shoppers, because most of the foods we eat (more than 90 percent) contain one or more of these ingredients. Even ingredients labeled "USDA Organic" may contain GMOs, but if foods are not labeled organic or non-GMO at all, then they are almost guaranteed to be GMO by default. What's worse is that Congress recently passed a bill to restrict GMO labeling. That bill makes labeling voluntary and says companies may not need to warn people if the FDA believes that a product causes no harm—thus no GMO labeling is required, even if the states and the majority of the public vote in favor of it. This is shameful, and in my opinion it's a subtle act of terrorism. This will lead to continuing harm to Americans' health and quality of life; it's a gross infringement of their right to have clean and harmless food and water. Our Congress has been hijacked by corporations, and those members who voted in favor of the bill will have to face the new challenges of what to do with their constituents as they get smarter on the subject and learn about the direct and indirect health risks they have been exposed to. Soon the public will become more aware that Congress does not represent the people but only big business.

I predict that as more GMO foods are added to the above list, we will see an increase in GI, skin, autoimmune, and other serious health conditions. The problem will be highlighted in two specific populations: infants and seafood consumers. Since infants consume their body weight in food in short periods of time because they need to feed constantly and grow, in my opinion, they are at the highest risk. Apples (and bananas and rice) are the base in many baby foods. This large amount of GMO exposure from an early age will place them at the highest risk for adverse reactions. Those who choose to eat salmon for its higher omega-3 and lower mercury content are also at risk, since this is a major source of their animal-protein intake.

Many of my patients who move toward a plant-based diet and avoid eating foods that cause specific inflammatory reactions (food allergies) still have symptoms because they still experience the damage that GMO foods can cause. Even I have noticed this effect. When I go out to eat, even though I eat a plant-based diet and avoid the foods that I am allergic or sensitive to, I too can still have GI complaints. When I look at what I consumed, my symptoms almost always correlate to eating GMO foods. For example, I might go to a

Mexican restaurant and have a vegan-type meal, with no meat, cheese, or sour cream (and none of the foods that I specifically am sensitive to), but still have GI complaints. That is because I am eating GMO corn chips and corn tortillas that are fried in GMO canola oil. When I eat the same exact meal at home, but using only organic, non-GMO ingredients, I have no symptoms whatsoever.

Be careful of grocery-store tactics that lead you to choose unhealthy GMO foods. When I walk into my local grocery store, the first items I pass are doughnuts and premade coffee drinks. Then I pass chips, sodas, and cereals. That's a lot of temptation! To combat the pull to make poor food choices, I advise you to try to eat something prior to grocery shopping. You will notice that you will make better food choices and avoid snack foods, since you are already satiated.

Here are some simple tips to help you choose healthier foods when you go grocery shopping:

Tips for Healthier Shopping Choices

1. **Shop veggies and fruits first.** Go to the fresh-produce section first and fill your cart with fresh organic, non-GMO vegetables and fruits before you visit the rest of the store. Avoid products that are placed near the entry, such as packaged doughnuts, coffees, and cereals. These "foods" are not the healthiest, but because of their placement, they easily entice us to buy them.

2. **Create a rainbow of color!** I like to call it the Rainbow Diet. Try to get as many colors of fruits and veggies in your cart as you can: all shades of green, red, yellow, orange, purple, etc. These colorful foods tend to have the highest amounts of antioxidants and phytonutrients, which are important for preventing and healing many diseases.

3. **Purchase smaller quantities.** This ensures that you consume a variety of foods. It also prevents you from stocking up on unnecessary amounts of food. When we shop at big-box grocery markets, we tend to purchase bulk convenience foods in large quantities because it is cheaper to buy in bulk. Unfortunately, many of these foods are unhealthy processed foods sold to us in bulk because we would not normally keep that much in our household.

4. **Look for clean labels.** The fewer ingredients the better. Avoid packaged foods that have dozens of ingredients on the label. A longer list of ingredients means chemicals, fillers, additives, flavor enhancers, preservatives, artificial colors, etc. For example, corn tortillas only require organic corn, lime, and water—that's it. Tortillas should not have twenty ingredients!

5. **Don't drink your sugar.** Avoid colored and sugary beverages and juices. Many of the fluorescent-colored beverages contain glycerol oil of wood rosin to stabilize the blending of artificial colors and flavor ingredients. Avoid electrolyte drinks (sports drinks), vitamin waters, energy drinks, sodas, and premade juices (even if organic). These drinks are full of sugar (usually GMO sugar—beet sugar), high-fructose corn syrup (GMO corn), colors, and other additives that are terrible for your body. Even "healthy" sodas and fruit juices can contain large amounts of sugar. Stick to filtered water or other organic beverages such as kombucha, teas, and green drinks. (A great sugar reference guide for packaged foods and drinks can be found at SugarStacks.com.)

6. **Avoid highly refined carbohydrates.** Choose organic, 100 percent whole grains or sprouted grains as much as possible. Avoid white tortillas, white bread, white sugar, and other highly refined packaged and processed foods.

7. **Avoid frozen or premade meals.** Frozen meals contain large amounts of refined foods, fats, and salt. Frozen meals usually contain more than *half* your daily salt intake in one serving! See section, "The Question of Salt."

8. **Reinvent the concept of dessert.** Most cultures have desserts that are real foods, instead of the highly refined and processed foods we typically think of as dessert. Many healthier substitutions for sugar-laden treats can be very satisfying. For example, for those who like yogurt, replace your sugar-packed flavored yogurt with organic unsweetened coconut yogurt with fresh berries, seeds, and nuts to taste. It can take a little creativity, but making a few changes like this gives you healthy nutrients in addition to satisfying your sweet tooth.

9. **Make a grocery list to avoid impulse buys.** The snack foods at the end of the aisle at the grocery store are there to tempt you into

impulsively purchasing them. Make a list of the groceries you need prior to heading out to the store so you are not tempted to fill your cart with junk. Consider cart size as well; the larger the cart, the more you will feel as if you need to fill it (and they want you to). The smaller the cart (or basket), the easier it is to fill it appropriately and avoid impulse items.

10. **Keep it local when you can.** Shop at a local co-op, farmers' market, or health-food store instead of big-box stores as much as possible. These stores encourage you to buy fresh and seasonal foods, which are healthier for you and your family. Eat as much locally grown organic, non-GMO foods as possible, and even grow a garden. You and your body will thank me later.

These ten steps are just a few simple suggestions that will change the way we eat for the better. It can feel like a big shift, but once we acknowledge the simple truth that food is *the* biggest contributing factor to our health, for better or for worse, rethinking our food choices also becomes easier.

You're probably familiar with the famous quote from Hippocrates, the father of Western medicine: "Let food be thy medicine and medicine be thy food."

But food in the United States is no longer our medicine; it has turned into our poison. What are we eating that causes us so much unnecessary suffering? Is our food today the same food our grandparents ate? Let's take a closer look.

What Are We Eating?

> And the food just ain't no good?
> The macaroni's soggy, the peas are mushed,
> And the chicken tastes like wood...
> With this ugly food that stinks,
> So you bust out the door while it's still closed
> Still sick from the food you ate,
> And then you run to the store for quick relief
> From a bottle of Kaopectate.
> —THE SUGARHILL GANG

The data below is from 2010.[22] You can get the idea very clearly about the poor dietary habits of the average person. Here's how it breaks down:

- Each year, Americans eat 85.5 lb. of fats and oils. They eat 110 lb. of red meat, including 62.4 lb. of beef and 46.5 lb. of pork. Americans eat 73.6 lb. of poultry, including 60.4 lb. of chicken. We also eat 16.1 lb. of fish and shellfish and 32.7 lb. of eggs.
- Americans eat 31.4 lb. of cheese each year and 600.5 lb. of noncheese dairy products. We drink 181 lb. of beverage milks.
- Americans eat 192.3 lb. of flour and cereal products, including 134.1 lb. of wheat flour.
- We eat 141.6 lb. of caloric sweeteners, including 42 lb. of corn syrup.
- Americans consume 56 lb. of corn each year, 415.4 lb. of vegetables, and 273.2 lb. of fruit.
- Americans consume a combined total of 24 lb. of coffee, cocoa, and nuts annually.
- Processed food consumption every year includes 29 lb. of french fries, 23 lb. of pizza, and 24 lb. of ice cream.
- Americans drink 53 gallons of soda annually, averaging about one gallon each week. We eat 24 lb. of artificial sweeteners in a year.
- Americans consume 2.7 lb. of sodium every year, which is 47 percent more than recommended.
- We also consume 0.2 lb. of caffeine each year, which works out to about 90,700 mg annually.
- In total, Americans eat an average between 2,700 and 3,790 calories each day.

Here's how all that works out on a daily basis:

- The average American consumed about one pound of animal protein per day.
- Americans consumed about two pounds of cheese and dairy products a day.
- We consumed half a pound of refined flour products every day.
- Those four hundred pounds of veggies we eat every year? About 95 percent of that total is in the form of french fries. Conventional

potatoes are the crop with the heaviest use of pesticides, herbicides, and chemicals.[23] Ketchup is now the second most common "vegetable" consumed.

Is it any wonder we average between 2,700 and 3,790 calories each and every day?

While these numbers from 2010 are shocking, current numbers point only to a continuation of these trends. We are eating nutrient-deficient calories, and we are "lovin' it."

According to the Centers for Disease Control (CDC) map **(see fig. 7)**, there has been a drastic increase in obesity in the United States from 1990 to 2009. In 1990, most of the country had a body mass index (BMI) between 10 percent and 15 percent. The most current data, from 2010, shows many of the states range from grey to dark grey, meaning the average BMI is between 25 percent and 30 percent. A more recent CDC study showed that "the average man's waist grew from 38.9 inches to 39.7 inches," and the average woman's waist grew "from 36.3 inches to 37.8 inches." More worrisome is that there has been an increase in abdominal obesity, which "starts at 40.2 inches for men and 34.6 inches for women." The study found "43% of men and 64% of women are in that zone," which is "up from 37% of men and 55% of women in 1999."[24] Since the editing of this book, there has been an update to the data from 2013 **(see fig. 8)**. If you look closely, the BMI ranges have changed to add a "greater than 35" level on the legend. We are getting so big that not only are our weight scales changing but also the scales on the maps! Now approximately 24% of the US population is considered normal weight (BMI less than 24.9), 35% is overweight (BMI between 25 and 29.9), 35% obese (BMI between 30 and 40), and about 6% morbidly obese (BMI above 40).[25]

In the southern states, the dark-red area is called the "stroke belt," meaning the people who live in these states are more likely to have a stroke or a heart attack than those in the rest of the United States. This is thanks to the fact that we have definitely "supersized" ourselves, not just our food.

Related to all this, I have identified an inverse-ratio phenomenon that I call the "body-weight to television-thickness effect." Think back to the 1990s, when people were thinner but television sets were thicker. The only things that have gotten thinner since then are our television sets; we have only gotten thicker **(see figs. 7, 8, and 9)**.

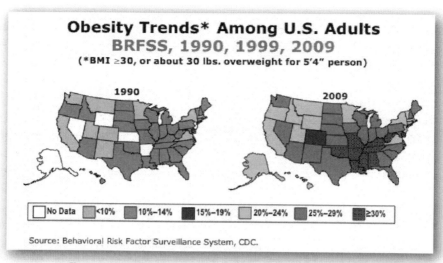

Figure 7: CDC: Obesity trends from 1990 to 2009 in the United States

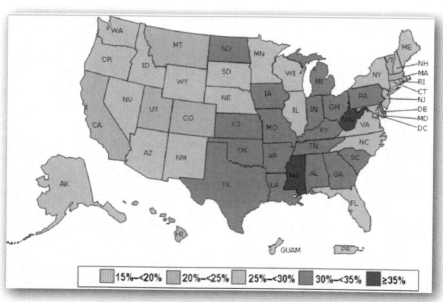

Figure 8: CDC: Obesity trends in the United States 2013

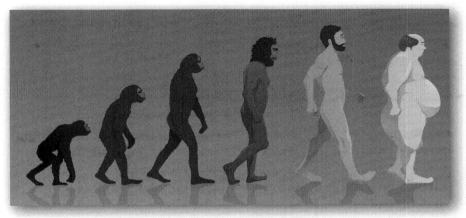

Figure 9: Evolution of modern human

Pro-inflammatory (Animal Proteins) vs. Anti-inflammatory (Plant-Based Proteins)

> *I like my steak well done, my taters fried*
> *Football games on Monday night*
> *It's just who I am*
> *A meat and potato man.*
> —ALAN JACKSON

Understanding the general types of foods that increase inflammation and the general types of foods that decrease inflammation is crucial to understanding why we are "supersizing." Controlling inflammation is as important as controlling our caloric intake.

The difference between such foods is actually pretty simple, although the idea is pretty unpopular with the average American.

Animal proteins cause inflammation, and plant-based proteins do not (unless there is a specific, individual allergic inflammatory reaction—such as to soy, corn, or wheat—which will be discussed later). That's the root of it, and here's why.

Anti-inflammatory Proteins = Plant-Based Proteins (Have No Cholesterol and Contain Protein, Fiber, Antioxidants, and Phytonutrients)

Plant-based proteins are the best for you to consume. Believe it or not, many plants are abundant sources of healthy proteins! Certain vegetables, whole grains, some fruits, and legumes (both beans and lentils) have abundant protein for a healthy body. Plant-based protein has *no* cholesterol and does not cause inflammation (unless it is GMO, or one has a food allergy—more on that later). Therefore, if you have a cholesterol problem and are taking prescription drugs or supplements to lower it, you can give your body a hand simply by eating more plant proteins and fewer or no animal proteins. Switching from animal to plant protein also helps if you have any of the two hundred or so "itis" diseases or conditions.

By a making a shift toward a plant-based diet (anti-inflammatory foods) and reducing animal proteins (pro-inflammatory foods)—and avoiding what our body has an allergy or sensitivity to—we are putting ourselves in the best state of health not only to recover from normal day-to-day inflammatory activities but also to live in a state of optimum health where we can reverse and prevent chronic inflammatory diseases down the road.

Highly trained professional athletes understand this concept the best. When pro athletes work out, they spend most of their day training at high intensities and pushing their bodies into ranges that make them into elite athletes. After each workout, training session, and event, they spend a great deal of time trying to recover faster by getting massages, stretching, and taking anti-inflammatory drugs. Over the past twenty years, it has come to light that some of the most competitive and famous athletes were and are actually vegan. Yes, vegan.

Some of these vegan athletes include Carl Lewis, Martina Navratilova, Jim Morris, Patrik Baboumian, Rich Roll, Brendan Brazier, and Mac Danzig, to name a few. Just search the Internet for vegan athletes, and you will be surprised.

Why would professional athletes eat a plant-based diet? What happened to glasses of raw eggs and platefuls of steaks for breakfast?

Pro athletes go vegan because they know that if they reduce the amount of inflammation they get from their diet by avoiding animal proteins, then they can recover faster—which helps them to train quicker. This in turn gives them an edge and makes them better athletes, since they are training and practicing more than their counterparts who take longer to recover after their activities.

It's not just professional athletes who have chosen to be vegan. Famous people throughout history have understood the value of eating mostly plants. Here are just a few to take note of: Gandhi, Einstein, Voltaire, Leonardo da Vinci, Pythagoras, Newton, Plato, Socrates, Buddha, Emerson, Thoreau, Confucius, Benjamin Franklin, Lincoln, and Cesar Chavez.

Today, successful entrepreneurs and Hollywood stars alike are moving toward a plant-based diet. Why? Staying on top of their game—whether that is in the academic, technology, or entertainment industries—requires them to be very competitive. When one doesn't feel well or is unhealthy, it shows up mentally, physically, and even spiritually.

Here is a list of some of the top entertainers and those in Hollywood who eat more plant-based diets: Madonna, Ellen DeGeneres, Justin Timberlake, Moby, Anne Hathaway, Jason Mraz, Mike Tyson, Russell Brand, Kristen Bell, Woody Harrelson, Carrie Underwood, Rosie O'Donnell, Ozzy Osbourne, Reese Witherspoon, Leonardo DiCaprio, Dr. Dre, Prince, Steve Martin, Michael Franti, Ted Danson, Bryan Adams, Alicia Silverstone, Jennifer Connelly, Russell Simmons, Jay Z, and Beyoncé, to name a few.

I ask my patients, if you were a Hollywood actor or actress who made tens of millions of dollars, wouldn't you like to keep your money and status for as long as possible? Even if they are motivated by selfish or financial reasons, the result is still positive: people are moving toward eating healthier foods. Although becoming healthier may not be on the top of some of my patients' lists of priorities, I do know that preserving their financial health is supremely important—not only to them, but to almost everyone. It's not my place to judge my patients' motivations when they choose to eat healthier; I just need to discover their motivating factor and use it to encourage them to change their health for the better.

Plant-based proteins also have fiber, which is important for your colon health and for lowering blood-glucose and cholesterol levels. Fiber is not the buzzword it once was, but it is still crucially important. Fiber not only lowers blood sugar by slowing down digestion and reducing the glycemic spike; it also lowers cholesterol while binding to toxins and excess hormones, removing them from the body. When we eat fiber, which is found *only* in plants, it binds to these unwanted elements in the GI tract and removes them from our bodies safely and effectively.

Optimally, one should consume about 40 g (or more) of fiber daily; the average American consumes 7–12 g of fiber per day. When there is less fiber in the diet, cholesterol, environmental toxins, and hormones (both those produced internally and those from outside exposure) are then reabsorbed through enterohepatic circulation. Therefore, when our diet lacks fiber, these unwanted elements, which can cause disease and increase our risk of developing cancer, continuously recirculate throughout our body. This bears out through disease statistics: those individuals in countries that consume the highest amount of fiber have very low rates of colon cancers and chronic health conditions; the United States has one of the highest rates.[26] In addition, a study showed a 46 percent reduction of breast-cancer risk for those women who had three bowel movements a day versus just one, and another study showed constipated women are at higher risk for the reasons mentioned above.[27]

In addition to fiber, plant-based protein sources also contain abundant antioxidants and phytonutrients, which are not found in animal protein. You need to have all four of these categories—protein, fiber, antioxidants, and phytonutrients—in your diet in order to achieve and maintain optimal health. Animal proteins on their own just don't cut it.

Pro-inflammatory Proteins = Animal Proteins (Contain Cholesterol, Cause Inflammation, Have No Fiber, Have Few Antioxidants, and Have No Phytonutrients)

Those who consume animal-based proteins such as beef, pork, lamb, chicken, eggs, and dairy actually trigger more inflammatory reactions in their body. Animal-based proteins, especially red meat (beef and pork—yes, pork is a red meat even though they advertise it as "the other white meat"), are the protein sources that contain the highest amount of omega-6 fatty acids. These omega-6 fatty acids actually trigger inflammation. As I have mentioned before, if there is trauma, pathology, or overuse, or if the immune system is fatigued, then these omega-6 inflammatory triggers can cause even more dysfunction and damage in the body.

The most obvious disadvantage of animal proteins is that they contain cholesterol, whereas plant-based proteins do not. So, if you have a cholesterol problem or heart disease and are taking medications for it, if you want to lower your cholesterol, you must first move toward a completely plant-based diet (more on this later).

If you have constipation and have to take fiber supplements (e.g., Metamucil, Benefiber, or FiberCon), stool softeners (e.g., Colace), or laxatives (e.g., Dulcolax), then you are eating too much animal protein and not *nearly* enough fiber.

Remember, average Americans get only 7–12 g of fiber in their diet every day (mostly through highly processed foods), and we need about *six times* that amount!

Most of us are not getting enough antioxidants and phytonutrients in our diets. So many people suffer from poor wound healing, diminished vision, and poor immune function. We are sick and feel tired all the time because we are not feeding ourselves enough antioxidants and phytonutrients. This is why stores carry aisles of antioxidant (e.g., vitamins A, C, and E), mineral (e.g., magnesium), phytonutrient (e.g., resveratrol, grape seed, broccoli seed, green tea, lycopene, and lutein) supplements—most people don't consume much (if any) in their diet because they are eating a majority animal-protein diet. Generic supplements simply aren't adequate; they are usually synthetic, microdosed (very low doses that do not provide adequate clinical benefits) vitamins and are not potent across the full spectrum (using only single isolates of nutrients which limit the efficacy). They therefore don't offer complete health benefits. For those tired of taking products like those, eating more plant-based foods is an easy, cost-effective, and clinically proven way to improve your health.

Omega-6s: The Pro-inflammatory Cascade

> *I'm gonna roam this highway*
> *Till my dying day.*
> —STEVE MILLER BAND

"How can foods be inflammatory?" you might ask. I'll explain it to you the way I explain it to my patients.

When I educate my patients about food, I like to start off by telling them about what I call the "highways" (pathways) of pro- and anti-inflammatory cascades. After gaining just a basic understanding of the way these pathways work, you will easily see how every food that you ingest can either worsen your physical condition or help your body heal.

I call the omega-6 pathway the "highway to inflammation." Some of my patients with chronic, painful medical conditions call it the "highway to hell." On this inflammatory pathway, certain foods start down a metabolic highway, and they end up along two specific routes of major inflammation enzymes called COX (cyclooxygenase) and LOX (lipoxygenase). There are hundreds of highways to inflammation, but COX and LOX are the major interstates. Decreasing the amount of travel down these interstates leads to less pain, less degeneration, and a reduction in chronic disease, and it can even mitigate the risk of developing cancer.

The highway to inflammation **(see fig. 10)** starts at **linoleic acid (fig. 10: #1)** and heads directly for the major intersection with **arachidonic acid (fig. 10: #2)**, the main inflammation hub. From there, it's on to the interstates of inflammation—COX and LOX—which lead to dozens of pro-inflammatory off-ramps (factors) that worsen every health condition.

Two main traffic sources feed directly into this inflammation cascade. One is **refined cooking oil,** and the other (a more direct and stronger link) is **animal products,** including **animal proteins, animal fats, shellfish,** and **mollusks.**

As you can see, the primary stimulators of the initial inflammation pathways are refined cooking oils like canola, safflower, corn, soybean, and peanut. You ingest these oils every time you eat french fries or fried foods, especially at fast-food or chain restaurants, many of which use cheap GMO oils. As most of my patients and I myself can testify to, when we first switch to a mostly plant-based diet and eventually become vegan, we tend to become french-fry junkies. Why? Well, before one learns to cook at home and make wonderful real meals with real foods, we rely on the quick-service food industry just like anyone else. Chain-restaurant or fast-food salads usually leave much to be desired. When we go out to eat with family and friends, avoiding meat usually leaves us with little more than french fries or other fried veggies (like zucchini sticks, which are also GMO) to fill us up. This itself, for new vegetarians or vegans, can be the single biggest inflammation-triggering factor as they ease into their new way of eating.

The next big inflammation traffic source is the major trigger point in the hub of inflammation, arachidonic acid. Animal-based proteins like beef, pork, lamb, eggs (whites and yolks), chicken (regardless of dark or white meat), and organ meats produce arachidonic acid. These foods directly feed into the main inflammation hub and trigger both COX and LOX pathways of inflammation. This means that if you already have a place in your body that is inflamed—whether by pain, chronic disease, or dysfunction—eating animal proteins will make your conditions worse! Adding insult to injury, many meals eaten in a restaurant in the United States consist of both meat and french fries. Thus the average combo meal is a "double-double"—a combo meal for double the pain and double the inflammation!

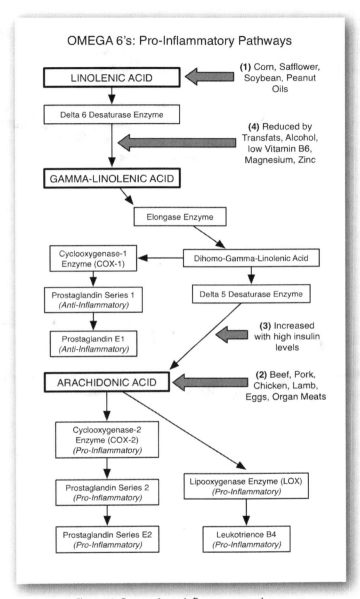

Figure 10: Omega-6: pro-inflammatory pathways

Another important item to note is that higher levels of insulin or blood sugar tend to increase this inflammation cascade **(fig. 10: #3)**; therefore, if you have insulin resistance or diabetes, your body is automatically more prone to have inflammatory health problems and its consequences. Diabetics have four times the risk of heart disease—a disease that is now better understood as an inflammatory disease. In addition, trans fats and alcohol **(fig. 10: #4)** reduce the conversion of gamma-linolenic acid (GLA). Gamma-linolenic acid (GLA) is an essential fatty acid derived from plants such as evening primrose, borage and black current seed oil which is a natural anti-inflammatory. It is important to eat an anti-inflammatory diet, take natural anti-inflammatories regularly, keep blood sugar under strict control, avoid trans fats, and limit alcohol consumption.

Omega-3s: The Anti-inflammatory Cascade

Cool the engines.
—BOSTON

Unlike the omega-6 fatty acids with their highways of inflammation, omega-3 fatty acids instead are anti-inflammatory. Thus, omega-3s decrease inflammation, help lower inflammatory-disease conditions, and confer numerous other health benefits. Omega-3s predominantly come from plant sources, such as soybeans, walnuts, hemp, perilla, and flaxseeds, but they are also found in certain fish, like mackerel, sardines, anchovies, salmon, and squid **(see fig. 11)**.

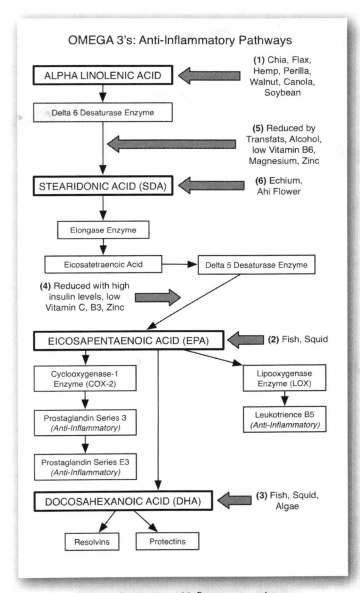

Figure 11: Omega-3s: anti-inflammatory pathways

As shown in figure 11, omega-3s start with plant-based proteins (**fig. 11: #1**). Further down the pathway, more abundant and direct amounts of EPA (eicosapentaenoic acid – which is beneficial for heart health and lowering inflammation) **(fig. 11: #2)** and DHA (docoshexaenoic acid – which is ben-eficial for neurological health) **(fig. 11: #3)** are derived from fish, squid, and algae. In short, the anti-inflammatory effects of omega-3s can help cancel out the pro-inflammatory effects of omega-6s. Even more impressive are the health benefits that occur when one eliminates as many sources of omega-6s (animal proteins and cheap cooking oils) as possible and eats mainly omega-3s. It is best not just to balance out the ratios so they cancel each other out but to consume far more omega-3s to ensure an anti-inflammatory outcome from your diet.

Although many plant-based foods also naturally contain omega-6s, they have naturally higher amounts of omega-3s as well, making them anti-inflammatory overall. This is not the case with pro-inflammatory omega-6 foods, which predominantly come from animal protein and fats.

Thousands of published articles tell the benefits of omega-3s. Here are just a few of the things that omega-3s are good for:

- Children's health (improvement of ADHD, visual development, intelligence/learning, autism spectrum)
- Diabetes and metabolic syndrome (lowering blood sugar)
- Cardiovascular health (lowering lipids)
- Immune health (allergy, autoimmune)
- Joint health (arthritis, injury)
- Gastrointestinal health (digestion)
- Cancer support (lowering inflammation)
- Mental health (improvement of cognition, depression, mood disorders)

Here's a little-known fact about a person with insulin resistance or dia-betes: their body has difficulty metabolically converting omega-3s to both EPA and DHA **(fig. 11: #4)**. Without a change in diet, omega-3 supplemen-tation is critical. Reducing the intake of animal proteins and switching to a plant-based diet can initiate a huge reduction of omega-6s instantly. By mak-ing this simple dietary change, one can reduce the need for supplementation of omega-3s. Alcohol and low levels of magnesium, zinc, and vitamins C and B6 also reduce the conversion of alpha-linolenic acid (ALA) to EPA, therefore decreasing DHA **(fig. 11: #5)**. When you keep alcohol to a minimum and your vitamin levels up, your body can use plant foods for an anti-inflammatory effect and other health benefits.

Omega-3 supplements have grown into a massive industry since the beginning of the twenty-first century. Fish oil is the primary source, but there are safer and more sustainable plant-based forms of omegas available, along with, of course, the omega-3s found in a whole-food, plant-based diet **(see Side Notes: Omega-3 Recommendations)**. Remember, omega-3s are anti-inflammatory in nature, meaning they decrease inflammation; omega-6s are pro-inflammatory, meaning they cause inflammation—especially in the high amounts that most Americans consume on a daily basis.

Omega-3s: What about Fish?

To the Salmon chasing slew
Four straight days Jimmy trolled the jagged coast line
But the fish were far and few.
—PRIMUS

Conventional dietary advice tells us to eat more fish to increase our intake of omega-3s. In recent years, many respected doctors and scientists have encouraged the consumption of everything from sardines, anchovies, and salmon to fish-oil supplements. Unfortunately, the problems with fish are more numerous than their purported benefits.

Most recently, studies have shown that we are facing a shortage of fish in the near future due to the unsustainable fishing practices of generic fish-oil companies and fisheries. Also, many fish contain dangerous chemicals and heavy metals (e.g., mercury, PCBs, and dioxins), and thus one must be careful when eating fish. When seeking a reliable source of information on potential hazards in foods and consumer products, I recommend the Environmental Working Group (EWG.org). EWG is a nonprofit organization that protects consumers by testing foods, cosmetics, and a variety of products that we place on and in our bodies. They have a Consumer Guide to Seafood that lists the pros and cons of many types of fish—from the amount of healthy EPA/DHA to the fish that have the highest exposure to toxic contaminants.

They also have a Seafood Calculator that will list how much of each type of seafood you can safely consume based on your age, gender, weight, and other risk factors, such as heart disease.

With regards to the overall safety of fish, the rule is as follows: Dangerous chemicals that have been dumped into our oceans and rivers have contaminated our fish. The larger the fish, the more chemicals are absorbed. This is because heavy metals and chemicals collect in the protein of the fish. Bigger fish eat smaller fish, and that concentrates those chemicals in the bigger fish. Therefore, small fish such as anchovies, sardines, and mackerel have the least contamination; tuna has much greater amounts; and shark has the most.

According to the Environmental Working Group, consuming a single six-ounce serving of albacore tuna a week significantly exceeds the EPA's safe limit (reference dose) of methylmercury. Canned light tuna has less methylmercury, but it provides far less omega-3 fatty acids and thus is not a suitable alternative for pregnant women or children, who are most vulnerable to heavy-metal exposure. Pregnant women and children should not eat more than one serving of canned light tuna a week. (As time goes by, and the fish become more contaminated, I tend to be more conservative and tell my pregnant patients and children to avoid tuna altogether.) Again, check out EWG.org to help determine the risk you face from the seafood you consume.

An interesting side note is that shark attacks have steadily increased worldwide since 1900, and this increase has been attributed to humans spending more time in the sea.[28] Although that might be true, I believe since sharks have the highest exposure risk to methylmercury, this toxic level may influence how sharks act.

For hundreds of years, mercury poisoning has been known to cause changes in behavior, increasing aggression and leading to psychosis. While occasional exposure to mercury isn't good for anyone, it's unlikely to manifest in extreme ways; however, lifetime exposure can be extremely hazardous. When compared to other professions, dentists have one of the highest suicide rates, along with higher neurological and psychiatric conditions; this may be attributed to their exposure to the mercury fillings that they work with every day for years.[29]

So although we are spending more time in the ocean, maybe the sharks over time are becoming more toxic, and that may be affecting their behavior toward us. These toxins are not safe for sea life or for us.

Wild Caught vs. Farmed

Wild-caught fish are better for your health than farmed fish. Wild-caught fish have higher levels of omega-3s, higher protein content, and lower fat content; farm-raised fish have higher levels of omega-6s, lower protein content, and higher fat content.

Wild-caught fish may contain contaminants (such as methylmercury, which is more concentrated in some fishing waters than others), but they usually have far fewer than farm-raised fish, which are raised with antibiotics and pesticides and adulterated with synthetic coloring. Even though most integrative-medicine doctors and holistic health experts have been advocating the benefits of eating wild-caught fish, it is uncertain for how much longer the benefits will outweigh the risks.

With the continued increase in ocean pollution due to industries that are not held accountable for their malpractices, contamination is increasing. Environmental disasters only add to the pollution; the Fukushima nuclear reactor in Japan is still leaking over three hundred tons of "radioactive-contaminated" water daily—and has been since 2011. Far from being totally diluted by the Pacific Ocean, radiation was found in the tuna and seaweed off the coast of California in 2012. As of this writing, there is no definitive plan or way to stop this radioactive contamination. This is no longer an issue only for Japan; it is a global issue that is already affecting the entire ecosystem and the main source of food for millions. You can keep up with this environmental disaster, along with other topics of concern, with information from the Center for Research on Globalization (www.globalresearch.org). Given this risk alone, is it wise to continue consuming fish in an effort to get our essential fatty acids?

Following the Fukushima disaster environmental groups have tested and confirmed that most of the coastlines of Hawaii, California, Oregon, Washington, and the west coast of Canada have some radioactive contamination; by the end of 2015, this radioactivity may reach South American coastlines if the leaking continues. Although there will be continued debate about how much radioactive contamination is "safe," I prefer to avoid exposure to these contaminants as much as possible, as they could be just one more contributing factor to chronic disease and cancer.

Now, it's true that the smaller the fish, the fewer contaminants it has. But it takes dozens of fish to make a single fish-oil softgel. Eating one sardine is not a problem, but concentrating dozens of them into two softgels could potentially be a problem. On top of that, choice in wild-caught fish is becoming more and more limited.

A study performed by *Consumer Reports* in 2013 showed that 30 percent of the fish in grocery markets (including the higher-end gourmet food stores) had been mislabeled (due to wholesalers mislabeling their fish when selling to the grocery fish buyers). This mislabeling resulted in customers asking for wild-caught fish but getting different species—many of which weren't even wild caught but farm raised.

This is a symptom of a larger problem—the problem of supplying enough (relatively) uncontaminated wild-caught fish to an increasingly informed public, who want (but may not be getting) a healthier option. Even though I recommend that my patients reduce or avoid animal proteins altogether, those who choose to eat wild-caught fish are facing shortages that may force them to find other options for their essential fatty acids sooner than they think.

What about the Mediterranean Diet?

You were somewhere on a cruise in the Mediterranean.
—ELTON JOHN

Many integrative and holistic physicians have been attempting to educate the public about the importance of the Mediterranean diet. All the studies on the Mediterranean diet have shown that, compared to the standard American diet (SAD), it was able to reduce heart disease and related conditions by approximately 75 percent. Yes, the Mediterranean diet is better than the SAD at reducing heart disease, but it is still not ideal.

When I finished my fellowship training in integrative medicine, the Mediterranean diet was the standard recommendation for a healthy diet.

This recommendation still dominates health education today. Let's look at the data more closely.

The people in Lyon Diet Heart Study (in 1994 and 1999) not only consumed wild-caught fish that had abundant omega-3s, but they also engaged in frequent fasting and vigorous daily exercise (even those over eighty years old), and ate large quantities of root and green vegetables, nuts and fruits daily, and whole-grain breads. While they were getting some protein from fish, they also were obtaining large amounts of their protein from the rest of their primarily plant-based diet.

When the original Mediterranean-diet studies came out, most of the omega-3 fish-oil companies and commercial fish companies used the data to take advantage of a new market for their products—which they could now market as part of a "healthy diet." For the most part, conventional fish oil was beneficial because it was helping to reduce the omega-6 overload from the SAD.

As I started learning more about plant-based diets and even more about their benefits over diets that included animal proteins, I started to question the previous data on the Mediterranean diet, which we all thought was outstanding.

A 75 percent reduction in heart disease for those eating a Mediterranean diet versus the SAD is amazing. But it led me to wonder...what about the other 25 percent? Why did these people still get heart disease even though they were eating this incredibly healthy diet? Wasn't there a diet that could prevent heart disease for everyone? At a conference I attended recently, Dr. Esselstyn from Cleveland Clinic presented a slide with data that answered just that question **(see fig. 12)**.

Those who ate a plant-based diet experienced a reduction in heart disease and related conditions that was greater than 95 percent. So, why would anyone want to settle for a 75 percent reduction of heart disease when you can get up to 95 percent reduction on a plant-based diet? To me, this was a no-brainer, an easy decision for me to continue to recommend a plant-based diet to all of my patients—even those who have done well with their health on the Mediterranean diet. A plant-based diet can reduce their risk of heart disease even more by increasing their intake of plant-based proteins, reducing their intake of animal-based proteins (even seafood), and eliminating the heavy use of refined oils.

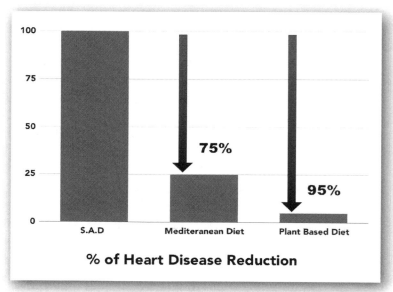

Figure 12: Risk comparison of heart disease with SAD, Mediterranean, and plant-based diet (Modified from Dr. Caldwell Esselstyn, 10th Annual Dr. Roizen's Preventive Care and Integrative Medicine Conference, December 7, 2012–December 9, 2012)

Omega-3s: What about Fish-Oil Supplements?

Manufacturing, marketing, pricing, packaging
—CEELO GREEN

Not all fish-oil supplements are the same, even if they all sound similar. Over the last sixteen years of practicing integrative medicine and studying the manufacturing, processing, and formulating processes of dietary supplements—and especially reviewing the clinical studies—I have learned many good and disturbing things about the dietary-supplement industry. Some companies have done very well in providing good products, and some have taken advantage of consumers.

The fish-oil industry is a great example of good concepts gone terribly wrong.

I talked a bit about my concerns with fish oils earlier in this chapter. The continued popularity of fish oils nationwide exacerbates these concerns. Over the past ten years, fish-oil supplements have been in the top-selling

categories of dietary supplements. This is due to the over eight
studies (a database of research is available at www.omega-research.com)
that have been conducted on the roles of EPA and DHA in a variety of health
conditions. This overwhelming data, coupled with savvy marketing, means
that most people understand the importance of omega-3s. But most people
don't know the differences in the processing, manufacturing, potency, and
purity of fish oils. Let's first start with the basics of fish-oil processing.

Fish-Oil Processing

The majority of generic fish-oil supplements that go to big-box and pharmacy chain stores rely on fish oil sourced from the larger fish like tuna and
cod. One of the biggest suppliers of generic fish oil sold to grocery stores
derives its oil from the tuna that it sells to the same stores. In fact, this
supplier makes more money selling fish oil than the actual tuna fish (for
legal reasons, I have chosen not to mention the name of this supplier).

Fish oil should always come from smaller fish species, such as sardines,
anchovies, and mackerel—not only for safety reasons (as described previously), but also for sustainability reasons. Beware of fish-oil supplements
that say their oil is derived from "marine lipid concentrate" or just "fish oil"
instead of listing their fish sources. Such generically labeled ingredients mean
these fish oils can use any type of fish or sea creature and, therefore, contain
the cheapest form of sea life available—throwaway sea-life products that
do not make it into the food supply. Is that what you want to be ingesting?

According to a 2012 report from the Food and Agriculture Organization
of the United Nations, an estimated three-quarters of the planet's fish stocks
are now fished to their maximum limits or are completely exhausted.[30]
Therefore, it is of the utmost importance to the health of our oceans to know
how the fish you consume are caught. When generic fish-oil companies are
selling fish oil containing the byproducts of commercial fishing, they are not
looking at long-term sustainability, and they are not concerned with the quality of their products. While this is sadly the norm for fish oils, a few companies
have done an excellent job following sustainable fishing practices, working in
conjunction with regional governments that monitor sustainable fisheries (in
the Antarctic and South America, in particular). But most companies do not
follow sustainable fishing practices, as doing so is not mandatory—nor is it

mandatory to disclose how they obtain their fish oil. For your health, and the health of our oceans, I strongly recommend only supporting companies that describe their sustainable practices and contribute to environmental organizations that also help preserve those invaluable ecosystems.

Fish-Oil Potency

In addition to understanding the sustainability of a particular fish-oil source, one needs to understand the ideal potency for fish oil.

Most fish-oil products state something like "total fish-oil concentrate equals 1,000 mg." Do not be fooled by totals! The label must state in milligrams (mg) exactly how much EPA and DHA are in the fish oil—not just total fish-oil content. For example, a generic big-box brand will list 1000 mg of total fish oil and then list 300 mg of EPA and DHA combined. You want to see EPA and DHA broken out into milligrams for *each*. Most generic fish oils will only give you a total amount and not specific milligrams of EPA and DHA. Some don't even mention that they have EPA and DHA, but only omega-3s. They do this to hide the fact that their fish oils do not meet efficacy standards. If your fish oil doesn't give you specific amounts (in milligrams) for EPA and DHA, then you shouldn't waste your money on it.

For fish oil to provide clinical benefits for a variety of health conditions— especially for those who do not eat a plant-based diet—I recommend these minimum dosages:

- EPA—750 mg/day
- DHA—500 mg/day

For those with severe lipid problems, inflammatory conditions, or neurodegenerative conditions, I recommend that they double those dosages so that they get approximately 1,500 mg EPA and 500–1000 mg DHA every day. Those who have insulin resistance or diabetes should also take higher doses, as they do not convert as much EPA and DHA from their food sources as do those without blood-sugar problems (see fig. 11). But if one were to eat a plant-based diet only, his or her blood sugar and cholesterol problems would usually resolve, and thus he or she would not need high doses of EPA and DHA from fish oil.

Fish-Oil Purity and Safety

> *Now there ain't no rules and regulations.*
> —THE DOOBIE BROTHERS

Now that you have an understanding of sustainability and sourcing of fish oil, along with the necessary potency to seek out, let's break down the specific issues you should be aware of regarding fish-oil safety.

Most of my patients ask the same question regarding fish-oil safety: "But isn't that what the FDA does—ensure the safety of products like fish oil?" No, it doesn't. The FDA only regulates drugs, and fish oil is a dietary supplement. Thus there are no current mandatory guidelines for fish-oil safety. That's a little scary, isn't it?

There are many organizations such as GOED (Global Organization for EPA and DHA Omega-3s), IFOS (International Fish Oil Standards), and my favorite, CRN (the Council for Responsible Nutrition). These organizations provide the guidelines for environmental-toxin limits (dangerous chemicals such as PCBs, dioxins, and dioxin-like PCBs), oxidation limits (determining the level of fish-oil rancidity through peroxide, anisidine, and total oxidation [TOTOX] levels), and heavy metals (such as mercury, lead, arsenic, and cadmium).

It shouldn't shock you to hear this by now, but only a few companies actually follow these safety guidelines. Most generic companies may list "purity tested" on their labels and come up with their own stamps to show some sort of quality measure, but these self-certifications don't tell you their testing standards. So, in essence, they can say they test for purity, and even though their numbers may not meet the recommendations for safety from the CRN, they still can state on their label that their fish oil has been "purity tested" or "purity certified." In my opinion, this practice is unethical and incredibly misleading, yet this is *standard practice* for many fish-oil companies. It's all profits first, consumer safety last. This is why it's so important not only to pay attention to labels but also to know how to read them—or, in this case, read through them.

For the last decade and a half, I have worked closely with a variety of supplement companies, all of whom provided me with their assurance of purity and safety testing. Some of these companies had products in both professional and retail markets. When one of these companies was first starting out, they focused on a few really great products that were not only pure but also highly potent. But as they became more successful, they began to increase the number of products (SKUs) they made in order to grab customers shopping for a variety of price points and health conditions. Although I recommended the products and admired that they invested in clinical research and helped pioneer the industry, their expansion from a few products to dozens of products shifted their focus. Growth and profitability moved them away from their original intention of providing high-purity and high-potency products.

You might wonder why this would bother me so much and why I would even bring it up as an issue. After all, what's wrong with being successful and profitable?

As an integrative-medicine expert, I work closely with my patients and am deeply involved in helping them choose and support their use of natural products, so long as these products provide health benefits. But over the years, I started to notice that most patients do not pay close attention to the details of their fish oil, opting to purchase based on brand name and, understandably, price point. They would tell me, "I take two of my fish-oil pills daily as you recommended." When enough routine testing didn't bear out the inclusion of fish oil in these patients' diets, I decided to investigate.

Once I looked more closely at these generic products, I discovered that potencies varied significantly from product to product—even within the same brand. The difference? It all came down to the price point at which they were sold. My patients thought they were getting a discount on price, but they were also getting a discount on potency of EPA and DHA. On top of that, most patients were taking a variety of products within the same brand, not knowing that each product varied in potency and, therefore, in clinical benefit. It was a confusing situation for a time, which is why I now recommend that my patients know not only what brand they buy but also the amount of EPA and DHA they take daily. I suggest they look for those milligrams consistently. To simplify the process, I like to recommend companies that have limited products and that instead focus on potency and purity.

Further complicating the situation, however, are the many "doctor brand" companies not offered in retail markets. These "doctor brands," marketed to health-care practitioners, state that their exclusivity ensures better manufacturing standards and quality for patients. Inevitably, however, just like other small-small providers who found market success, some of these once-trusted companies got larger and larger. Some were bought out by corporate conglomerates seeking to increase the presence of the nutraceuticals sector in their investment portfolios. Thus the companies that once provided excellent products shifted focus from product quality to increasing market share. To these conglomerates, fish oil and vitamins were just another part of a product portfolio that also contained multilevel-marketing companies, hotels, cosmetics, and IT companies. But a larger market share and improved marketing materials don't improve quality, and they don't drive sustainability.

I believe strongly that knowledge is power. So, I decided to cut to the chase and simply ask all these fish-oil companies for their test results. I told them I wanted to compare them to similar brands and see how they stacked up. Not surprisingly, I ran into roadblocks. Some would show me a purity test on a batch that was done months to over a year previously. When I asked them, "Well, what about the bottle that I have in my office? Or the bottle that my mother takes or my nieces take? What about *those* purity-testing results?" Every company told me that they conduct testing on various batches throughout their processing, but they *never provided the result for each batch*. Furthermore, they would not provide me test results for the bottle I was taking, even if the relevant batch data was "on file." Some companies stated that they do purity testing before processing, meaning they don't test after the production of the product. But fish oil that passes purity testing could easily fail rancidity or oxidation testing, as many products on the market would. These are the fish oils that have that fishy taste or smell, and their manufacturers are the same companies that won't disclose actual potency; such fish oils do not give you what you're supposed to get.

That's right—fish oil should never taste fishy. If it does, it means that the oil is rancid or off in some other way. For those who eat sushi, think of the "sushi rule," which is that good sushi does not taste or stink like fish. That's because good sushi is so fresh that the oils in the fish have not become rancid. Once the oils in the fish oxidize, they release the stinky fishy smell that we are all familiar with.

Here's a simple freshness test you can conduct on your fish oil: if you have a softgel, you should be able to chew it without having to spit it out because of its fishy taste. Companies that advertise "enteric-coated" fish oils tend to have the highest level of rancidity (fishy taste). Enteric coating prevents the oil from opening in the stomach, causing customers to notice, thanks to that familiar fishy burp aftertaste, that the fish oil was already rancid. Not all enteric-coated products are being used to mask poor ingredients, however. Most doctors have rightfully educated their patients that enteric coating is better when it comes to medicines (such as aspirin) because it prevents irritation to the stomach lining and decreases risk of ulcers. Unfortunately, companies are misusing this excellent idea to mask subpar fish oils. Fish oil never requires an enteric coating (or a capsule that is opaque); you should absorb fish oil just as you would absorb real fish: through the normal digestive process. The idea of bypassing the stomach absorption is a trick to hide bad oil, period.

Ethyl Esters vs. Natural Triglycerides

Synthetic overload
—Black Sabbath

Most people who take prescription fish-oil products or highly concentrated fish-oil supplements may be taking synthetic ethyl esters. Ethyl esters are used to increase the concentration of EPA and DHA in fish oil, but this is not an ideal process. The problem is that most companies do not convert the fish oil back into a natural triglyceride form (as nature intended) because of cost, thus keeping the synthetic ethyl-ester bond. Research has shown that the body does not efficiently absorb these ethyl esters. This same research shows that the body absorbs the natural triglyceride forms of EPA and DHA between 30 percent and 70 percent better (depending on which clinical research you're reading).[31]

Quality trumps quantity, always. You should only take fish oil in the natural triglyceride form, even if it is a high concentrate or high potency—especially in light of emerging research that suggests that ethyl esters may be causing increased oxidation in the body.

Most generic extra-strength fish oils use ethyl esters unless they state specifically that they are in natural triglyceride form. Even prescription fish oil is in ethyl-ester form, and of course, drug companies try to market that as a benefit, demonstrating that prescription fish oil is just another way for a pharmaceutical company to charge ten times the amount, bill your insurance company, and collect a co-pay.

Let me give you an example of how pointless and subpar ethyl-esters fish oil is. One of my patients in his early forties has elevated lipid levels. He exercises, generally eats well, and when he takes the right fish-oil supplement, his lipids are within normal limits. When I saw him after a few months for a follow-up and repeated his testing, all his bad cholesterol numbers had gone up. When I asked him if he was taking the fish oil that I recommended, he told me that he had switched over to another brand. His physical trainer at the gym had recommended another brand, which claimed to have four times higher levels of EPA and DHA. If it was four times stronger, he reasoned, he should have even better cholesterol results. I asked my patient to contact this fish-oil company and have them send me purity and potency testing on their product. Sure enough, he was taking ethyl-ester fish oil. On top of that, this fish oil had a much lower percentage of EPA and DHA than was printed on the label—up to 70 percent less! My patient was very upset, as he felt he had been completely misled, even though the marketing for the brand (to athletes) was very good. I told him most product information is just that—marketing. If he had taken what I recommended, his numbers never would have gone up. After a simple switch back to the fish oil I recommended, his lipids went back to normal. Now he is eating a plant-based diet, so he does not need to use fish oil at all.

What about Salmon Oil?

> *River runs to the sea*
> *Salmon runs to the sea.*
> —CARLY SIMON

The Mediterranean diet is largely responsible for the perception of salmon as a health food. Out of all the fish in the sea, wild-caught salmon has one of the highest amounts of omega-3s. Yet fish like tuna, cod, sardines, mackerel, and anchovies have always dominated the fish-oil market as more economical sources of omegas. Although one of the healthiest species of fish to consume, salmon is also one of the more expensive types of fish to buy when wild caught. Imagine my surprise, then, upon seeing "wild-caught salmon oil" in health-food stores. When I noticed how *inexpensive* these "wild-caught-salmon" oil products were, I knew I had to figure out why. When I started to investigate more closely, I discovered some shocking revelations.

Some seafood companies sell salmon oil that is certified to contain only salmon and natural flavoring. This isn't too bad, but you have to take, on average, three capsules to get approximately 240 mg EPA and 220 mg DHA. Remember, I recommend adults get at least 750 mg EPA and 500 mg DHA daily. But at least these companies are selling what they claim.

Many other companies do something that, in my opinion, is unethical. I found out that many companies that sell so-called wild-caught-salmon oil are using salmon oil from farm-raised fish. You might be wondering, How can these companies do this? Isn't that deceptive advertising? Here is what I found out.

First, many of these companies purchase farm-raised salmon from fish farms in East Asia, in countries like Indonesia, Thailand, Vietnam, and China. Companies source fish from these countries to get cheap sources of seafood while avoiding oversight and regulations. Salmon raised on these farms are fed corn and animal waste products. Feeding salmon things they would normally never encounter in nature—much less actually eat—elevates their omega-6 content, making the salmon more inflammatory (as described earlier). In addition, these salmon are raised in overfilled tanks that are crowded with fish, necessitating the use of high levels of antibiotics and pesticides to prevent infections and diseases that occur with unclean water in the tanks.

If you think this is bad, we haven't even gotten to the trickery employed by the companies that put the foul oil from these fish into their products.

Since farmed salmon are not as healthy as wild-caught salmon, their flesh is a very light pink to a sort of grayish color—not the deep orange and pink that we associate with wild-caught salmon. (The natural bright orange and deep pink of wild-caught salmon comes from the microalgae that the salmon eat in their natural habitats.) In order to rectify this color problem, the fish farms add astaxanthin to the fish feed.

You have probably heard of astaxanthin; it's an antioxidant that is very good for our eye health, like lutein. Astaxanthin is commercially collected from shrimp-processing waste. When fish farms go to process their shrimp, they extract astaxanthin from shrimp shells for use not as an antioxidant (carotenoid) but as a colorant. Twelve thousand pounds of wet shrimp shells can yield six to eight gallons of astaxanthin/triglyceride oil mixture. The FDA has approved the use of astaxanthin as a natural colorant that can be added to seafood and animals, so there is nothing specifically questionable going on as far as its intended use.

Many people take astaxanthin for its antioxidant and eye-health benefits, but research shows that it takes about four or more milligrams to obtain full clinical benefits. You might see these amounts in a good astaxanthin supplement, but the fish factory farms only need to add a small amount into the fish (about 16 micrograms) to turn their grayish flesh to a bright orange and deep pink. For those who need a visualization of how much that is, it's about five grains of sand—yes, almost a negligible amount.

Here's how these companies get their "wild-caught salmon": Once the farm-raised salmon are fed the astaxanthin, their flesh instantly appears healthier than it really is. Then a machine moves the salmon from their fetid tanks to the local river (most fish farms are located next to a natural water source), drops them into the water, and then picks them up just a few feet away. Voilà! "Wild-caught" salmon!

This is how most of the industry gets away with selling cheap "wild-caught-salmon" oil legally—on a technicality. It only takes a quick dunk in a river. This is a clear example of how industry finds loopholes to cheat the consumer while still complying with labeling laws. "Wild-caught-salmon" oil is just one of hundreds of examples of how the discount-dietary-supplement industry exploits consumer trust. *Buyer beware* has never been more apt.

Krill Oil vs. Fish Oil

> *Getting smaller and smaller.*
> —NINE INCH NAILS

Krill oil's popularity has grown exponentially since 2000. Krill are even smaller than anchovies, sardines, and mackerel, so in general they contain less contamination than most other marine life. If you listen to marketers, they are also the most sustainable ocean source of essential fatty acids. The explosion of krill-oil supplements has not brought about an equal explosion in regulation (or conclusive oceanographic data on the environmental impact of krill harvesting). For this reason, I tend to avoid krill oil. More than anything, I am not convinced that we can deplete a major ocean food source from the top of the food chain without negative effects.

Take a look at some of these facts about krill:[32]

- Krill is one of the most abundant species in the ocean, and it is the foundation of the entire food web.
- Krill is the main food source for whales, penguins, seals, and fish.
- Krill are tiny creatures, measuring no more than sixty-two millimeters long.
- The Antarctic supports 50 percent of all the krill biomass on earth and is the primary location where krill is fished.
- Both Canada and the United States have decided not to allow krill fisheries in their waters.
- Krill has declined in the Antarctic by 38 percent to 80 percent over the last thirty years. Along with the decline of the krill population has come a decline in the animals that depend on krill for food.
- In the Antarctic, krill reproduce under the sea ice. Diminishing sea ice (occurring from climate change) means fewer krill.

Antarctic scientists believe that fishing for krill is taking an unnecessary risk with an entire ecosystem. They provide three key reasons:[33]

1. Krill forms the base of the entire food pyramid in the ocean. Most large sea life, such as whales, penguins, seals, and other species, relies on krill as a major food source;
2. Because no population survey has been conducted, we really do not know how much krill there is. The basic data needed for management of fisheries has never been compiled. Most of the krill estimates have been based on calculations over a decade old, and we know that the ocean life is constantly changing because of environmental changes. Since krill live in swarms, they are easy to overfish, causing depletion;

3. Climate and sea-ice changes affect krill population. Climate change is happening very quickly in the Antarctic.

I side with the science and choose not to support the krill industry. In addition, many krill-oil products are adulterated; some contain not only krill oil but also fish oil. A consumer group recently tested one of the most popular brands selling "pure Arctic krill oil" and found that fish oil was the first ingredient and then krill was added as the second ingredient!

Furthermore, krill contains very small quantities of EPA and DHA—too small to provide the entire full benefit of their cardiovascular, neurological, and anti-inflammatory effects. For example, a popular krill-oil product on the market, Omega-Red, is advertised heavily on TV. It contains 50 mg of EPA and 24 mg of DHA per softgel. Remember, I recommend minimum dosages of 750 mg EPA and 500 mg of DHA *per day* for real clinical benefits. To achieve those benefits with Omega-Red krill oil, you would have to take *fifteen* softgels to get enough EPA and *twenty* softgels to equal the DHA of two softgels of high-quality fish oil (my specific brand recommendations are coming).

Therefore, although krill oil is marketed as easier to swallow (due to the smaller softgel), consuming enough krill oil to achieve real clinical results is both difficult and expensive. On average, a bottle of sixty krill-oil softgels costs about thirty-three dollars. Extra-strength krill oil only provides 64 mg of EPA and 30 mg of DHA per softgel, and it comes in bottles of forty-five softgels that cost approximately thirty-five dollars. With a suggested serving size of one softgel daily, it's impossible to get full omega-3 clinical benefits. To obtain full clinical dosages and benefits, a bottle of sixty regular softgels would only last you about four days, and extra-strength softgels would last you about three days. That starts making things very costly.

Again, this industry is providing a product that *could* be helpful. But instead of providing clinical doses, many manufacturers microdose krill oil potencies to make more profits. Unfortunately, such small doses will never provide full clinical benefits. Krill oil is heavily marketed to consumers who eat the standard American diet (SAD), take prescription medicine for cholesterol (e.g., a statin like Lipitor or Crestor), and then believe that taking krill oil will act as the magic bullet to help lower their cholesterol and heart-disease risk factors!

Fishy Labeling

> *There must be something fishy going on.*
> —DOLLY PARTON

When independently tested by third parties, 30 percent to 70 percent of fish-oil supplements don't meet their label claims of EPA, DHA, and other ingredients! That means that whenever you purchase conventional fish oil, you're likely to get 30 percent to 70 percent less EPA and DHA in the bottle than is stated on the label. Since many companies take advantage of the fish-oil craze, be on the lookout for the following deceptive marketing claims:

- *Pharmaceutical grade*: This term means nothing; the FDA has not defined this term, but companies use it to lend an air of quality and standardization when none usually exists.
- *Tested in FDA-approved laboratories*: The FDA does not approve labs but may register or inspect them.
- *Daily Value of Percent EPA and Percent DHA*: No daily value for essential fatty acids has been established, and this wording is not approved for health claims. Companies may list only milligrams of EPA or DHA, not percentages.
- *Free of*, or *void of*, or *no detectable*, or *purity tested*: These are excellent "weasel words," as they cannot be verified unless your manufacturer provides the actual test results of each batch.

So, how to ensure you get what you pay for?

- Read the ingredients carefully: Remember, many oils contain fish other than what the label discloses—like "wild-caught" salmon (often a mix or farm-raised fish colored with astaxanthin); while

so-called "pure Arctic krill oil" can actually be fish oil instead of krill, or a mix of oils.
- Do a label-claims test: Find out if your fish oil meet its label claims of EPA and DHA. Request testing data from the manufacturer and make sure it matches what's listed on your bottle!

Omega-3 Supplements: What to Avoid

I can't go for that.
—HALL & OATES

- Avoid enteric-coated pills: Enteric coatings mask the rancidity of bad oils.
- Remember the "sushi rule": Make sure the pills have no fishy taste or smell—chew them!
- Avoid fillers such as sodium laurel sulfate (SLS), propylene glycol, preservatives, and colors.
- Ingredients should be fish oil (or other source of omega-3s) and natural antioxidants only! Specifically, look for green-tea extract: green-tea extract is 40 percent more effective at keeping peroxide levels in check than lemon oil or rosemary oil, which are the standard in the industry. Green-tea extract is 100 percent more effective than the synthetic antioxidant BHT.
- Avoid GMO ingredients like vitamin E from GMO soy.

What about Omega-3s for Vegetarians or Vegans?

Because of the exponential growth of the fish-oil market worldwide, lax regulations, and the near-universal use of unsustainable fishing practices by fish-oil suppliers, I prefer to recommend a plant-based omega-3 to my patients.

It can be a challenge to implement a plant-based diet, but many of my patients find it easy to switch to omega-3s that are not fish based. Inevitably they ask me what vegetarian (or vegan) sources of omega-3s I prefer. Here's what I tell them.

Flax oil is a popular choice for many, but I do *not* recommend it. Flax is not a good source of omega-3s, as it only has about a 3.8 percent conversion to EPA and less than 1 percent conversion to DHA. Here's why these conversions matter: If you're taking one tablespoon of flax oil—which contains about 5000 mg of flax oil—you only get about *170 mg EPA and 15 mg DHA*. However, flax is not without its merits! I highly recommend taking organic flaxseed or flax meal, as you'll obtain the full benefits of its high-protein content and high fiber. But as a source of omega-3s (EPA and DHA), flax is woefully inadequate.

So what are the best sources of plant-based EPA and DHA?

One can find a fantastic source of EPA in Ahiflower oil (*Buglossoides arvensis* seed oil, which will be available in the marketplace soon) and eschium oil (*Echium plantagineum* seed oil). Both are sustainable plant sources of omega-3s that grow in North America, Europe, and southeastern Australia. These plant oils contain the precursor to EPA, called SDA. In the body, SDA converts to EPA at a rate of 30 percent, (versus the 3.8 percent with flax oil). That means you can obtain clinical doses of EPA from these healthy, sustainable plant sources. These renewable, non-GMO natural sources of omega-3s have a higher potency of EPA than flax, black currant, hemp, and SDA-enhanced soybean oils. I recommend products grown according to Crop Assured 365, which ensures the plant identity and preservation and checks to make sure there are no heavy metals, PCBs, or other harmful materials.

The best plant source of DHA that I've found comes from algal oil (an algae called *schizochytrium sp.*). This source of DHA is sustainably harvested and processed—something that cannot be said for most sources of DHA. Most major retailers and generic brands use DHA that is processed using hexane and other chemical solvents, which are dangerous to your health. One major supplier has dominated the marketplace by adding their hexane-extracted "DHA-enhanced" product to infant formula (even the infant formula used in neonatal ICUs) a practice to date has gone unquestioned by healthcare providers. Everything from soymilk to other plant omega-3 supplements uses this hexane-extraction process, which has (rightly) been criticized by many health-advocate organizations. Therefore I recommend my patients use *none* of the generic "DHA-enhanced" products on the market unless the product's manufacturer guarantees that they used no hexane in processing. Some companies use water-extraction methods to remove the DHA from algae, but that method costs slightly more, and many companies choose to use a cheap chemical solvent instead of thinking about their customers' health.

Because of my frustration with the major players in the fish-oil industry, I researched and located a company that has solid sustainability practices and clinical potency. This company derives its oils from sustainably harvested wild stocks that are closely regulated and monitored by government authorities. They even utilize energy conservation measures as well as help donate to environmental organizations. Finding a company that met my standards and surpassed my expectations of purity was a huge relief. This company not only tested each batch of their oil, they also developed an innovative gold standard for the industry that has challenged many companies (most of whom are afraid of raising their standards to this level). This system is called Pure Check, and it is the standard by which I measure all other omega-3 oils.

With Pure Check, each bottle (liquid or softgel, fish or plant-based oil) has a *lot number* on it. At the Pure Check website, you can enter your product's lot number and see the results of the purity testing for that lot. The test results cover everything from standard toxins to heavy-metal and oxidation levels and more—all from a third-party source posted in real time on every bottle. They even test for the amounts of EPA and DHA in each bottle and almost always exceed their label claims. Pure Check guarantees potency and purity, taking the guesswork out of the omega-3 industry. They preserve their products using a green-tea antioxidant, which is better at lowering the potential for oxidation than rosemary, lemon oil, or ascorbyl palmitate. For details on the above, see **Side Notes: Omega-3 Recommendations**.

SAD = Inflammation Overload

You know it's sad but true
—Metallica

The standard American diet (SAD) is incredibly "sad." It would be laughable if it weren't so dangerous to our collective health.

Americans have loaded our diets with enormous amounts of omega-6 fatty acids. Let me give you an example of why this is.

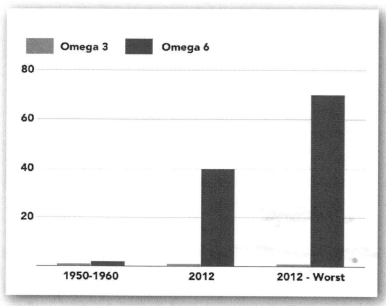

Figure 13: Ratio of omega-3 to omega-6 in SAD

In the early half of the last century, Americans consumed a diet that was pretty much balanced with regards to omega-3s and omega-6s. This ratio was approximately between 1:1 and 1:2 **(see fig. 13: 1950–60)**. Thus, for every food that Americans consumed that was high in omega-3s (e.g., fish, nuts, and seeds), we simultaneously consumed roughly the same amount of omega-6s (e.g., beef, pork, chicken, animal fats, and refined vegetable oils). Why is this important? With an approximately equal ratio between the anti-inflammatory and pro-inflammatory foods, they basically canceled each other out, and Americans ate a balanced diet in regards to the fatty acids. This almost-balanced ratio was due to the high cost of animal-based proteins. At that time, all but the wealthiest Americans ate steak, pork chops, or a roast on a very limited basis—say, for example, when someone had a pay raise or a birthday, when grandparents came over, or after church.

Unfortunately, industrialized factory farming and the commercial food processing of animal-based proteins have driven the cost of animal protein down significantly. Now we can have a Baconator—a hamburger that consists of three beef patties, three cheeses, and six pieces of bacon—for just a few dollars! While this was unheard of even fifty years ago, large amounts of inflammatory, animal-based proteins can now be consumed for very little out-of-pocket cost (except for the high cost of omega-6s to our health).

Over the past decade, several robust studies have indicated that these omega fatty acid ratios have changed dramatically due to our lifestyle and diet. Today, Americans have an omega-3 to omega-6 ratio anywhere from 1:7 all the way up to 1:40 **(see fig. 13: 2012)**. This means for every anti-inflammatory omega-3 food that we consume in our SAD, we consume up to *forty times* more pro-inflammatory omega-6s. Even worse, as I mentioned earlier, an entire swath of the United States (mainly southern states like Mississippi, Louisiana, and Alabama), called the stroke belt, has the highest incidences of strokes in the country. This is because the stroke belt consumes up to *seventy times more omega-6s than omega-3s* **(see fig. 13: 2012 Worst)**. In this area, they even fry the green tomatoes! It's no surprise that this region is responsible for a new junk-food craze that boasts about a Twinkie stuffed with a Twix candy bar, wrapped in bacon, and then deep fried. "Stroke belt" indeed!

What all this translates into is that we are *An Inflammation Nation*.

Cheap Food: The Common Denominator for Expensive Health Care

Done Dirt Cheap
—AC/DC

When the economy is down, it almost forces people to choose (or they have been aggressively marketed to look for) cheaper fast-food items, like a sixteen-piece bucket of fried chicken with sides and biscuits—marketed as a family meal for four for under thirty dollars. But these foods are not nutritious. As of 2013, a simple cheeseburger, french fries, and soda accounted for 80 percent of a person's daily recommended calories and 139 percent of their recommended sodium.[34] Although these foods are cheap, the long-term costs of fast-food decisions are much greater.

Let's explore this more closely. In the last forty years, there has been a dramatic increase in chronic diseases—especially those that are based on or triggered by inflammation—such as obesity, heart disease, diabetes, arthritis, colitis, headaches (including migraines), autoimmune diseases, and especially cancers. The World Health Organization (WHO) recently released a warning statement that eating processed meats, such as bacon, sausages, hot dogs, and red meats can cause cancer. The International Agency for Research on Cancer (IARC), which is part of the WHO, reviewed more than eight hundred scientific studies that looked at possible links between the consumption of processed or red meat and cancer. The review was conducted by a panel of twenty-two international experts examining meta-analysis data collected from a range of cultures, races, and diets from around the world. In particular, most of the studies focused on associations with colon, pancreatic, and prostate cancers. The results were so shocking that it prompted the WHO to classify processed meat as a carcinogen as deadly as tobacco, asbestos, and diesel fumes. Eating processed meat products increase your risk for cancer as much as smoking.[35] Yes, as much as smoking! The studies suggested that an additional 3.5 oz. (100 g) of red meat per day raises colon cancer risk 17 percent, while eating a smaller amount of processed meat 1.7 oz. (50 g) raises colon cancer risk by 18 percent. I remind you that these are not large amounts to begin with. The average meat topping pizza provides 12–18 g of protein per slice.[36] Most people eat three slices of pizza.[37] That's a total of 36–54 g of processed animal protein. This should be of grave concern for those who are eating processed meats and red meats, particularly as this does not include what else we may have eaten that day. Some claim that an organic plant-based diet is too expensive for American consumers; today's popular "meat lovers" pizza, however, will you more than you bargained for.

At a recent cancer conference, I learned that current data indicates that *one out of two males and one out of three females in the United States will get cancer over their lifetime.* This statistic is *only for the United States.* Over half the foreclosures of homes in the United States stem from financial crises caused by rising health-care costs.[38] In 2010, the initial cost of treating cancer for males and females ranged from $5,000 to $115,000, ongoing costs ran $1,000 to $12,000 a month, while costs during the last year of life reached $62,000 to $140,000.[39] At certain specialty hospitals, costs can exceed *tens of thousands of dollars per week* for courses of treatment *that can last for years*. How does that compare to spending slightly more for local organic fresh foods?

I say the same thing to my patients over and over: you need to invest in your health daily with the foods you consume. It's a sound investment. You are what you eat—both literally and figuratively. I suggest simply that the food you eat might be making you sick. Think about it.

The ugly truth is that our poor eating habits have led us to be a very sick nation, struggling with escalating health-care costs and poor outcomes. We pay more and get less than ever before. Buy cheap food and medications now, and you'll pay more later—much more.

I try to explain to my patients that it costs far less to see an integrative-medicine physician; use natural therapies, such as Bosmeric-SR; and make lifestyle changes, such as eating an organic, non-GMO, plant-based diet and practicing yoga or another type of movement therapy or exercise, practice mediation or stress reduction techniques, than it costs to see oncologists and undergo surgery, chemotherapy, and radiation. This does not even include the time (uncompensated) you will have to take out from your job during the several months of treatment. Your first bout with cancer might not be your last. Even after the most successful treatments, a cancer patient has a greater than 50 percent risk of reoccurrence over the next five years. Repeating treatment means going through all of it again—surgery, chemotherapy, and radiation—in addition to again paying, at a minimum, the initial and ongoing costs described above, and then adjusted upward for inflation. Of course, that's *if* you survive until the second time around...and that is a big *if*.

We are not healthy because we are not eating healthily. It's that simple. Although many people don't like to hear it, in my opinion, health is a choice. It is not a right. You choose to eat healthily or not. You choose to smoke or not. You choose to exercise or not. You choose to reduce stress in your life or not. You are not guaranteed that right; rather, it is a choice that you make, and hopefully, you make the right choice for all of us. We pay for poor choices every day with our taxes and through increased health-insurance premiums. Savvy marketing has coerced all of us to make certain choices, choices that may be not in *our* best interest but in someone else's. Did you know that eleven large insurance companies that sell life, disability and health insurance own $1.9 billion of stock (as of June 2009) in the top five fast food chains which include McDonald's, Burger King, KFC, Pizza Hut and Taco Bell?[40] This translates to them making money on food that makes you sick and the insurance policies they sell you for the consequences of your actions that they have influenced (eating food from those fast food companies). Hopefully this book will help you make the choices that are best for you—not for the corporations who try to sell toxic foods, dangerous medications, and unfavorable health policies.

Omega-6 fatty acids dominate our diets. We have all seen the increase in fried foods, processed foods, junk snack foods, and foods cooked with cheap, omega-6-rich oils. Our animal proteins come from GMO-grain-fed, hormone- and chemical-injected, diseased animals. This brings us to another key component in our omega-6 overload.

When animals are fed corn and other grains instead of natural grasses, the omega-3 fatty acids in their protein are diminished. Thus, although I strongly recommend eating a plant-based diet and avoiding animal proteins as much as possible, if one were to eat animal proteins, then one should only eat grass-fed, organic sources. Most animals that we consume eat a plant-based diet. Our largest animals—elephants, horses, rhinos, blue whales, and even gorillas—eat only plant-based proteins.

Does it sicken you that factory-farmed US beef cattle are forced to eat other animal proteins or corn, when they have evolved naturally to eat grass? These animals graze on grass and plants; fish "graze" on plankton and other sea plants. It almost demands the question: if all these animals don't need animal proteins to grow and to be healthy and strong, why do we? The answer is simple and sinister: because we have massive food industries that have successfully convinced us that we need to eat animal proteins, even though enormous amounts of conclusive scientific evidence prove just the opposite. For an extensive look into this concept, I recommend reading *The China Study* by Dr. T. Colin Campbell.[41] It is the largest nutritional study done worldwide. It will change the way you eat forever and improve your health outcomes overall. Another more recent favorite book is *How Not To Die* by Dr. Michael Greger[42] which covers the top fifteen causes of death and provides evidence based scientific data on plant based diets can prevent and reverse these diseases (usually better than prescriptions drugs and surgical interventions).

Farm Raised vs. Factory Farmed

Let me tell you about the farm.
—HANK WILLIAMS JR.

The average human diet has almost always included animal protein of some kind. Here are some examples of how farm-raised and factory-farmed foods have increased our intake of omega-6s (pro-inflammatory) and decreased omega-3s (anti-inflammatory).

Free-range chickens eat vegetables, insects, and fresh green grass, which is high in omega-3 fatty acids. Farm-raised chickens are predominantly fed corn. Free-range eggs have an omega-3 to omega-6 ratio of 1:1.5, so they are still slightly pro-inflammatory. But compare them to supermarket eggs, which have an omega-3 to omega-6 ratio of 1:20. Yes, that's twenty times more omega-6s than omega-3s! **(See fig. 14.)** Modern agriculture's emphasis on increased production has led to the development of grain-based, GMO chicken feed. This cheap, toxic feed is reflected in the out-of-balance ratio of fatty acids in the supermarket egg. Thus, the cleverly marketed "perfect protein" is now the perfect inflammatory food.

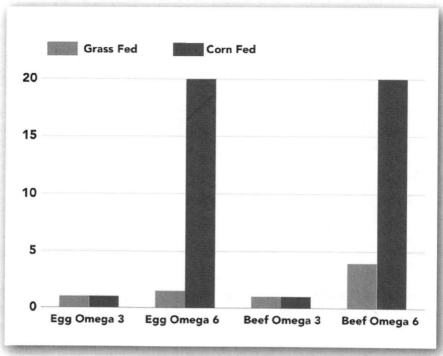

Figure 14: Ratio of omega-3 to omega-6—grass fed
(farm raised) vs. corn fed (factory farmed)

The next time you order an All-American Slam breakfast, you will get just that—a grand slam of inflammation, cholesterol, saturated fat, and calories. It will take you out of the park and directly into the cardiologist's office!

Here's what you'll get from the All-American Slam breakfast meal: 990 calories (almost half of your daily calories with 740 of those calories from fat); 83 g of fat (your total daily amount of fat); 26 g of saturated fat (6 g more than your daily amount); 680 mg of cholesterol (2.3 times your daily amount); 1,870 mg of sodium (more than 80 percent of your daily amount); 40 g of protein (71 percent of your daily amount); and only 3 g of fiber (only 7 percent of your needed daily amount).[43] In addition, because of the factory farming of animals, you may get over seven times the amount of inflammation per egg and animal-protein source, such as sausage, bacon, and ham. To make things worse, this is only a typical breakfast meal; we haven't even touched our lunch and dinner!

The real picture, however, is likely still more grim. The above figures come from restaurant company laboratories. Recently many consumer groups who tested similar foods from such restaurants found cholesterol and fat levels that ran 30 percent to 70 percent higher, since actual restaurants use more grease than the food company's laboratory does.[44] In addition, a series of studies in the journal *Preventing Chronic Disease* showed that over the past eighteen years, not much has changed with the nutrition in fast foods. In fact, some of them have gotten worse. Roughly 44 percent of foods tested actually showed an increase in calories over the years, and 33 percent showed increased amounts of sodium.[45]

Taking that into consideration, ordering an All-American Slam will get you ejected you from the game of healthy living. With a breakfast like that, you're well on your way to sitting on the bench for the rest of the season.

Although I highly recommend eating only a plant-based diet with no eggs at all, if you must eat eggs, then look for certified cage-free, organic eggs. When you eat cage-free, organic eggs, you will notice not only that the egg tastes better than conventional factory-farmed eggs but also that the yolk is a much darker orange and the shell is much thicker. Supermarket eggs have light-yellow yolks and thin shells. However, even these characteristics can be misleading. Savvy egg eaters have noticed this over the years, so, of course, many factory-farmed-egg producers have since learned a trick to make the yolks from a factory-farmed chicken turn dark orange.

The secret is marigolds.

When I was traveling near my hometown near the south coastal region of India, I saw near the docks veritable mountains of marigold flowers. Each radiant, dark-orange mountain of flowers must have been two to three stories high! When I asked the people outside what all the marigolds were for, they replied that they ship them to the United States (the largest importer of marigolds) for the factory farmers to feed to their chickens. When the marigolds are placed into the *corn* feed, their natural color darkens the egg yolks, creating the illusion of a healthier yolk. There is no significant nutritive value to marigolds; their use is strictly aesthetic.

Supermarket eggs are marketed as "fresh" to imply that they are healthy, but that is far from the truth. According to the USDA, eggs cannot be marketed or advertised (if using federal funding from the American Egg Board) to say the words "safe", "nutritious" or even "healthy".[46] This is because eggs do not meet the basic criteria for those definition of those words! So if those are words they can't say, what about the words they can say? Sadly, deceptive practices have become so commonplace that even the very specific label of "cage-free" can be misleading. This marigold deception seems minor, but it is yet another example of the factory farms of industrial food companies tricking the consumer. Supporting local farmers who raise free-range chickens is good for your local economy and helps to ensure that you are purchasing a more sustainable and humane form of animal protein.

The following comes from the Humane Society's website:[47]

The vast number of consumer labels affixed to egg cartons can leave a shopper feeling dazed and confused. One carton may label its eggs "Natural." Another carton may call them "Free Range," while yet another may claim its eggs are "Certified Organic." How are thoughtful consumers supposed to know what these labels and claims really mean?

The truth is that the majority of egg labels have little relevance to animal welfare or, if they do, they have no official standards or any mechanism to enforce them.

The Labels
Certified Organic: The birds are uncaged inside barns, and are required to have outdoor access, but the amount, duration, and quality of outdoor access is undefined. They are fed an organic, all-vegetarian diet free of antibiotics and pesticides, as required by the US Department of Agriculture's National Organic Program. Beak cutting and forced molting through starvation are permitted. Compliance is verified through third-party auditing.

Free-Range: While the USDA has defined the meaning of "free-range" for some poultry products, there are no standards in "free-range" egg production. Typically, free-range hens are uncaged inside barns and have some degree of outdoor access, but there are no requirements for the amount, duration, or quality of outdoor access. Since they are not caged, they can engage in many natural behaviors such as nesting and foraging. There are no restrictions regarding what the birds can be fed. Beak cutting and forced molting through starvation are permitted. There is no third-party auditing.

Cage-Free: As the term implies, hens laying eggs labeled as "cage-free" are uncaged inside barns, but they generally do not have access to the outdoors. They can engage in many of their natural behaviors such as walking, nesting, and spreading their wings. Beak cutting is permitted. There is no third-party auditing.

Free-Roaming: Also known as "free-range," the USDA has defined this claim for some poultry products, but there are no standards in "free-roaming" egg production. This essentially means the hens are cage-free. There is no third-party auditing.

Vegetarian-fed, Natural, Farm Fresh, Fertile, Omega-3 Enriched, Pasteurized: Designations with no relevance to animal welfare.

Now that you are educated about the differences in how chickens are raised for eggs in factory farming, it is my recommendation that you reduce or more importantly eliminate eggs from your diet. When you stop eating eggs, your cholesterol levels will decrease since eggs contain very high amounts of cholesterol (i.e. two eggs contain 423 mg of cholesterol) and you will also lower your overall inflammatory exposure. If however you still choose to consume eggs then you should seek out local farmers and obtain certified organic eggs and verify the conditions of their chickens.

What about free-range bison or free-range beef? Are there differences in their omega-6 content and their fatty acid ratios? Let's have a look at the studies.

In 2001 North Dakota State University conducted a study on the nutritional differences between grass-fed and grain-fed bison, the results of which closely mirrored the egg studies.[48] The grass-fed bison had omega-3 to omega-6 ratios of 1:4, and the grain-fed bison had omega-3 to omega-6 ratios of 1:21. Additional studies by other entities continuously show that the longer cattle are fed grain, the greater their fatty acid imbalance. For instance, after two hundred days in the factory-farm feedlot, grain-fed cattle have omega-3 to omega-6 ratios that exceed 1:20.[49] **(See fig. 14.)** Corn-fed beef has over *seven times* more inflammatory omega-6s than grass-fed beef!

With all the scientific data that has been published concerning omega-3 and omega-6 fatty acids, if one were to consume beef, it would be wise to choose organic, grass-fed beef over grain-fed beef. But even though grass-fed beef has less omega-6 than grain-fed beef, it still is a pro-inflammatory food that also contains cholesterol and has few antioxidants, no phytonutrients, and no fiber. Therefore, avoiding beef as much as possible and eating an anti-inflammatory, mostly plant-based diet (which contains protein, antioxidants, phytonutrients, and fiber) is still the best and easiest answer for reducing inflammation in the body.

The Grass Is Not Greener on the GMO Side

> *Take me to the other side.*
> —AEROSMITH

Spoiler alert! Coming soon to farms everywhere is the thing that we all have feared: GMO grass. Just when you didn't think GMOs could filter down into every part of your life, Monsanto—through their Scott division—will soon bring GMO grass to farms and lawns near you. This is a perfect opportunity to advance GMOs. There is no federal regulation from the FDA on grass because it is not considered a food. Blockbuster idea, right?

Wait a minute...isn't grass a food for your grass-fed beef, chicken, pork, and bison?

Although we do not yet have any scientific data on GMO grass, if history repeats itself (as it usually does), we will likely see the same health problems in the animals eating the GMO grass that we see in the animals eating GMO corn. That means eventually we will also see those problems in the people who eat those animals. Remember, you are what you eat, and now knowing what you are eating means also *knowing what whatever you are eating is eating*. Those who follow the Paleo Diet and those who choose organic, grass-fed animal proteins will soon be cheated of the concept of "clean food." Again, eating a whole-food, plant-based diet can easily eliminate the risk.

"Where's the Beef?" Not in Your Burgers!

You don't know what beef is.
—NOTORIOUS B. I. G.

The last twenty years have seen fast-food chains advertising larger and beefier burgers, with options including double, triple, and quadruple patties. However, although burgers have gotten bigger, that doesn't mean there's more beef!

A study published in the *Annals of Diagnostic Pathology* studied the top eight fast-food chains and discovered the following.[50]

- The average beef content per burger ranged from 2.1 percent to 14.8 percent!
- A half-pound burger patty or two quarter-pound burgers may contain less than 5 g of actual meat (this is equivalent to about the weight of one nickel or five small paperclips).
- Some burgers contained harmful bacteria, parasites (such as sarcocystis), and ammonia hydroxide (from washing the meat).

In addition to the above, fast-food burger meat often contains MSG or autolyzed yeast extract, along with dimethylpolysiloxane, a silicone product used in breast implants and Silly Putty.

If nothing else, you should be upset at these establishments for not providing what they market. Doesn't it make you wonder what the other 85.2 percent to 98 percent of the "beef" is? Unfortunately, when it comes to fast-food Dollar Menu or Value Meals, you get what you pay for: cheap chemicals and preservatives, along with fillers such as GMO soy, GMO corn, and wheat, plus "pink slime." If you do not know what pink slime is, do some research on the Internet and prepare to be shocked. I don't recommend eating before you do.

Many health-conscious people are taking part in the high-animal-protein diet craze. Many patients who come to see me are baffled by the fact that even though they eat just the burger and not the bun, they still have inflammatory symptoms. What they haven't considered are their unique food sensitivities. If they are sensitive to soy, corn, or wheat, they will get more of their allergens in the beef patty than in the bun! And most likely those ingredients are also GMO.

Now that you know what's really in your hamburgers, it may remind you of an old advertising campaign, which is more relevant today than it was in the 1980s: "Where's the beef?"

No, really. *Where's the beef?*

Keep Your Eyes on the Fries

> *Do you want fries with that?*
> —TIM MCGRAW

Now that you have learned that there is not much beef to your burger, what about the fries that go with that? As I mentioned before, most of us who transition to a plant-based diet may start to eat more french fries because of the convenience and availability in almost every restaurant. However, french fries are not as healthy as you may think.

Michael Pollan gave a lecture titled "How Cooking Can Change Your Life," which was posted in an article titled "The Big Food Discrepancy: Why Are American Foods Routinely More Toxic Than European Versions?" on Dr. Mercola's website.[51] The lecture and the article both describe how french fries in the United States come to contain many chemicals, such as TBHQ (tertiary butylhydroquinone), a preservative used to extend shelf life that is also found in cosmetics, lacquers, varnish, and even pet foods. Animal studies suggest this chemical may be associated with a number of health hazards, including liver effects at very low doses, positive mutation results from in-vitro tests on mammalian cells, biochemical changes at very low doses, and reproductive effects at high doses.

In addition to this preservative, fries also contain other chemicals, including color stabilizers and antifoaming agents such as the aforementioned dimethylpolysiloxane, which is used in products like breast implants and Silly Putty—meaning you get that chemical in *both* your burger and your fries.

French fries are also made with wheat and milk derivatives to create a beef flavor. Because the fries contain these other foods, they carry an allergy warning for those with dairy and wheat sensitivities. This creates a problem for those with wheat allergies who avoid eating the highly refined carbohydrate bun on the burger but still eat the fries.

According to Dr. Mercola's article and Michael Pollan's lecture, McDonald's french fries use only russet Burbank potatoes, which give them their unusual long shape. That shape allows the restaurants to place them into the red box packaging and present a "bouquet" of fries, which makes them more appealing. However, in order to provide the best-looking potatoes, perfect without any defects or natural dark spots, the farmers have to spray a highly toxic pesticide called Monitor. These pesticides do not wash off, and they enter the potatoes, even through their skins. Because that spray is so toxic, farmers avoid entering a farm for five days after spraying. Even worse, after harvesting them, farmers must "off-gas" the potatoes for *six weeks* in atmospheric-controlled warehouses the size of football stadiums. During this period, while farmers wait for some of the pesticides to dissipate, the potatoes' toxicity is so high that they are inedible. According to the Environmental Working Group's (EWG) "Complete Guide to Pesticide and Produce Dirty Dozen Plus 2015" report,[52] potatoes are among the top twelve pesticide-exposed foods and have more pesticides by weight than any other fruit or vegetable. Therefore, when eating french fries (and the average American eats almost 400 lb. per year), try to choose only organic potatoes with non-GMO oils. You can purchase these at any health store or make them fresh yourself.

"When Pigs Fly"—Is Your Pork from China?

Pork salad is my bread and meat.
—JOHNNY CASH

Now, where's the bacon?

Have you noticed the explosion of bacon on everything at fast-food restaurants? Everything is wrapped in bacon or comes with a pile of bacon. Why are restaurants adding bacon to all these foods as a topping?

The answer is probably not something you want to hear: a large Chinese corporation now owns and controls most pork production in the United States. That isn't bad in and of itself, but when we factor in how factory-farmed pigs are raised, things start to get ugly.

Pigs are extreme omnivores that have been known to eat everything under the sun—including waste of themselves and other animals and trash when not given access to their normal diet. When pigs are factory farmed, waste and trash are commonly mixed into their feed. This waste and trash are metabolized into their protein, which people then consumed whenever they eat pork.

What makes matters worse is that the pigs are raised here in the United States, shipped to China for processing, and then shipped back to the United States.

Wait a second. How are they able to ship pigs back and forth to China and produce pork that's in any way affordable?

Think about it. The only reasons to ship a product out of the United States are to reduce labor costs and, most importantly to factory-farm conglomerates, to avoid regulation and stricter health standards. (There are regulatory agencies in China, but their methods are questionable, and they can be paid to look the other way.) How is our pork being processed? Nobody seems to know, and what's worse, nobody seems to care.

Yes, pigs are raised on the farms here, shipped to China, "processed," and then shipped back to us—and the cost of bacon has dropped more than ever. You don't have to be an economist to see that some part of this equation is missing or is being replaced by something else. If we can't find the beef in this country, how can we find the bacon on the other side of the world?

If there are questions about bacon, you might ask, "What about hot dogs?" Hot dogs are such a classic American food with that regions of the country have their own distinctive styles, such as the New York–style hot dog, the Chicago dog, and the Kansas City dog. Unfortunately a recent study by Clear Food examined 345 samples from seventy-five brands obtained at ten major retailers and found some results that are difficult to swallow.[53] They found that 14 percent of the samples had problems with what was actually in them. For instance, 10 percent of so-called veggie hot dogs were found to contain meat ingredients, and 3 percent of chicken or turkey products were found to contain pork. Even worse, 2 percent of the hot dogs were found to have *human* DNA. Yes, human DNA. It takes more than just a few fingernails to make that amount—not trace amounts but 2 percent! That should ring alarm bells for everyone who eats hot dogs. We should never have human DNA in any food. Cheap foods have definitely changed our standards of ethics, morals, and hygiene. With these suspicious factory-farmed food practices, I hope that we are not moving toward Soylent Green.

Sadly, pork processed in the United States may not be much better, but at least we know how American pork is processed. Let's start in an unlikely place: the world-famous Las Vegas buffets.

Many of us have visited Las Vegas casinos and eaten at the all-you-can-eat buffets. If you haven't, they are an amazing display of almost every imaginable food—hundreds of items in massive dining areas, provided to patrons almost around the clock.

Various groups, including the National Resource Defense Council, have calculated that between 40 percent and 90 percent of Americans throw away food unnecessarily. This unfortunate habit prevails at buffets, where people can pick and choose, eat as much or as little as they like, and throw out the rest. Recognizing this pattern, many of the big casinos recycle their food waste. "How do they do this?" you may ask. They provide it to local pig farms. That's right: all the partially eaten food, from appetizers (breads and muffins) to main courses (beef, chicken, fish, lamb, seafood, and pork—yes, pigs are fed pork) to desserts (filled with artificial flavors and colors, high-fructose corn syrup, and hundreds of food additives), is delivered to a local pig farm. Las Vegas goes through approximately sixty thousand pounds of food daily (twenty-two million pounds a year), so you can imagine how much is thrown away. Just one of the major casinos discards around eight thousand pounds of food daily. This waste food is then taken to the pig farm and sorted to remove the plastic bags, glass bottles, and bones. The pig farmers then place this food-waste slurry into a big cooker and boil it into "food" for the pigs. The pigs that eat this "food" are then slaughtered and processed, and they end up back at the casino buffets as bacon, ham, and other pig-protein items.[54]

You really are what you eat.

While we're on the subject of "you are what you eat," let's take a brief look at the famous McRib sandwich. According to *Time* magazine, the McRib bun contains azodicarbonamide, which is a flour-bleaching agent most commonly used in the manufacture of foamed plastics like yoga mats and the soles of shoes. Yes, you read that correctly; the McRib sandwich shares ingredients in common with a yoga mat. Europe and Australia have banned azodicarbonamide as a food additive, classifying it as a "respiratory sensitizer" that potentially contributes to asthma. But this yoga-mat compound is just one

enty ingredients in what is supposed to be a *sandwich*. In addi-
:arbonamide, the McRib contains chemicals like ammonium
sulfate, polysorbate 80, and sixty-seven other ingredients (thirty-four in the bun alone). This "restructured meat product" (the appetizing technical name for the highly processed McRib patty) contains pig heart, scalded stomach, and tripe. This, by the way, is all according to the restaurant's own website.

Even though the McRib contains no bones, the patty is molded to resemble a miniature rack of ribs. According to those who helped create the McRib, "When cooked together with salt and water, proteins are extracted and act as a form of 'glue' that helps keep the reshaped 'rib' meat together." Even without regard for the "Frankenfoods" content of the McRib, the sandwich is incredibly unhealthy to consume. At a whopping 500 calories (a quarter of your daily calories), the McRib contains 26 g of fat (40 percent of your daily total fat), 44 g of carbs, and 980 mg of sodium (41 percent of your daily sodium)![55]

I don't bring up buffet-waste pig food and the ingredients of a highly processed fast-food sandwich to offend you, but rather to help demonstrate how all the food you've been led to believe is real is in fact manufactured parts, chemicals, fillers, and flavors. Factory farming and overprocessing have skewed our concepts of what food is and what it should cost. This immense demand for cheap animal proteins has reached a point where food production is in the realm of science fiction movies.

Ditto Foods

Help I'm steppin' into the twilight zone
The place is a madhouse, feels like being cloned
—GOLDEN EARRING

Do you remember Dolly the cloned sheep? Now we really have entered the Twilight Zone because cloned animals will soon be coming to a table near you. Recently, a large company in China announced that it will be able to clone animals for food production on a massive scale. Starting with 100,000 cloned cows per year (more than six times the largest American cattle farms) and cloned pigs up to one million per year.[56] Even more troubling is that the FDA has concluded that meat from cloned animals is safe and would not require any additional labeling to be sold commercially.[57] Yet we have no long term real population data or human clinical studies to justify its safety. Just as we are not federally mandated to label our foods if they are GMO, we will not be allowed to know if they are cloned. I believe we must have a serious debate on these issues as many companies will profit from these technologies but at what cost to our ethics, morals and most importantly to our health? Unsound manufacturing practices doesn't stop with beef and pork, but also includes seafood and chicken.

Colorless, Odorless, Tasteless

I want red, there is no substitute for red
—SAMMY HAGAR

When I worked in the emergency room and a patient was brought in uncon-sciousness, a classic diagnosis of their problem could be instantly given by viewing the color of their blood as it was being drawn. If their blood was a bright cherry red color (versus the normal darker red color of blood), the cause of the patient' s unconsciousness was due to carbon monoxide poi-soning (most commonly due to malfunctioning exhausts from stoves and portable heaters or lack of carbon monoxide detectors working properly). Carbon monoxide binds more effectively to hemoglobin than oxygen does and forms carboxyhemoglobin that causes the cherry-red color.

Now you might be wondering, "why is Dr. Pai bringing up this topic when he is discussing issues with food production?" Because the use of carbon monoxide is how the food industry keeps animal proteins looking fresh. It is estimated that the meat industry loses over $1 billion a year due to meat looking unappetizing.[58] Many studies have shown that meat color is the most significant appearance factor that determines whether meat eaters purchase it or not.[59] With this in mind, many food companies (along with approval from FDA) take meats and fish and vacuum seal them with carbon monoxide through a process called "modified atmosphere packaging." This makes the ground beef and other meats as well as fish such as tuna look "fresh" due to the enhanced bright red color that is produced from blood and flesh treated with carbon monoxide.

The problem with this bright color is that it stays long after the meat and fish has spoiled. So the consumer can not tell when the food is not safe to eat. Tests have shown that the carbon monoxide exposure to ground beef, loin steaks, and pork chops lasted 21 days beyond the time of spoilage and even up to 2 years.[60] This may be a contributing factor to food borne illness and other health problems in many Americans and another reason to start eating more of a plant based diet.

Winner, Winner, Chicken Dinner?

Chickity China, the Chinese chicken,
You have a drumstick and your brain stops ticking.
—BARENAKED LADIES

Many health-conscious consumers have been moving away from pork and beef products and eating more chicken, thinking it's healthier and safer. But is it really?

With over nine billion chickens consumed annually in the United States, that is twenty-three million per day and 269 per second.[61] Processing such a huge number of birds in so short a period of time requires faster production at processing plants, which in turn may cut corners to meet demand.

Chicken is the most consumed meat in the United States, and it's making us sick more often than you might think. According to the Center for Science in the Public Interest, from 2000 to 2012, chicken was responsible for more foodborne illnesses, hospitalizations, and deaths than any other food, followed closely by ground beef.[62]

With the increase in public awareness of the overuse of antibiotics in chicken, certain fast-food establishments have started to remove them because of bad publicity and public-health concerns. McDonald's—the largest fast-food chain, with over twenty-two thousand restaurants—has announced it will remove antibiotics from their chicken by 2018 (although the plan applies only to chicken served in its US restaurants). However, they are removing only the human antibiotics; McDonald's will continue to serve chicken treated with veterinary-type antibiotics, such as ionophores, which have led to controversy regarding their safety. As the antibiotics controversy continues to attract attention, other fast-food-industry leaders such as Chipotle have banned their suppliers from using both human and animal antibiotics.[63]

Aside of food borne illness problems from eating chicken and antibiotics used in factory farming chickens, an even more shocking problem is that the FDA found that over 70% of chicken in the U.S. has high arsenic levels.[64] This was discovered from the FDA testing chicken exposed to a Pfizer drug called Roxarsone, which is given to chickens to increase weight gain. This drug is also used to give store-bought chicken the semblance of healthy coloring and plum appearance. Arsenic is known to cause cardiovascular diseases and high blood pressure, neurologic problems, developmental disorders, skin hyperpigmentation, keratosis and cancer. It also causes DNA methylation, a biological process that causes many crippling and fatal diseases. Finally arsenic causes male fertility problems.[65] Health concerns with chicken is not limited to the U.S. but may be also overseas.

Interestingly, the USDA is now allowing chicken to be processed in China. Upon learning of this new development for his industry, a spokesman for the National Chicken Council stated, "A Chinese company would have to purchase frozen chicken in the United States, pay to ship it 7,000 miles, unload it, transport it to a processing plant, unpack it, cut it up, process/cook it, freeze it, repack it, transport it back to a port, and then ship it another 7,000 miles. I don't know how anyone could make a profit doing that."[66]

He only needs to look to the beef, pork, and seafood industries (large seafood companies also process Pacific salmon, Dungeness crab, and other fish in China) to understand how it is not only possible but also incredibly profitable—and with animals far bigger than chickens.

These types of food practices are abhorrent. In a petition to Congress that I supported, public health activists Bettina Siegel and Nancy Huehnergarth stated that "Good economic sense should never trump valid concerns about food safety. And China's food safety system, which is decades behind ours, can only be described as horrific, as evidenced by just some of the more recent food safety scandals in that country."[67] Their petition helped positively change the language in an appropriations bill negotiated by both parties in Congress. That bill now includes a provision that would bar the federal funding of any poultry processed in China for use in the National School Lunch Program or any other federal child-nutrition program. Hopefully, this bill will be signed into law in the future. However, it will first need to get past the lobbyists for foreign corporations and the food industry that continue to influence our government, and more importantly our health outcomes, to their advantage.

Chicken of the Sea: Is Seafood a Healthier Option?

You see, beneath the sea is where a fish should be.
—DAVE MATTHEWS BAND

I would like to educate you about why most of our seafood is very cheap. Do you remember when seafood was considered an expensive form of protein? Many Americans could not afford lobster, shrimp, crab, or fish on a regular basis (unless they lived coastally), so they reserved these foods for special occasions. Now almost every large city and small town in the United States offers all-you-can-eat seafood buffets. How can they serve this expensive source of animal protein so cheaply? The answer is slave labor. Over the past few years, numerous international agencies and consumers' organizations have found that many large seafood suppliers from Indonesia are using human slave labor. Doing so lowers the costs of the produce, increases the sale of seafood, and makes it more profitable for everyone involved.[68]

So what about the seafood that is not harvested using slave labor—is there a problem with that? Unfortunately, there is a growing problem with both fresh and farm-raised fish because of the environmental pollution of plastics.

A recent study published in February 2015 estimated that five to thirteen million metric tons of plastic litter are dumped into the world's oceans every year.[69] This enormous amount of waste is equivalent to five plastic grocery bags filled with plastics for every foot of coastline. Plastic is not biodegradable, but over time it breaks down into smaller and smaller particles called microplastics. Sea creatures then ingest these tiny particles, and they become part of the animals' protein. These plastics contain harmful chemicals such as xenoestrogens, which can affect our hormones and potentially harm us in other ways. Eventually these chemicals end up on our dinner plates.[70] With all the information presented on fish and other types of seafood, I recommend that you avoid seafood altogether.

Moo Gloo

I'm going to stick like glue.
—ELVIS PRESLEY

You may be thinking to yourself, "OK, I can avoid processed meats and fast food pretty easily." But are whole cuts of meat—such as fillets, steaks, and chops—actually better? Some of my patients tell me that they eat "real meat," not processed meats. But if they buy their steaks at a big-box store for cheap or go to an all-you-can-eat buffet, I have to ask them if they really think this "unprocessed" meat is safe. If you think it is, think again.

Let me introduce you to an industry and restaurant secret called "Moo Gloo: Meat Glue for the Modern Cook." Moo Gloo is glue for meat. Glue... for meat. Here's how it works.

Moo Gloo is a powdered compound used in most restaurants and food-processing plants, and it's even sold on online. Moo Gloo is primarily made of blood-coagulation enzymes taken from a cow or pig, powdered and mixed with other ingredients. It costs between $12 and $144 per pound, depending on what other ingredients are mixed in (such as milk, wheat, gelatin, or maltodextrin; some contain a pH buffer to extend usage time) and whether it is kosher or not. (I would really like to meet the rabbi who blessed this idea, as I find it utterly offensive that they would even consider approving such a product.)

Restaurants and food vendors take (often the undesirable) scraps of meat—like beef tips or pork pieces that would otherwise be discarded—combine them with the Moo Gloo, wrap the "glued" meat in cellophane, and refrigerate it for a few hours. The blood enzymes start to "glue" the pieces of meat together, and after a few hours, the process results in a reformed, new-looking piece of meat. This reformed meat can now be cut into fillets, steaks, chops, etc.

So, when people go to an all-you-can-eat steak buffet or buy cheap steaks at the big-box stores, they may not be getting an authentic cut of meat; they

ng the throwaway meat scraps, glued back together. If you
' eaten, search the Internet for Moo Gloo and related meat
продукты to see how widely it is used in the food industry.

But what's the big deal, if using meat-glue products are safe? According to the FDA, Moo Gloo is *generally recognized as safe* (GRAS), but the EU and other countries don't agree. They banned the use of meat enzyme "glues" in the 2010.

When we cook meat, we are trying to make sure there are no bacteria (from processing and handling) left on the meat when we eat it. Thus, we place our steaks or chops on the grill to cook, even if just for a short time. The interesting fact is that if we are cooking a real piece of meat, the inside is actually sterile—without any bacteria—even if it is bloody and not well done. The same is not true for meat processed with meat glue products.

If you're eating meat with glue, you're eating dozens of pieces of scrap meat with multiple surface areas, all glued back together and reformed to appear as an expensive cut of meat. Thus, dangerous bacteria can get stuck between the pieces. When only the outside of the food is cooked, the bacteria between the pieces remain intact, causing illness. This is why the EU banned meat glue products—it increased foodborne illnesses. The United States is behind the times, so be careful when choosing your meat by price. Remember that the everyday low-price food is usually not what you think or hope it is.

Food modifiers like Moo Gloo are not limited to cheap meat; they can also appear in high-end organic products thanks to food-manufacturing loopholes. Companies do not have to list these sorts of products on the ingredients panels, as they are used in processing and are thus not classified as actual ingredients. Pretty sneaky, right? In addition, the blood-coagulation enzymes used to make Moo Gloo into a powder can contain ingredients that certain people may not want (e.g., pork-blood products for those who eat kosher, milk, wheat/gluten, soy, or corn) without disclosure. This is especially problematic for the "organic" meat consumer, who assumes a certain level of quality. Such "oversights" can cause problems for those with food allergies, who are coming into contact with common allergens even though they think they are eating clean food that is grain or dairy-free.

Again, the above example is not meant to shock you, but to inform you. We can no longer refuse to care about our food and just ignore where it comes from, how it is grown and processed, and what it takes to get it to our table. You are what you eat, and this matters more than ever before, thanks to the fact that the foods we eat today are not the same as they were a generation ago. Today factory farming, hormones, and antibiotics for the animals are *de rigueur*, as are a multitude of chemicals, fillers, preservatives, and cancer-causing ingredients. These items are standard in almost all food we eat today. How often do you think about what it takes to make a boneless chicken breast or a chicken nugget, a fillet steak or McRib, with the same cookie-cutter shape and size, each and every time, in every restaurant nationwide?

Factory Farms: A Clear and Present Danger

Highway to the danger zone
—KENNY LOGGINS

Human health is inextricably tied to the health of our farmers, the animals, and the environment. Factory farming is the number-one contributor to CO_2 emissions—more than all the cars, trucks, and airplanes combined! **(See: Side Notes: Books and Movies.)** Eating more plant-based foods is the least expensive way to mitigate the effects of climate change; it only takes cutting down the number of burgers you eat per week. The planet will thank you, and so will your body.

Data taken from a variety of environmental, economic, and agricultural groups show that the average American now eats about three burgers per week, or about one hundred fifty burgers per year.[71] Regardless of how you feel about climate change, the facts are irrefutable: the amount of diesel, gas, and coal used in the process of producing a burger comes out to about 7.7 lb. (3.5 kg) of CO_2—per burger. Your average car produces 6.6 lb. per day (3 kg per day) of CO_2; clearing the rainforest to produce beef for one hamburger requires 165 lb. (75 kg) of CO_2. For reference, eating one pound of hamburger does the same damage to the environment as driving your car for more than three weeks.[72] Therefore, the average person contributes approximately 1,200 lb. of CO_2 per year—just by eating burgers—or 15 percent of the average car's yearly CO_2 emissions! Bear in mind that this does not take

double, triple, or quadruple burger, or the multiple strips of
ese, or the buckets of chicken nuggets, wings, and hot dogs!

With climate change bringing us more drought in many states in the United States, conservation of water is also extremely important. Many hotels, restaurants, and even cities are placing restrictions on the usage of water. According to the US Geological Survey, the average household uses 98 gallons of water daily, and the use of industrial goods (such as clothes, paper, and cotton) consumes another 44 gallons.[73] But have you thought about how much water is used for your food? Just producing a pound of beef takes about 1,799 gallons of water, whereas pounds of rice, soy, and potatoes respectively take 449, 216, and 119 gallons. So again, when you choose to eat a plant-based diet, you are helping conserve water as well as improving your health.[74]

We have had such a massive change in food production, not to feed more people but to allow big corporations to reap bigger and bigger profits each year—at any cost. In order for the multinational food industry to maximize their profits and production, they feed their animals GMO corn and soy (e.g., marbleized corn feed) which increases the fat content (including cholesterol and saturated fat) of the meat produced. They also feed livestock other unhealthy ingredients (including animal parts, even of their own species), antibiotics (which leads to antibiotic resistance in humans), and hormones (which increases our risk of hormone-related health conditions). All of this decreases the nutritional content of the meat, depleting vitamins, minerals, and omega-3 content, and making factory-farmed meat a pro-inflammatory food, not to mention a vehicle for smuggling excess hormones and antibiotics into our bodies.

Foodborne Illness: More Common Than You Think

What's the time? It's time to get ill.
—Beastie Boys

It's obvious that factory-farmed-animal proteins are not good for us, but it's important to understand that they are actually hazardous to our health.

The most recent data (from the CDC and other organizations) shows that foodborne illness affects forty-eight to seventy-six million Americans every year. That means that from one in four to one in six Americans get sick each year from our foods. Our food causes 328,000 hospitalizations and approximately five thousand deaths each year, costing us $152 billion annually in Superbugs have gained resistance to antibiotics thanks to their humans, and now antibiotic use in food production is contributing t   ᴖsis-tance. These superbugs contribute to twenty-three thousand deaths per year.[76]

More people die each year from foodborne illness than died on 9/11. And even though we have done everything we can since 9/11 to protect ourselves from another attack, spending trillions on security and defense, the true unspoken terrorist attack occurs at our dinner tables, potlucks, buffets, and barbeques every day. Maybe we should have a "war on food" to protect us from the daily threat that is at our dinner tables.

Another disturbing fact about foodborne illnesses is that sources (such as the Environmental Working Group and *Consumer Reports*) estimate that between 39 percent and 90 percent of beef, pork, chicken, and lamb now contain two antibiotic-resistant bacteria. Yes, that means up to two different bacteria—such as *E. faecalis* (which is the third leading cause of infection in ICU), *salmonella*, *E. coli*, and *campylobacter*—are present in our meat supply. But even I found it hard to believe that data, even though it came from independent consumer and watchdog groups. Then I read the USDA/FDA report that showed that in 2013, 100 percent of store-bought meat had up to five antibiotic-resistant bacteria. That's right—100 percent of all types of meat. Factory-farmed chicken had 100 percent contamination with between two and five antibiotic-resistant bacteria. Sadly, 84 percent of organic chicken was also contaminated; this has been attributed to the fact that eggs are injected with antibiotics before they go to organic farms. Cross contamination also commonly occurs when organic farms use the same meat-processing facilities as conventional chicken.

You might ask, why are there bacteria in my meat? The answer is somewhat complicated.

Most cities across America have chain pharmacies like Walgreens or CVS, where millions of antibiotics are prescribed daily. As alarming as antibiotics distribution on such a large scale of might seem, the numbers really aren't all that shocking. Why would I make such a statement? Because the truth is that even though the US medical system prescribes and sells millions of antibiotics to Americans every day, that quantity is nothing when compared to the amount of antibiotics being used in factory farming.

You'll probably be just as surprised as I was to learn that 80 percent of all antibiotics used in the United States goes to factory-farm feed lots. Yes, animals use four times the total amount of antibiotics that humans are prescribed. The poor conditions that the animals are subjected to cause high infection rates, and farmers use antibiotics to keep these rates down. Despite the heavy use of antibiotics in factory farming (which causes antibiotic resistance), 328,000 people will be hospitalized and about twenty-three thousand people will die annually from eating chicken wings, hamburgers, bacon, and other factory-farmed meat.[77] The number of deaths attributable to secondary causes may be many times more. (Secondary causes include going to the hospital with diarrhea, fever, or vomiting and dying from pneumonia or other complications while there.)

If you eat factory-farmed meat, even if you haven't had many antibiotics in your lifetime, you can still develop resistance to antibiotic treatment. Every factory-farmed animal you've eaten has been treated all its life with antibiotics. The bacteria that they carry are already resistant to most of the common antibiotics you would need to fight infection to save your life. Scary, right?

Factory farming in the twenty-first century has increased its production to unprecedented numbers of animals being slaughtered per day. This, inevitably, leads to inappropriate handling and cutting of corners to meet demand and increase profitability.

Consider the raw numbers: every day in the United States over twenty-three million chickens are slaughtered. That means nine billion chickens are slaughtered per year—an almost impossible number to imagine. Incredibly, this number keeps going up every year, increasing the incidence of foodborne illnesses, inhumane farming practices, and labor exploitation just to maintain the "everyday low prices" of poultry that will be marketed as "healthy" animal protein.

According to the CDC, populations at the highest risk for antibiotic-resistant illness are those receiving chemotherapy, those who have undergone surgery (e.g., joint replacement), those suffering from rheumatoid arthritis (thanks to the pharmaceutical drugs that lower immune function), those on dialysis or with end-stage renal disease, and those who have undergone organ or bone-marrow transplants.[78] Knowing this, and knowing how conventional meats contribute to antibiotic-resistant illnesses, you might be shocked to learn what foods hospitals serve nationwide.

To me, the idea of a person dying from foodborne illness and antibiotic resistance is unacceptable, outrageous, and completely un-American. No one in this country (or any country, for that matter) should ever die directly or indirectly from foodborne illnesses, especially with the regulations and safety measures that are supposed to be in place.

Dietary Protein and Cancer

If U really wanna find the answer 2 this cancer, then we must rewind.
—PRINCE

Diet is one of the most important factors for good health, yet medical doctors and health-care professionals have little if any training in nutrition. We need to change that.

We used to think in the 1980s and 1990s that low-fat foods were better for us and would help decrease cancer rates; however, scientific data has proven just the opposite. Eating low-fat food actually correlates to higher animal-protein intake, even if the calories are the same. Low-fat foods like low-fat cheese, low-fat milk, skim milk, and very low-fat cottage cheese and cheesecake actually have higher amounts of animal protein. The greater the animal-protein contents in food, the greater the increase in cancer rates—especially breast cancer.[79] Long-term outcome studies—like the Harvard Nurses' Health Study, which tracked almost two hundred thousand nurses over a decade—found the amount of protein consumed was about 20 percent greater in low-fat diets. In addition, although these low-fat diets had fewer fat calories, they were actually higher in cholesterol as well as animal protein, both of which are pro-inflammatory and significantly increase the risk of developing cancer.[80]

But if low-fat diets aren't good for you, what diet is? Remember comprehensive, short-term, and long-term clinical trials and prospective large epidemiological studies demonstrate that whole-food, plant-based diets result in better health outcomes in all categories, including cancer, diabetes, heart disease, blood pressure, and obesity.[81]

Research from as far back as 1968 demonstrates that certain types of protein stimulate cancer growth.[82] This Indian study showed that animals fed a low-casein (dairy protein is 80 percent casein), low-protein diet and exposed to carcinogens to elicit tumor growth showed little to no significant additional growth in the tumors. But when these animals were fed a diet of just 20 percent protein, all of the animals showed tumor growth **(see fig. 15)**. The study showed a dose relationship here as well, meaning the higher the animal-protein intake, the higher the rate of cancerous growth.[83] **(See fig. 16.)**

Dietary Protein %	Animals with tumors and hyperplastic nodules
20% (regular)	30/30 (100%)
5% (low)	0/12 (0%)

Modified **From:** Madhavan and Goplan, 1969
Confirmed by Wells et al. 1974
Confirmed by Campbell et al. 1982, 1987, 1981

Figure 15: Increasing protein (casein)—increasing cancer?

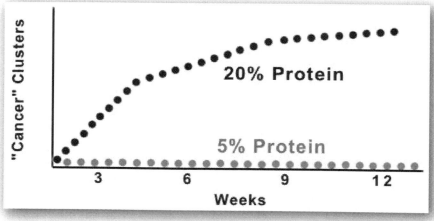

Figure 16: Dose relationship with dietary protein and cancer (Modified from LD Youngman and TC Campbell, J Nutr, 121, no. 9 (1991):1454-61; LD Youngman and TC Campbell, Nutrition Cancer, 18, no. 2 (1992):131-42).

The link between dietary protein and cancer was confirmed in 1974[84] and then again twenty years later when Dr. T. Colin Campbell reviewed this information and reproduced similar results.[85] He demonstrated that when a hepatocellular carcinoma is induced in mice—from aflatoxin, for example—and one group of mice is fed just 5 percent protein, tumor cells do not grow significantly. Once that same group of mice is fed 20 percent protein, cancer-cell growth is definitive. But while raising the dietary proportion of protein to

20 percent turns on the cancer-growth factor, switching the diet of the same animal back to 5 percent protein decreases cancer growth. Further, switching back to 20 percent protein causes the cancer to grow again **(see fig. 17)**.

The results of this study tell us that animal-based proteins (specifically casein) promote cancer growth. It does not mean, however, that casein *causes* cancer. What the study demonstrates is that, if you do have cancer cells, then consuming amounts of animal protein in excess of a critical percentage of your diet will stimulate the growth of those cells **(see figs. 17 and 18)**. There is an amount of animal protein that one can safely consume (below 8 percent of total calories), but the average person in the United States gets 15 percent to 30 percent of his or her calories from protein (mainly animal proteins) and 45 percent to 65 percent of his or her calories from highly refined carbohydrates and sugar **(see fig. 19)**.

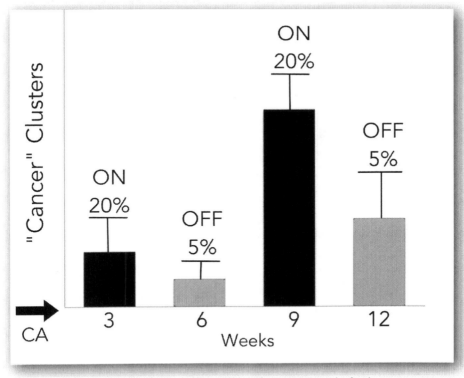

Figure 17: Increasing amount of protein (casein) increases growth of early cancer cells (Modified from LD Youngman and TC Campbell, J Nutr, 121, no 9. (1991):1454-61; LD Youngman and TC Campbell, Nutrition Cancer, 18, no 2. (1992):131-42).

Dietary Protein and LATE Cancer
(Youngman and Campbell, Carcinogenesis, 1992)

Chemical effect = cancer <u>INITIATION</u>

Protein effect = cancer <u>PROMOTION</u>

Protein %	# of Animals	Tumor Severity*
5% - all **LIVING** at 100 weeks	60	248
20% - all **DEAD** at 100 weeks	58	3321

* % incidence x tumor weight

Figure 18: Dietary protein (casein)—a cancer promoter (Modified from LD Youngman and TC Campbell, Carcinogenesis, 13, no. 9 (1992): 1607-13.)

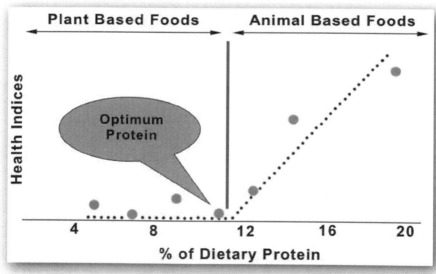

Figure 19: Optimum amount of protein needed for health (Modified from T Campbell and TC Campbell, The China Study, (Dallas, BenBella Books, 2006).

Two problems in general are occurring with protein. People are consuming too much and the wrong type. The Institute of Medicine Food and Nutrition Board recommends about 46 g per day for the adult female and 56 g per day for the adult male.[86] However, the average female consumes about

75 g and the male about 100 g.[87] This is the average. Let me explain w type of protein you consume makes a difference.

According to Dr. Campbell and multiple scientific laboratories, casein is now viewed as the most relevant chemical carcinogen ever identified. When we consider mitigating our cancer risk by eliminating BPA from plastics, reducing as many chemicals as we can from our environment, and eating certified organic foods, we are probably not thinking about casein from dairy products. Nothing promotes cancer growth as fast and in such a clinically relevant way as casein. As early as 1997, casein was shown in scientific literature to increase IGF-I 5 (insulin growth factor-1), which is a trigger for cancer cells, prompting the cells to obtain more glucose to "feed" them. This in turn promotes cellular dysfunction. For example, high casein intake (over 20 percent of daily calories) increases progression from hepatitis B to liver cancer faster than when the casein intake is kept to a minimum at 6 percent.[88] In addition, studies have shown that the dairy protein also triggers growth of cancer cells through other mechanisms, especially in the prostate for men.[89] Therefore, one can view casein as one of the most relevant chemical carcinogens, especially if there is already a disease or dysfunction in the body. Casein affects the way the cancer cells grow; therefore, I always advise my patients to avoid it as much as possible—especially patients with cancer, risk factor for cancers, or cancer-reoccurrence risks. Interestingly, soy and wheat protein, at a level of 20 percent intake of daily calories, did not increase precancer development of tumors.[90]

Remember, we consume dairy to promote growth. For example, a baby calf drinks its mother's milk in order to grow. Yes, it's the baby calves' milk, not ours. Yet once a calf drinks enough milk over a short period of time, it stops and moves on to eat grass throughout its life to maintain its 2,500-pound weight. The same goes for us as humans. We all should have been breastfed or should breastfeed our babies, but in all cultures around the world, by the age of four the child has grown enough not to need breast milk. Unfortunately we continue to eat another mammal's (mother's) milk. The average American is consuming about two pounds of dairy products per day. This is neither normal nor healthy for us. This obsession (and addiction) with dairy consumption also correlates with the growing incidence of diseases such as obesity, diabetes, heart disease, inflammatory conditions, and cancer.

Casein affects the way cells interact with carcinogens, the way our DNA reacts with carcinogens, and the way cancer cells grow. Nutrients from animal-based foods increase tumor development, while plant-based foods decrease tumor development. The science bears this out again and again. However, this does not account for soy or wheat sensitivities due to the genetic modification of foods, which can also trigger increases in bodily inflammation. That is a different situation altogether (which I will talk about later).

The thought of eliminating meat and dairy in the diet causes many people to ask the universal question, "Where do you get your protein?" The answer is, simply, from plants.

All plants—yes, all plants—contain protein **(see fig. 20)**. Although those educated in nutrition understand this, for the average person it comes as a complete shock (don't worry if you did not know this; most likely neither does your doctor). I first like to answer that all plants have protein, and there is never a lack thereof. The abundance of protein in plants enables many large, powerful animals—such as horses, rhinos, hippos, giraffes, elephants, and cows—to eat plants *exclusively* **(see fig. 21)**. These animals do not need animal protein to be big, fast, strong, and healthy.

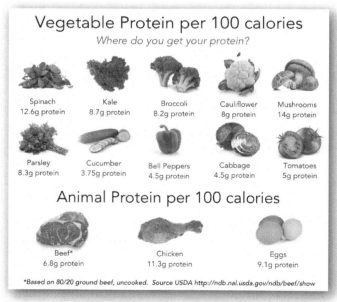

Figure 20: Top ten sources of veggie protein

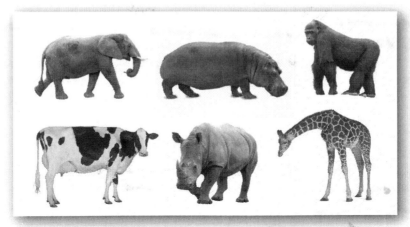

Figure 21: The universal question—"Where do you get your protein?"

Food	Amount	Protein (grams)	Cholesterol (mg)	Fat (grams)	Fiber (grams)	Calories
Seitan	1 cup	75	0	2	1	370
Soybeans	1 cup	68	0	37	17	830
Lentils (raw)	1 cup	50	0	2	59	678
Kidney Beans	1 cup	44	0	1	46	607
Black Beans	1 cup	42	0	3	30	662
Tuna (canned)	4oz	30	35	9	0	210
Ground Beef Patties	4oz patty	26	95	27	0	333
Peanut Butter (chunky)	1/3 cup	24	0	50	8	589
Salmon	4oz	23	62	15	0	235
Steak (porterhouse)	4oz	23	64	17	0	252
Tofu, Firm (raw)	1/2 cup	20	0	11	3	183
Tempeh	1/2 cup	19	0	11	?	193
Chicken (uncooked)	1/2 breast	18	56	8	0	150
Ham (deli slices)	4 slices	18	64	10	2	183
Turkey Breast (deli slices)	4 slices	14	36	1	0	87
Eggs whole (raw)	2 eggs	13	423	10	0	143
Bacon	4 slices	11	62	34	0	351
Walnuts	1/2 cup	9	0	38	4	383
Brown Rice (cooked)	1 cup	5	0	2	4	216

Source: USDA FOOD NUTRITION INFORMATION (www.nal.usda.gov/fnic/foodcomp/search/)

Figure 22: Comparison of protein, fiber, cholesterol, and fat in plant protein vs. animal protein

There is no cholesterol in plants; there is no fiber in animal proteins; and we get just as much protein from plants—especially when we eat a variety of them **(see fig. 22)**. Fiber is important for keeping the colon healthy, for reducing the risk of colon cancer (as well as other cancers), and reducing blood-glucose intake, thereby reducing the risk of insulin resistance, metabolic syndrome, and heart disease. Doctors prescribe cholesterol medications without a second thought, when it is by far safer and just as effective to simply reduce the amount of animal products in the diet. By including more vegetables in our diets instead, we can enjoy a multitude of health benefits, not the least of which is a proven, significant reduction in the risk of developing serious illnesses.

According to the Physicians Committee for Responsible Medicine, people should be encouraged to eat the "Power Plate" **(see fig. 23)**—dividing their plate into four categories: fruits, legumes (beans and lentils), vegetables, and whole grains. People can usually eat as much organic, non-GMO, plant-based foods as they like—without the risk of obesity or disease (with the exception, of course, of foods that people have sensitivities or allergies to). Eating a healthy plant-based diet is easy; one does not need to count calories, monitor grams of fat, or check cholesterol, since plant-based foods are low in caloric density and "bad" fats and contain no cholesterol.

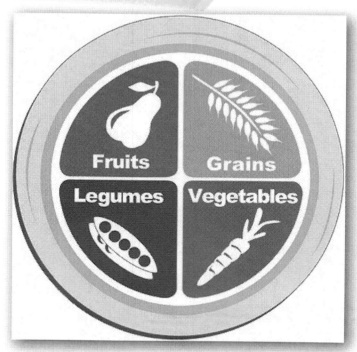

Figure 23: The "Power Plate" from PCRM.org

I talk a lot about "diet" in this book, but it has nothing to do with changing what you eat for a short time to lose weight. It's about empowering yourself to feel better by making sustainable changes in what you choose to eat.

For additional guidance, I recommend that all my patients read certain books and watch certain movies **(see Side Notes: Books and Movies)** that help reinforce their decision to embark on a healthier, plant-based diet as much as possible. We now have decades of clinical studies, epidemiological data, and clinical experience that proves without question that diet is *the* major factor contributing to diseases and that diet alone can improve and even reverse disease. Medical pioneers such as Dr. Dean Ornish, Dr. Colin Campbell, Dr. Caldwell Esselstyn, Dr. Joel Fuhrman, and Dr. John McDougall have clearly demonstrated the benefits of a good diet and have published dozens of studies in medical journals and books detailing the science behind this revolution in medicine and nutrition.

Not only have these physicians published this data but they have results to back up their data in hundreds and hundreds of patients over the years, all of whom improved their health conditions by simply changing how they ate. All of my patient recommendations for further reading and viewing on the importance of sustainable agriculture, the choice of plant-based foods, and the dangers of becoming a "fast-food nation" are listed under **Side Notes: Books and Movies**.

CHAPTER 4

STEP 2: Testing What Is Triggering Inflammatory Responses in Your Body

When it comes to inflammation related to allergies, there are three primary allergy categories: contact allergies, inhalant allergies, and food allergies.

1) Contact Allergies: The Inflammation That We Touch

Can't touch this.
—MC Hammer

Contact allergies arise from our direct contact with chemicals (and irritant compounds) such as fabric softeners, detergents, perfumes/fragrances, or jewelry/metals. Contact allergies usually elicit what's called a "local" response, meaning these irritants cause a direct inflammatory reaction at the site of contact. These reactions include acne, eczema, rashes, or hives wherever the chemical irritant touches the skin.

Most of my patients come to me with some understanding of what it means to eat healthily and why they might take natural dietary supplements when necessary. But many forget about the chemicals our body-care products expose us to on a daily basis. This everyday chemical exposure is called our "body burden." Our environment exposes us to these chemicals without our knowing it; we absorb them into our skin, and they build up over time. These everyday chemicals on their own can cause immediate problems (contact allergies). Together they contribute to cumulative cellular damage and cause low-grade, chronic dysfunction of our organ systems, which can lead to chronic diseases and cancers.

You don't have to have contact allergies to be concerned about what comes in contact with your skin every day. Given that our skin is our largest organ, maybe we need to take a closer look at what we have been putting on our skin for most of our lives. And maybe we should also look at the water we are ingesting and bathing in.

Water from bathing is our skin's primary source of chemical exposure, followed closely by body-care products and then the water that we drink. Everyone should use some type of home filtration for his or her water. The water in homes, no matter where you live, is not as healthy as it used to be. Remember, water that comes from your local municipal plant has been disinfected so that we do not get sick from various types of bacteria and waste products. That is a good public-health practice, since the World Health Organization's (WHO) data states that 80 percent of all diseases in the world are caused by an unsatisfactory quality of drinking water and violations of sanitary and hygienic standards in water supplies. Luckily we in America rarely have to worry about those diseases that pass through unsanitary water. However, our water sometimes contains higher amounts of chlorines and other chemical agents that we use to kill microorganisms but which are not necessarily good for ingestion or absorption through your skin. When traveling to different cities or hotels, you might have noticed that the water smells chlorinated, like a public pool. It may also be heavy in minerals such as iron, copper, manganese, and heavy metals, which leave red rings in the toilets and showers.

Our water doesn't just contain the chemicals used to treat it or the metals and minerals that it leaches from the pipes it flows through. Many people and health-care institutions unfortunately dump their prescription pills down the toilets (which you should not do), and these medications then end up back in our municipal water system. Because the water systems do not filter them out, they return back to the population. Recent studies have found that sewage treatment plants only removed half the prescription drugs, and these medications were found in the drinking-water supplies of twenty-four major US metropolitan cities.[91] Those studies found traces of herbicides, hormones such as estrogens (from birth-control and hormone-replacement drugs), antibiotics, antibacterials (e.g., triclosan), antiseizure drugs, mood stabilizers (e.g., antidepressants and antianxiety medications), and anti-inflammatories (e.g., diclofenac and other NSAIDs). Although the studies found only trace amounts, no safety studies have been performed to see the effects on humans. But not only do we lack data on the effects of chronic trace exposure to each of these drugs individually, we also lack data on chronic exposure to their combination in this toxic soup. Even as health-care practitioners recommend drinking more water daily—about half your weight in fluid ounces for an adult— we still do not know the side effects or long-term health risks of drinking unhealthy water. Nor do we know the effects populations who might be at greater risk, such as pregnant women and young children, who drink a greater percentage of their body weight on a daily basis than do adults.

One of the answers to this problem is to take extra steps to ensure that your water has adequate filtration to eliminate common chemicals such as chlorines, chloramines, and others that are found in the municipal water that supplies our homes. In addition, many municipalities have upped fluoride levels in municipal water, piling on the chemical load. There are many affordable systems that you can use to help reduce these contaminants and also soften your water without salt or other additives **(see Side Notes: Water Filtration)**.

Home filtration is a must. You should also take steps to improve the energetic qualities of your water by structuring and harmonizing it, even more so after filtration. Many people think that water is simply H_2O, but it's not. It has its own unique energetic properties. A new science of water is transitioning our understanding from a simple molecular level to a complex quantum physics and even consciousness level. This new field of research is based on the principles of quantum electrodynamics developed by Italian physicist Emilio Del Giudice and experimentally confirmed in Russia, France, and the United States. Scientists like Luc Montagnier (Nobel Prize winner), Gerald Pollack, Alexander Konovalov, Vladimir Voeikov, and many others are developing theoretical and experimental foundations of a new science of water. Every year top-level scientists involved in water research meet for an annual international conference (www.waterconf.org); for those who wish to study in more detail I recommend both the conference and the large amounts of data published in the multidisciplinary periodical *Water Journal* (www.waterjournal.org).

Although many people are starting to learn about the amazing energetic qualities that water may possess, many do not understand the unintended consequences that result from various types of filtration and reverse osmosis; filtered water is "clean" physically but also "dead" energetically. (Some of you may have learned about the energetic qualities of water—e.g., from Dr. Masaru Emoto's work, as well as others—or read the dozens of published studies researching and demonstrating these principles.[92]) Water that has undergone the processes of filtration and reverse osmosis loses its unique and inherent energetic properties. Think of the difference between water from a bubbling spring racing over the rocks of a riverbed and water pumped from the municipal plant and then through your home filtration system. It is no longer active but static, and this phenomenon has been studied for decades. Therefore, obtaining clean water as clear of chemicals and prescription drugs as possible is the first goal but not the final answer. After improving your newly cleaned water, you need to structure it.

I recommend a simple device that is not only effective but also affordable. In order to change the pH and energetic qualities of your water, you do not need to buy expensive machines that require electricity and replacement parts and cost thousands of dollars (like the products usually sold by multilevel-marketing companies). Instead, you need a Crystal Blue Water Structuring Unit. I use it in my home and office and on the go, and I offer it to my patients at Sanjevani. Not only will you notice an improvement of your health while using this simple solution, you will also see changes to your environment, including an improvement in the yield of your garden and plants **(see Side Notes: Structured Water)**.

I finally recommend adding trace minerals from humic and fulvic acids, if possible, which can provide even more benefits to your filtered, chemical-free, and structured water. Remember that the municipal water supply, after proper filtration and reverse osmosis, removes chemicals, but it also removes the trace minerals that are essential for optimum health. That is why many people around the world drink natural spring or mineral water that comes from the source. Unfortunately, most of the world's water supply is now owned by a handful of corporate giants who take water from our communities and then sell it back after "purifying" it at a higher cost. Many people in the United States think that the bottled water that they are buying is spring or mineral water, but it is just filtered municipal water with clever marketing.

Some of those products have the minerals added back in, but these companies use the cheapest and most synthetic forms to keep their profits higher. When you use the humic/fulvic acid products that I recommend, you get the best natural sources of what nature has intended with appropriate ratios and amounts of trace minerals. These trace minerals improve cellular function and also enhance absorption of other nutrients, helping to improve our intake of vitamins and herbs **(see Side Notes: Humic and Fulvic Acids)**.

As your skin is your body's largest organ it is important to be aware of what you put on it. For example, as part of a daily routine, the average male uses eleven body-care products, and the average female uses thirteen body-care products. That means most of us expose ourselves to well over one hundred chemicals before breakfast! If you use body-care products, as almost everyone does, then I suggest you review the **Side Notes: Cosmetics and Body-Care Products** section to learn more about how to protect yourself from unnecessary chemical-microdose exposure. A little goes a long way when it comes to your skin.

It's easy to ignore how a generic lotion or toothpaste might affect your health. After all, you're never using a large amount of these products at any one time. But microdosing with hundreds of chemicals every day has a cumulative effect. That is why I ask all my patients to research the products they use on their skin or mucosal membranes—everything from toothpastes, shampoos, and conditioners to deodorants, makeup, shaving creams, and more.

The Environmental Working Group (EWG) provides a great consumer guide at their website, www.ewg.org. The EWG's Skin Deep guide and app makes it easy to review all the products that you use daily. The guide categorizes them into colored-coded zones based on their levels of chemical ingredients. I try to only use products in the green zone; I minimize my exposure to products in the yellow zone and avoid those in the red zone.

Although I try to follow a purist lifestyle to the best of my abilities, I am also a realist. I know certain products and choices are out of reach for many of my patients. So, instead of telling my patients to throw out everything that fails the EWG criteria, I encourage them to try to buy one item at a time that is on the green zone. Over time, this makes the products in their home greener and safer, helping to decrease their body burden significantly.

An important part of Ayurvedic medicine are the tandem ideas of Hitayu (public/environmental health) and Sukhayu (personal health). These ancient but wise concepts describe how an individual and the environment influence

2) Inhalant Allergies: The Inflammation That We Breathe

> *Take my breath away.*
> —BERLIN

Inhalant allergies, the type of allergies caused by what we breathe in, (along with food allergies or sensitivities) are the major triggers of your *individually specific* internal inflammation. Inhalant allergies create the classic seasonal allergic symptoms thanks to histamine release. Triggers include grasses, weeds, trees, molds, dust mites, cats, dogs, and cockroaches. Inhalant allergies result from your immune system's unique response to your environment.

In Albuquerque, New Mexico (known as the "land of enchantment"), we have the most beautiful sunsets and 360-degree views of the horizon that can be seen year-round. But our panoramic vistas make New Mexico one of the worst places to live for those with inhalant allergies. For a three-hundred-mile radius—from Colorado above us down to southern New Mexico and El Paso, Texas—dust and pollens can travel freely, unobstructed by the varied topography and air pollution typical of other parts of the country. Unlike the distinct allergy seasons created by extreme temperature swings in other regions, the allergy season in New Mexico is almost year-round.

Inhalant allergies cause inflammation in the upper airway. This inflammation makes our noses become runny or congested, our ears itch, our lungs fill with mucous (or constrict as in asthma), and our eyes watery and red. These symptoms affect how well we sleep and think, and they can affect our overall energy level throughout the day.

It's easy to confuse inhalant and food-allergy symptoms, since they can mimic each other. If you experience allergy symptoms during the spring, summer, and fall, then you probably have inhalant allergies. But if you *also* have allergy symptoms—such as runny nose and congestion—in the winter, then you may also have food allergies or sensitivities. We'll talk about those a little later.

When it comes to inhalant allergies, it's all about the respiratory part of the mucosal tract (I'll talk about specific allergy testing later). When we breathe in pollens, dust, and a variety of allergens that are specifically irritating to our immune system, our soldier cells send out inflammation signals in the blood (i.e., cytokines and interleukins). These signals act in your bloodstream like bullets, targeting and striking what are called mast cells, which explode and release histamines. Histamines cause the familiar allergy symptoms of itchiness, congestion, and mucous production.

Although allergy symptoms make us miserable, the release of histamines and, in turn, mucous production serves a purpose. Believe it or not, the histamine response is a protective mechanism, designed to block more exposure to allergens. For example, if you encounter certain weeds or animals and start sneezing, your body's telling you that you should not be near those things. What about all that mucous? That's your body trying to prevent you from continuing to breathe in anything that's causing inflammation or irritation.

The release of histamines is actually an inflammation-triggered response; therefore, if you can block or lessen the triggers, then fewer inflammation signals are sent, and fewer histamines are released. By taking an inflammation-reduction approach, we can help decrease inhalant-allergy symptoms by addressing the underlying mechanisms that exacerbate the release of histamines. This approach allows us to do something that Western medicine doesn't do very often: treat the cause and not just the symptoms of inhalant allergies. When you consider that the body's response to inflammation (triggered by numerous different factors) elicits most diseases, you can see why I felt compelled to write this book!

Let's look more closely at an extreme inhalant-allergy reaction. When allergens stimulate soldier cells (immune cells), inflammation can become so severe that the sinus's mucosal cells start to divide and create polyps, which are fatty grapelike tissue clusters. Upon developing polyps, most people would see an ENT doctor for surgery. Surgery can, of course, help to remove any obstruction blocking our airways, but in this case it is only a temporary fix. If one does not address the underlying allergic inflammation that caused the polyps to begin with, they are likely to grow back in the future. If you have chronic sinusitis, sinus problems, or nasal polyps, see **Side Notes: Sinus Polyps and Surgery**.

But surgery is an extreme treatment for an extreme allergic reaction. As mentioned previously, people use antihistamines or steroids far more often, but these too only treat the symptoms and not the underlying cause of allergies (inflammation). So many people are stuck taking antihistamines and steroids whenever they have allergic symptoms that it's seen as normal.

Fortunately, there are integrative-medicine approaches to allergies that improve the overall function of your respiratory tract and your immune system: sublingual immunotherapy (SLIT) or Soliman Auricular Allergy Treatment (SAAT). These two treatments are far better options because they were developed to resolve allergies—not just manage symptoms forever.

Let's start with a look at sublingual immunotherapy.

Allergy-Drops Therapy: Safer, More Accurate, and More Convenient

I feel that they are safer.
—REO SPEEDWAGON

Although we can treat inhalant, food, and contact allergies, in general I tell my patients that, while you can usually control what you eat or touch, you can't always control what you breathe. I offer my patients a unique and targeted treatment called sublingual (under the tongue) immunotherapy (SLIT), or in simple terms, Allergy-Drops Therapy. SLIT has been used successfully for over sixty years in Europe and for over thirty years in the United States. Over a hundred clinical studies have concluded that SLIT is *more clinically effective, more cost-effective, and safer* when compared to other forms of immunotherapy such as allergy shots.[93]

SLIT or Allergy Drops Therapy is safer than subcutaneous immunotherapy (allergy shots that require injection into the tissue in the arm or buttocks). Allergy shots carry a 5 percent chance of anaphylaxis every time you get the shot. Whether it is your first or hundredth time getting the shot, you always have a 5 percent chance of anaphylaxis. Allergy shots are a serious commitment of time, as they are administered weekly—that's fifty-two times a year for four to five years on average. With allergy-drops therapy, there has not been a reported incidence of anaphylaxis in over sixty years—worldwide! The reason for this is that with Allergy Drops Therapy, you take a small physiological dose that is specifically made for you (*not* a tincture or homeopathic dose which is a standard calculated dilution) of what you are allergic to three times a day underneath the tongue. That's it. No going to the doctor's office every week. A metered-dose pump spray underneath the tongue at your own convenience is far easier and, most importantly, far safer.

Unlike allergy shots, which contain phenols (chemicals that patients can be sensitive to), Allergy Drops Therapy are mixed with a natural vegetable glycerin and do not need to be refrigerated. Allergy Drops Therapy is custom tailored to each patient, and each drop can contain over a dozen different allergens. Each dose of antigen (what you are allergic to) is titrated to your exact allergic response based on accurate blood testing (RAST), thus delivering a more precise dose compared to shots.

Skin-Prick Testing vs. Blood Testing

The pins and needles prick the skin.
—OZZY OSBOURNE

The major benefit of blood testing for allergies is the elimination of the pain, discomfort, and inconvenience of skin testing. Skin testing has been the standard for over a century, but we now have a deeper understanding of the mechanism of allergic reaction. We know now that an allergy is an inflammatory reaction and that many extraneous factors can affect how the skin responds to the skin-prick test, resulting in many false positives and negatives. We can avoid these false results through blood testing.

With the blood test, we don't have to worry about which medications or supplements the patient is taking (as long as they have not had a recent immunosuppressive infusion). Skin-prick testing, on the other hand, is affected by a litany of foods, supplements, and medicines:

- Antihistamines (natural, OTC, or prescription)
- Steroids such as prednisone
- Anti-inflammatories like ibuprofen, naproxen, or acetaminophen
- Antioxidants like vitamin C and E
- "Super fruits" like acai, goji, and mangosteen
- Antidepressants

- Antianxiety medications
- Blood-pressure medications
- Thyroid medications
- Muscle relaxants
- Painkillers

A person's hydration status and even their skin type can skew the results of skin-prick testing as well.

Considering all these factors that can influence the accuracy of the skin test—factors that affect almost everyone who has allergy symptoms—skin-prick testing is not as accurate as people think. The tests return too many false results, meaning that while you might test positive for substances to which you have no actual allergy, you can also test negative for the very allergies that affect you the most.

So why do doctors still perform the skin-prick test? In simple terms, it makes more money for the physician and insurance company. Conventional medicine created a system that allows insurance companies to bill for each individual skin prick; therefore, the more skin pricks, the more money they make. You might have experienced the result of this billing practice yourself. Or maybe you have taken your children to get allergy tested and watched them receive dozens of skin pricks on their back and arms. (I have personally witnessed and experienced over one hundred skin pricks carried out at one time.)

On top of the discomfort of the skin-prick test—and the risk of common foods, drugs, and supplements causing inaccurate results—another complication makes this test even more unreliable.

Since forty-eight hours elapses between the skin test itself and the follow-up viewing (when the doctor will charge your insurance for reading each individual skin prick), this delay introduces another factor that can affect the accuracy of test results. This factor is called interreader variability. Simply put, interreader variability means that there can be differences in how the person actually reads the swelling, or "wheel" sizes, at the sites of the skin pricks. One person may read a result as a "+1," and another person may read it as a "+2." The same individual may also read different results depending on the time of day or the day of the week (e.g., Monday morning versus Friday afternoon). Skin-prick tests require subjective judgment.

This is why I prefer blood testing for allergies. These tests measure the blood's immune reaction and thus are very accurate. Results are calculated through a computer, virtually eliminating human error. However, there are differences in the types of blood tests available (e.g., those carried out by regular laboratories versus specific allergy laboratories), as well as insurance coverage. Insurance usually covers skin-prick testing, and that is why most people have it done. In the end, however, those who get skin-prick tests typically receive the same medications that they were using when they went to the allergist to begin with; the only difference is that they now have a list of what they are allergic to. Their treatment remains the same—addressing the symptoms only, not the cause of the allergies.

With Allergy Drops Therapy, I can tailor treatments based on the individual's specific results, specifically titrating each allergen based upon more accurate blood-test results. Allergy Drops Therapy allows the body to desensitize itself against its specific allergens. In other words, it makes your immune system stronger so that it will not overreact when exposed to allergens, thereby decreasing the signaling that kicks off the inflammation cascade. In this way, Allergy Drops Therapy stops allergic reactions in their earliest stages instead of waiting until *after* allergy symptoms present themselves and then treating them with antihistamines, steroids, or supplements.

I have successfully treated hundreds of patients using Allergy Drops Therapy. Those who choose this form of treatment are not only very happy with the outcome but also almost universally without allergy symptoms. Patients start experiencing relief within six weeks, with continued improvement thereafter. Based on individual testing results, an average course of treatment runs three to five years, or until the person does shows no significant symptoms for over a year on the maintenance (lower) dose. Since we address complete lifestyle changes along with using Allergy Drops Therapy, most patients have shortened the duration of treatment to between two and four years.

Allergy Drops Therapy means fewer doctor's office visits, no painful injections, no waiting to see if you have an anaphylactic reaction, and no exposure to harmful phenols. Allergy Drops Therapy do *not* need to be refrigerated. You simply take one pump under the tongue *at your convenience,* three times a day. If you're used to taking pills or shots on a regular basis, this option saves you time and hassle, and treating the cause is far more effective than managing symptoms for years. Even better, it is more cost-effective. Allergy Drops Therapy costs less than a cup of coffee a day, which, of course, is nothing compared to the cost of weekly visits to the doctor, copays for the shots, copays for prescription meds such as Singulair, OTC medications such as Benadryl, Claritin, or Zyrtec, nasal sprays such as Afrin or Flonase, and countless other allergy medications.

There are, however, a couple of caveats when it comes to Allergy Drops Therapy. First, we can treat for all inhalant allergies, but we cannot treat all food allergies—specifically allergy-drops therapy does not treat nut allergies, wheat/gluten/gliadin sensitivity, and celiac disease. However, most people with wheat/gluten/gliadin sensitivities have other food allergies (usually soy, corn, or eggs) that we *can* treat to help make their dietary restrictions a little easier.

We have all been taught to take medications when we feel sick, but very few of us have been taught to take supportive therapies that not only treat symptoms immediately but also prevent further symptoms. That brings me to the other caveat with Allergy Drops Therapy—they only work if you take them for the full course of your treatment. That seems like a simple concept, but it can be difficult for some patients to continue taking their drops when, after a few months, their symptoms are minimal or completely gone.

The best responders to Allergy Drops Therapy are those who have fewer medical conditions and young children. Some of my favorite patients are the kids who come in when they are, say, seven years old and stop being the "allergic" kid in school by the time they are nine or ten. Most of my patients who have treated their children with allergy drops report that they are effective and help both their children's health and their behavior. Because a healthier kid is a happier kid. They are able to breath better, have more energy, sleep better and thus improve focus and concentration in school as well as other activities. This is an added bonus for parents and kids alike.

If you are tired of suffering from your inhalant allergies and want to learn more about sublingual drops for your allergy symptoms, please visit **www. allergydropstherapy.com**.

SAAT (Soliman Auricular Acupuncture Treatment)

In my ear
—THE ROMANTICS

For those who have trouble with managing daily regimens or who prefer a different approach to treating their allergies, there is another easy and effective option called Soliman Auricular Acupuncture Treatment, or SAAT. SAAT is a specialized form of auricular (ear) acupuncture that involves auricular bio-energetic testing (ABT). ABT is a subsection of energy medicine that focuses on the effects of electric fields both inside and outside the human body. Once I receive a patient's allergy blood work, I have the patient select which allergens (either inhalant or food) they would like to be desensitized to. SAAT is largely successful because it uses methods to eliminate direct and indirect bias on the parts of both patient and provider (unlike other forms of testing like "muscle testing"). Dr. Soliman, an internationally recognized medical doctor specializing in auriculotherapy, with whom I trained, developed this unique protocol.

Once the allergies to be treated have been identified, the SAAT protocol applies a specialized instrument (neuro-electric therapy or microcurrent device) to a zone of the ear shown to be related to the liver (the organ in your body that is responsible for the metabolism of foods and histamine production). A specific point in the ear zone is then identified and confirmed using ABT or Nogier pulse reflex (a vascular autonomic signal). A tiny sterile acupuncture needle (2 mm in size) is placed into the surface of the skin and covered by a small bandage (or Steri-Strip). The patient then avoids the allergens as much as possible over the next three weeks, after which they remove the needles (up to two different allergens can be treated at one time). Following treatment, the patient is more tolerant of the allergic triggers. Response rates for SAAT treatments are about 90 percent successful.

While this protocol may sound improbable at first blush, Dr. Soliman has accumulated over ten years of experience, published clinical data, and successfully treated thousands of patients with this method. This type of treatment is a great option for those for whom daily Allergy Drops Therapy would be difficult or who just have a few allergies (or even dozens) that they would like to become more resilient to without having to remember to take drops daily.

For more information, please visit **www.SAATacupunture.com.**

3) Food Allergies: The Most Important Triggers of Systemic Inflammation

And the same food you eat to live / Can make you die.
—SLY AND THE FAMILY STONE

The third type of allergy—and the most important to your overall health—is food allergy. Since approximately 80 percent of your immune system resides in the GI tract, it is important to understand that certain foods cause inflammation in everyone, and other foods cause specific reactions that are unique to each of us.

Food allergies (sensitivities), in my opinion, are the most overlooked underlying causes of the inflammation that triggers or worsens all negative health conditions. Many people have both inhalant and food allergies. For example, in the summer months their symptoms worsen because they are outside, exposed to inhalants, while eating foods that are also problematic (e.g., barbecue and potluck dinners on the Fourth of July in the park). Let's first take a look at the foods that cause specific reactions in individuals.

We all have seen and heard of the severe food allergies that cause anaphylaxis (trouble breathing, swelling of lips and throat, and cardiovascular collapse) in movies and on TV, or even from personal experience or people you know. Severe, life-threatening allergies to peanuts, melons, and shellfish get a lot of press, but these allergies only occur in less than 2 percent of the population. Western medicine has developed acute-care drugs that have not only saved thousands of people worldwide. (They even saved my life, and I'll talk more about my personal experience with severe allergies soon.) This is where Western medicine shines—treating acute or life-threatening conditions.

But for chronic conditions (which include most health problems in the United States, such as heart disease, diabetes, arthritis, colitis, and asthma), Western medicine treats the symptoms—not the underlying cause. When it comes to food allergies, Western medicine has done wonders for acute emergencies (for example, my EpiPen can save my life instantly). But when people have allergic reactions that do not threaten their lives, physicians tend to ignore them, since resolving chronic health concerns doesn't require our heroic medical intervention. Once symptoms become chronic, it's almost a relief; we tend not to worry as much because we can send you on your way with a prescription or two.

Let's get back to the significance of food allergies to your overall health. While inhalant allergies cause inflammation to the respiratory tract, food allergies cause inflammation to the GI tract *and* to the body systemically (all over).

Food allergies (or inflammatory reactions) can be divided into two categories:

1. Immediate IgE responses, both acute immediate and regular immediate, and
2. Delayed IgG responses

The IgE response can be split into two reactions—one life threatening and the other not. Most people who have a life-threatening food allergy already know it; many have had a "crash," trouble breathing or swallowing, broken out in hives, or been hospitalized after eating a certain food. These life-threatening reactions cause some allergy sufferers to carry EpiPens, inhalers, or steroids to help prevent an emergency from exposure to their allergen(s).

Fortunately, most of the population (98 percent) does *not* have acute, immediate, life-threatening allergic reactions. They can, however, have regular, immediate IgE inflammatory reactions that do not threaten their life.

What does this mean? This means that after eating a certain food that causes an IgE reaction, you can experience immediate inflammatory symptoms that affect your upper GI tract, such as heartburn, reflux, and stomach pains. Then, once the food enters the lower-GI tract, symptoms such as gas, bloating, diarrhea, and constipation occur. This reaction can start up within an hour after consuming the offending food; what you ate for breakfast could bother you within a few minutes of eating it or up to an hour later. Thus, if you are eating foods that cause inflammation daily, the symptoms can last all day and night. Now, the importance of the food allergy is not just as the trigger of the GI symptoms (some people will not have GI symptoms due to their *dosha* [mind-body constitution in Ayurveda], meaning some body types have stronger digestive capabilities and thus hardly ever complain of GI symptoms); once these food allergens are absorbed from the GI tract, the inflammation goes all over the body—and becomes systemic.

In addition to the IgE immediate-type reactions, there is a second type of food-allergy inflammatory response called IgG (specifically IgG4)—the delayed response. This inflammatory response occurs from a few hours to up to four days after the ingestion of the offending food. Therefore, while most people who keep a food diary or journal may be able to pinpoint their IgE (immediate reaction) foods, it is almost impossible for them to figure out their IgG (delayed reaction) foods. On top of this, the same person can have both an immediate reaction *and* a delayed reaction, which I call a "double whammy." This allergy hits you not only within the first hour, but also anytime thereafter over the next four days. This means that what you eat for breakfast on Monday can bother you by dinnertime, by breakfast on Tuesday, or even by breakfast on Thursday! Most people spend their lives on this constant allergic rollercoaster, not realizing that they are subjecting themselves to constant inflammatory reactions, one after the other, for years at a time.

My Personal Experience with Food Allergies

Allergies
Something's living on my skin.
Doctor, please
Open up, it's me again.
I go to a famous physician.
I sleep in the local hotel.
From what I can see of the people like me,
We get better
But we never get well.
—PAUL SIMON

Let me give you a personal example of the two different types of allergic or inflammatory reactions. As I mentioned before, I have a severe food allergy; specifically, I have an anaphylactic reaction (an IgE, immediate, life-threatening reaction) to peanuts. That means if I eat a peanut, within a few minutes I will go into cardiovascular and respiratory collapse.

I found myself in the hospital many times as a young child. After allergy testing and a thorough review of what I ate prior to these anaphylactic attacks, it was easy to see that peanuts were not for me. Thanks to the wonders of conventional medicine, acute-care treatments such as epinephrine and steroids and even a ventilator can be used to assist me through a crisis and heal me almost immediately. To this day, I am grateful to those doctors, nurses, and medicines that helped me have a normal childhood and that continue to help me if I have an unexpected exposure to peanuts. But the other aspect of food allergies or inflammatory responses, which most conventional training overlooks, is the delayed-response reaction, or the IgG/IgG4 reaction.

At the same time that doctors discovered my severe peanut allergy, I was also dealing with chronic eczema. Due to my severe peanut allergy, I was evaluated at the top Ivy League medical institutions. Unfortunately, they could do nothing for my chronic eczema, only for my acute peanut reaction. Those with eczema, or those with family members who have eczema, understand the extreme discomfort of dry and scaly patches on the elbows, backs of the knees, neck, and sometimes the face and elsewhere. Eczema is usually treated with topical steroids and occasional oral steroids for acute flare-ups. When I was growing up, I learned to deal with my chronic eczema by covering myself up with long sleeves and using steroid creams constantly. Although these tactics got me through the day, they also interfered with my confidence, and at times they made me feel embarrassed or humiliated. I dealt with eczema throughout high school, medical school, residency, and fellowship—all the way up till 2009, when something life changing happened to me.

As I read the book *The China Study* by T. Colin Campbell—the largest epidemiological study on diet published to date—I decided to switch from my vegetarian diet to a completely plant-based diet, without any animal proteins—not even dairy or eggs. Within two weeks of my switch, my eczema went away. I could not believe or understand why it did. For over thirty-five years, I had tried not only medications and prescribed topical treatments but also natural therapies—from almost anything that was published in a journal to products on the Internet and even home remedies, indigenous medicines, vitamins, superfoods, and homeopathics. Most of them did not work at all, and whenever I did get a somewhat positive response, it was only temporary. No cure was permanent. But after just two weeks of eating a plant-based (vegan) diet, my eczema cleared up. It felt like a miracle.

While I was making my switch to a vegan diet, Maureen Sutton, Sanjevani's health and lifestyle elder and medicine woman, asked me if I had ever been tested for an allergy or sensitivity to eggs. At first I scoffed at the idea. I told her that I had been eating an egg almost every day of my life, and some days even more than one. How could something I enjoyed on a daily basis not be good for me? I loved eggs so much that I would sometimes dream of opening an "Egg Shoppe" restaurant with eggs made dozens of ways in different types of foods. I was taught at a young age that the "American" breakfast was an egg, toast, and coffee or tea. That breakfast became a daily habit for me, especially as I went through my medical training; I could always pick up a breakfast burrito at the hospital or come home after a long shift and whip up an omelet or scrambled eggs quickly. Besides, I was told that eggs are the "perfect protein," so what could be wrong with them?

What was wrong was that my test for food allergies did confirm (as it has for many other people) that I had a very high delayed allergy (IgG4) to eggs. Because I did not have an immediate reaction (IgE) but a delayed reaction (IgG4), my eczema symptoms from my breakfast burrito would appear not at breakfast time but at dinner that evening or up to four days later. Since I was eating eggs daily, my symptoms were chronic, and I was experiencing constant flare-ups from things I had eaten up to four days earlier.

Again, I cannot express how much gratitude I have for being saved from my life-threatening peanut allergy, but how did the system miss the egg allergy that plagued me for decades?

As I mentioned before, conventional medicine is best for acute care, but when it comes to chronic conditions, it treats only symptoms. I would never have died from eczema, but it bothers me that I went through decades of having a "nuisance" allergy that interfered with my social life, my confidence, and my well-being. If someone had told me decades ago that I could get rid of my eczema by stopping my consumption of eggs, I would have done so in a heartbeat. But how would anyone discover such a delayed reaction unless the doctor knows to test for it?

The Factors That Contribute to Inflammation from Foods

The severity of the inflammation from individual food-allergy reactions depends on a few factors:

1. The amount of the food that is eaten,
2. The number of multiple allergic foods (if there is more than one) eaten together,
3. "Leaky-gut syndrome" and the strength of the GI tract and immune system, and
4. The overall health of the individual.

Let's start with the amount of food you eat. If a food causes inflammation directly (via a specific food allergy or sensitivity) or indirectly (as in the case of animal proteins that are high in omega-6s), the more of it you consume, the more your body burns with inflammation. Thus consuming a large amount of one food source can cause an inflammatory flare.

The second factor is eating multiple inflammatory foods. Think of each pro-inflammatory food as fuel for a fire. The more sources of fuel you add to the fire, the higher and longer it burns. For example, let's say someone has a food allergy to eggs, dairy, tomatoes, and wheat. If that person eats each of them separately in small amounts, they will still trigger inflammation, but on a small level. If the person eats a lot of just one, that can cause an inflammatory flare also. But if the person consumes all these foods in large amounts all together—as when eating multiple slices of pizza—that will cause the inflammation to flare the most, with some of the inflammation flaring immediately and some flaring on a rolling basis, over hours or days.

The state of the individual's GI tract and overall immune system can lessen or worsen the reaction to the above two factors. Since the GI tract is the point of entry for food, the type of food and the amount we eat are important. But the digestion, assimilation, and excretion of this food from the GI tract are equally important.

For example, if someone has taken multiple antibiotics or has IBS symptoms, then the foods he or she is sensitive to may cause symptoms of heartburn, reflux, stomachache, gas, bloating, cramping, and diarrhea or constipation. As I mentioned before, taking multiple courses of antibiotics or antimicrobial medications (and natural antimicrobial therapies), consuming alcohol and other drugs, or experiencing a large amount of stress can all cause worsening GI symptoms and lead to what is now known as "leaky-gut syndrome." This term has been around for over thirty years, but originally only holistic and naturopathic circles recognized the syndrome; conventional medicine primarily dismissed it. Over the past decade—as the understanding of GI health through immunology, physiology, and cell biology has advanced—even major conservative medical institutions have begun to embrace leaky-gut syndrome at their educational conferences. They are now referring this area of anatomy, physiology and immunology as the "gut microbiome."

So, what is leaky-gut syndrome exactly? It's a term that describes a chronic condition caused by the disruption of the good, probiotic bacteria in the GI tract through the use of antibiotics or other factors. With leaky gut, the intestinal villi (or crypts)—where food particles filter into the gut based on the size and type of particle—open up on a cellular level, allowing food particles to leak into inappropriate sites in the gut. This leaking causes dysfunctional symptoms like heartburn, reflux, stomachache, gas, bloating, cramping, diarrhea, or constipation. If we were to look at an endoscopy (upper-GI test) or colonoscopy (lower-GI test), we most likely would not *see* pathology or disease, even though the patient may be complaining of symptoms. That's because only *disease* can be seen, not *dysfunction*.

Once food particles leak from the GI tract, the immune system goes on alert. The immune system starts to attack or defend itself from the food particle invaders by creating inflammation. I give the following example to my patients at Sanjevani to make this concept easily understood.

At Sanjevani when my patients arrive for an appointment, they come in the front entrance and then proceed through different clinic doors to get to the appropriate treatment room. When I see them in their treatment room, I recognize them and greet them with open arms and a smile. Like in a healthy functioning GI tract, the system functions smoothly when everyone enters and exits as they should. A "leaky gut," however, is like a medical office where the patients are trying to enter through the windows. Although I recognize my patients when they walk through the front door, if they come in through a window, it might look very suspicious. I might call the police, thinking they are burglars. And once the police arrive, they might shoot the person to stop what looks like a break-in.

In this analogy, the police are like the immune system's soldier cells, responding to a threat; their use of force is like the body's use of inflammation. Similarly, when food leaks into inappropriate sites within our gut, our immune system goes on the defensive. And, in extreme cases, just as certain situations can cause police to overreact and inflict more harm than is necessary, conditions in our gut can cause our bodies to overrespond with too much inflammation, and this is how we develop chronic diseases and autoimmune disorders.

Finally, let's consider the fourth factor that determines the severity of inflammation caused by our body's reaction to a food allergy. If the person's overall health is good, he or she will have a stronger ability to defend and repair against inflammatory triggers. If, however, the individual is chronically ill, has multiple medical problems, is dealing with metabolic disorders, or is under a lot of stress, he or she will have a weaker response to allergic triggers and, therefore, experience more allergy symptoms. A person with a depressed immune system under constant, low-grade attack tends to have more chronic degenerative diseases. Over long periods of time, that can lead to cancer. For example, up to 43 percent of people who have ulcerative colitis for twenty-five to thirty-five years develop colorectal cancer,[94] and those who have active rheumatoid arthritis for more than ten years have a seventy-one-fold-higher rate of lymphoma than the general population.[95] Therefore, even low-grade food sensitivities can cause major problems over time in people with weakened immune systems and other inflammatory conditions.

Inflammation's Four Favorite Targets

That's my favorite spot.
—THE BLACK EYED PEAS

To understand how inflammation affects the body systemically, remember that when you eat food, all its different components—proteins, carbs, fats, sugars, vitamins, and minerals—are dispersed throughout the body. Each cell receives nutrients from food, and if you have allergies or sensitivities, they're also exposed to inflammation. So how does inflammation work on a cellular level?

Because I live in the Southwest, I use a desert analogy to explain how it works.

In the Southwest, especially in New Mexico, we have flat roofs that don't have the pitch or drainage systems you'll see on homes in other parts of the country because we don't experience the rain and snow of, say, the Midwest. Therefore, when it rains in New Mexico, the rainwater collects on most of the rooftops, and eventually it finds an area of weakness and causes a leak. Inflammation in the body does the same thing. To make matters worse, even if the roof is repaired, the next time it rains, the water will again tend toward the area of prior damage or weakness. This is because even though the roof was fixed, it will never again be 100 percent normal. It will always be slightly less than perfect (say 99 percent). Thus the water tends to go to the area that had previous damage before going elsewhere. Inflammation in the body behaves in similar ways.

Once inflammation is triggered in the body, it likes to go to four "weakened" places in particular:

1. Areas of trauma
2. Areas of pathology
3. Areas of overuse
4. Areas where the immune system is not strong enough or is not paying attention

In most people, inflammation likes to go to areas of trauma first.

To follow the analogy of the leaky roof above, once an area of the body is weakened by trauma, that is the place that is most likely to experience inflammatory flare-ups down the road. For example, let's say you had a knee injury in college. After the immediate pain and short-term damage, the body eventually heals itself. But on an immunological and cellular level, there is still a small amount of inflammation remaining from the injury—say 1 percent. Now, this is not enough to cause immediate discomfort or dysfunction, but if anything else comes into the body that is pro-inflammatory, like fuel to a fire, it will make the inflammation grow hotter and bigger. For example, take your kitchen stove. If it is a gas stove, it has a small pilot light that remains on. You will not feel much heat from the pilot light, as there is very little fuel to make it burn. However, if you have a gas leak in your kitchen, the stove is the first place that will light up. "Healed" trauma, even one from decades before, is like that tiny pilot light; it remains a sensitive area prone to inflammation.

When my patients state that their arthritis is flaring up, I always ask them, "So what did you do to make it so?" They always respond that it must be due to aging. But this is not necessarily so. Arthritis is a disease not of aging but of chronic inflammation to the joints.

Most patients experience inflammation symptoms not only when they are active but also when they are at rest. They can't figure out why, for example, on Sunday when they are not at work and they just went to church or stayed home watching the football game, their knees, back, or other body parts hurt. I explain to them that there is always a trigger to those "itis" areas, and it mainly comes from foods that produce immediate or delayed responses (or both). Again, they don't have to use those joints or muscles continuously or incorrectly; it's simply that once that area is sensitive, due to past trauma, it becomes the "roof leak" where inflammation likes to settle.

The second area that inflammation likes to go is an area of past pathology—which means any place where disease has triggered inflammation in the past. Once an area experiences chronic degeneration or acute aggravation of tissues, such as is seen in polyps (e.g., sinus or colon)—or even more seriously, benign or malignant tumors—inflammation immediately goes to those areas. When it comes to areas of pathology where disease is taking place (or has taken place), we aren't talking a small roof leak but a big tree falling on the roof and causing major structural damage. Therefore, all the rain (i.e., inflammation) will go to this area and cause major water damage.

The third area that inflammation likes to go is any place in the body that has been overused. Now, we all have places of overuse, so that doesn't mean that inflammation is dangerous for us. But over time such overuse can inhibit how we function physically and mentally. For example, if you were to increase your time on the treadmill or up the amount of weight you lift, you might be sore the next day. This inflammation, from working your muscles hard, is a good response. After the soreness departs, more muscle tissue builds up, thus making us stronger.

However, as time goes on, we might find that the time we take to recover after such workouts gets longer and longer, driving us to decrease the amount of exercise we do. Again, most patients will tell me that they can't exercise as much as they used to because they are getting older, but aging is not the reason they feel the way they do (although that is what they think). They feel that way because their body is getting exposed to more and more inflammation over time from other sources, making post workout recovery take longer than it used to. Some people—such as receptionists, computer

programmers, or retail workers who scan items all day long—exp
daily inflammation in the hands. Others experience inflammation in their
backs from lifting and moving heavy objects all day long, or sore legs from
standing on their feet all day. However, when our body continues to experience more and more triggers of inflammation, we naturally modify (reduce)
our activities and, in extreme cases, change our professions. Long-standing
inflammation leads us to take medications, like pain relievers, to feel better when we can't change our jobs. Taking pain medications only masks our
ability to perceive the pain. While decreasing inflammation may seem like
the chief effect of pain medications like NSAIDs, the severe side effects make
them a very risky choice **(see chapter 7)**.

Finally, the fourth area where inflammation likes to go in the body is
wherever the immune system is not strong enough or is not paying attention. This is a simple concept. If your immune system's soldier cells are tired
or exhausted— for instance, if you are recovering from an injury or undergoing chemotherapy— you will be more susceptible to chronic illnesses, which
are all caused by inflammation.

We are familiar with the role of vitamin D3 in our body and its importance in overall immune functioning. It is a reliable marker that show how
strong our troops (immune system) are from an overall standpoint; our
D3 level provides not a specific measurement but a general one. It tells us
whether or not we are strong enough to fight infections, fend off diseases,
and repair damaged tissues. Therefore, I recommend having your doctor test
for vitamin D3 levels, looking for an optimum level between fifty and one
hundred for a healthy person and between seventy and one hundred for
cancer patients. If you have had your levels tested and are currently taking
D3 daily, you will notice fewer flus and colds, and you will feel better overall.
There is more to optimum health than vitamin D3, of course, but it is a very
important factor in helping us along the way. Studies have shown that once
vitamin D3 is in its target zone, we get a 60 percent reduction in our risk of
developing future chronic disease—including cancer! Vitamin D3 is easily
one of the biggest preventative public-health measures. We could essentially
cut 60 percent of our total health-care costs if everyone's vitamin D3 level
was in the target range.

While I cannot overstate the importance of vitamin D3 in disease
prevention, one shouldn't overlook other important aspects that affect

immune-system function. Stress, lack of sleep, poor diet, and metabolic conditions such as diabetes can wear down our immune system. Once someone's immune system is down, that person is more likely to experience inflammatory conditions and illnesses, since the body cannot fight, fix, and repair as it should. When we experience severe illnesses or chronic stress, inflammation goes systemic with often devastating results.

So, now that I have described how inflammation works in the body, you may be wondering how it relates to some of our most serious current healthcare crises. Let me explain with a few examples how inflammation works as the triggering mechanism for almost all diseases.

Example 1: Alzheimer's disease = chronic inflammation of the brain.

> *I don't remember, I don't recall*
> *I got no memory of anything*
> *—anything at all.*
> —PETER GABRIEL

When one has had chronic inflammation in the brain for decades, memory problems become more common and pronounced. At this point, a person will see a neurologist, and a CT scan or MRI will show white plaques within the brain matter. This is a classic radiological diagnosis (along with the history and cognitive difficulties) to correlate with Alzheimer's disease. The problem with the conventional Western approach to this disease is that we are, again, not addressing the underlying cause; we're looking for ways to improve the existing state of the diseased condition, and at the time of diagnosis disease has already damaged the brain. In general, doctors prescribe pharmaceuticals to patients with Alzheimer's in an attempt to improve certain functions of the brain. Drug developers do not focus on what is causing the underlying dysfunction, or what triggers the protein plaques (e.g., beta amyloid and tau proteins) in the first place, but on delaying progression of the disease.

Why don't these pharmaceutical drugs *stop* the progression of this disease? Because these drugs are used to improve a neurological function, the function that has been disabled to the buildup of protein plaques. But the drugs ignore what causes those plaques to deposit in the brain in the first place—you guessed it—inflammation.

Just as the body responds to inhalant allergies by releasing histamines to prevent more exposure, the brain responds to inflammation by producing protein plaques, which, in the beginning, are used to calm the inflammation. While this helps at first, too much inflammation over time causes too much plaque buildup, which in turn causes the neurons in the brain to function abnormally. When neurons aren't functioning the way they should, memory loss and other dysfunctions occur—despite Alzheimer's drugs **(see Side Notes: Exelon Patch)**.

One can take steps to limit the progression of Alzheimer's disease and, possibly, even reverse mild to moderate cases. The reason for this will be explored in chapter 8, and that reason is related to the country with the lowest incidence of Alzheimer's disease: India.

Example 2: Heart disease = chronic inflammation of the endothelial lining of the coronary vessels.

In the burning heart
The unmistakable fire
—SURVIVOR

Heart disease is now viewed as an inflammatory disease. Certain inflammatory markers, such as hs-CRP (high-sensitivity C-reactive protein), are becoming part of standard diagnostic blood tests to demonstrate the risk of inflammation to the heart. The higher the level of inflammation, the higher the risk of heart disease. In fact, the main cause of heart attacks and strokes is not just an elevation in blood lipids (cholesterol, triglycerides, bad cholesterol, etc.) but also calcium/cholesterol plaques that are fixed onto the walls of the vascular system. How do these plaques appear in our arteries? The same way they do in our brains: via inflammation. Only the composition of the plaques is different; they appear for the same reason—to try to calm inflammation.

When the arteries in the body are inflamed **(see fig. 24)**, the endothelial lining thins over time. The body responds to this thinning by laying down calcium/cholesterol plaques to try to heal that inflammation. The body continues to create plaque as long as the inflammation remains in the vessel walls or as long as they are exposed to the triggers of inflammation (e.g., pro-inflammatory foods and food allergies). As more and more plaque is applied, these vessels constrict. This causes turbulence in the blood, and when the individual is also stressed, the blood platelets will get temporarily thicker **(see chapter 11: Sympathetic vs. Parasympathetic Response).** When these platelets bounce off the plaques, a clot can form in the restricted vessel and cause a blockage. Also, when the cholesterol plaque becomes supersaturated, crystals can form within it. Like frozen ice, these crystals expand and create tiny spikes that tear through tissue, causing the plaque to rupture and leading to blockage in the vessel.[96] These two mechanisms of blockage cause heart attacks and strokes. Again, treatment of heart disease using only lipid-lowering drugs or even just natural lipid-lowering agents is not the full answer. One must reduce the inflammation that is triggering this sequence of events.

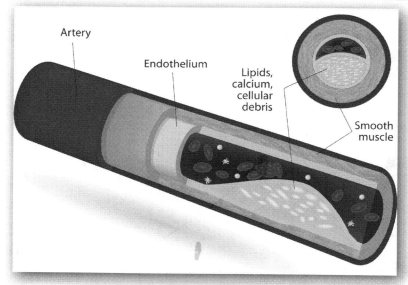

Figure 24: Plaque buildup in coronary arteries (atherosclerosis)

The top-prescribed drug class worldwide—by a wide margin and for over two decades—is statins (e.g., Lipitor and Crestor). That means that the overall rate of heart attacks and strokes should be going down, right? More and more people medicated with statins means fewer and fewer blockages. So, why have the rates of heart attacks and strokes remained static for over a decade? With such widespread use of statins, heart disease should

be nearly eradicated from the population if these drugs have been wc   g
as intended. Yet most people with heart disease over the past twenty years
have not only taken multiple types and doses of statins but also received
stents and undergone bypass surgeries! To further understand why this
class of drugs does not work as effectively as it is marketed, see **Side Notes:
Absolute Risk vs. Relative Risk with Statins and Other Medications**. The
missing piece in preventing and treating heart disease is not only lipids but,
more importantly, the inflammatory triggers that make these lipids stick to
the endothelial lining.

Here is a great example of the conventional medical disconnection
when it comes to lipids, inflammation, and heart disease. In August 2013,
former President George W. Bush, upon his annual physical, showed signs of
an electrical abnormality on an EKG. Without any symptoms after a stress
test, he had a CT angiogram that found an area of concern, and thus he had
a stent placed inside the artery in his heart—even though the most recent
studies have shown that stents have no better outcomes compared to medical therapy alone. In addition, there is no evidence stent treatment will help
President Bush live longer, feel better, or have fewer heart attacks. So why do
doctors push for this procedure when it's largely unnecessary?

While stent placement may allow immediate and sustained blood flow
to help heart-attack patients recover, for those who have not had a heart
attack, the benefits are not as clear—especially when a person is not having
chest pains or other classic symptoms. There is currently *no* evidence that
stent placement prevents future heart attacks; in fact, there is some data
showing that those who have had a stent and were asymptomatic when it
was placed might be at higher risk for having problems in the future.[97]

So, why did President Bush's doctors suggest he receive a stent? My guess
is that he has the best insurance (being a former president) and that the
hospital and doctors can bill a large amount for this treatment. The average
out-of-pocket cost for a stent procedure is between forty and fifty thousand
dollars. But why did he have narrowing of his coronary arteries in the first
place?

We all have come to know that President Bush is overall very physically
fit; we've seen him exercising and even mountain biking. So why, if he did
not have chest pain, did he have narrowing of the artery in his heart? My
guess is that he had lots of inflammation through his diet (and the stress

of being president of the United States) that made plaque build up in his arteries. But since he also exercises frequently, he developed a strong collateral microcirculation and thus did not have chest pain when physically active. Collateral microcirculation is the process by which the body develops and improves additional arterial blood flow due to the increased demand on the heart. If the heart tissue is not getting adequate blood flow, it will grow and strengthen the smaller vessels to carry more blood to wherever it is needed. Thus the body is constantly trying to maintain equilibrium, and if the requirement for an increase of blood flow is not excessive, then the body can reorganize itself, and the person will never notice the symptoms. But if demand for blood is high and the body cannot supply the demand, then the person experiences angina (chest pain) and may progress to a heart attack.

Since the 1980s, people have equated exercise with good heart health, but that is not necessarily true. *Exercise is a state of physiology, not a state of health.*

Most people think that if they eat cheeseburgers, steaks, doughnuts, and ice cream, they can simply increase their time on the treadmill to negate the negative effects. This is just not true. Health is not only about exercising more; it may be more about eating healthier.

In Texas, they take barbecue very seriously. I have to guess, then, that President George W. Bush has always eaten a diet with a lot of animal protein. Therefore, although he is fit and could ride a bike farther and faster than I can, his cardiovascular system is being exposed to more inflammation than mine. This is due to his diet—which is nothing other than the standard American diet (SAD): high amounts of animal proteins, refined oils, and copious quantities of highly refined sugars.

Now, some people might think that I am picking on President Bush, but everything I'm saying goes for former President Bill Clinton. When President Clinton was running for office, he was noted for eating Big Macs and visiting McDonald's while running. He too was victim of the SAD, probably more than President George W. Bush. Over time, President Clinton had to undergo bypass surgery for heart disease. But that was not enough to keep him healthy, as later on he had to have stents placed in his heart in order to keep those vessels open. At that time, his cardiologists and the White House doctors were quoted as stating it was all in his genes, and lifestyle had nothing to do with it.[98]

Most of you know by now that President Clinton is no longer using previous doctors, and one of his current cardiologists is Dr. Dean Ornish. Dr. Ornish, a cardiologist from Stanford University, has published dozens of studies over the past thirty years showing that blood flow can be improved through dietary measures to increase heart function[99] and heart disease can be reversed.[100] Yes, reversed! By eating a plant-based diet, doing yoga/meditation, and engaging in moderate exercise, you can reverse heart disease. It also shown to reverse disease in men with early prostate cancer and even diabetes Type 2 by positively changing gene expression in over five hundred genes.[101]

In fact, a recent study in *The Lancet Oncology*[102] showed that by following the Ornish Lifestyle Program participants increased their telomere length by 10 percent compared to the control group, whose telomeres shortened. That means that by following these healthy behaviors (plant-based diet, yoga, and stress reduction), you could lengthen your telomeres. That means this is the first study to show that, through lifestyle changes, you can actually slow down and reverse the aging of your DNA! No drug or surgical procedure has been able to do this so easily, so effectively, without side effects, and basically without any extra out-of-pocket cost. Best of all, you don't need an insurance company to get involved.

So, how did President Clinton reverse his heart disease and become healthier now than ever before? That's right: President Bill Clinton is now on a plant-based diet. His heart vessels are better than they have ever been. He looks healthier now than when he was in office; he looks statelier; he is thinner; his eyes are brighter and sharper; and his body is less puffy. During interviews, he has stated that he feels better now than ever before, thanks to eating a plant-based diet (see CNN—Sanjay Gupta's video "The Last Heart Attack," from 2011).[103]

That's two former presidents who have heart disease, both being treated with the conventional approach of surgical procedures and medications, one without changing his diet and the other changing to a plant-based diet. They both have access to the best health care and doctors, yet at the outset, none of these doctors talked about what was causing their disease or how to prevent it, only what could be done for their immediate concerns. You think that it would be in the best interest of our national security to keep our presidents as healthy as possible. The cardiology hospitals, drug companies, and conventional doctors (whose salary is based on the amount of procedures that they do each year) don't seem to want to slow down the disease-management industry. If only both President Clinton and President Bush had been told about plant-based diets earlier in life, they could have avoided their stents and surgeries! I am glad to hear that President Clinton has changed his lifestyle and now advocates plant-based diets. Maybe he could recommend his cardiologist to President Bush.

If you had a choice, which treatment would you choose? I personally prefer to go the noninvasive way, with changes to my diet and lifestyle.

Example 3: Colon polyps = chronic inflammation of areas of the colon.

Oh, should I take laxatives or have my colon irrigated?
—WEIRD AL YANKOVIC

Colon polyps are small clumps of cells (which look like grapes) that form on the inner lining of the colon. Although most colon polyps are harmless, some can become cancerous over time.

Anyone can develop colon polyps. But you're at higher risk if you're fifty or older, are overweight or a smoker, eat a high-fat, *low-fiber diet*, or have a personal or family history of colon polyps or colon cancer. Most of the factors—like being overweight, smoking, eating a high (animal) fat diet, and having chronic constipation—are inflammatory in nature.

A polyp is created when the colon cells try to wall off the inflamed tissue in the colonic wall by pushing it outside the rest of the colon. In essence, the body is trying to protect itself, just as it does in the airways (as in nasal polyps) and the heart vessels (as in plaque buildup). Again, most people, including GI doctors, tend to ignore or remove (if possible) the colon polyps without truly understanding the reason they occurred in the first place. It is good to remove polyps because, as with all chronic inflammation, over time some polyps can turn cancerous. If you've been paying attention, you know that chronic inflammation is a pathway to cancer; about 43 percent of colitis patients progress to having colorectal cancer within twenty-five to thirty-five years of their initial diagnosis.[104]

How do we prevent colon polyps? Again, it's pretty simple: people who eat plant-based diets have the lowest risk and occurrence of colon polyps and colon cancer. For those who have had colon polyps removed in the past,

AN INFLAMMATION NATION

it is never too late to change your diet and add natural anti-inflammatories **(see chapter 8)** to your routine to help reduce the occurrence of polyps and to shrink any existing polyps you might have. Remember, plant proteins also contain antioxidants, phytonutrients, and fiber. Animal protein has little to no antioxidants, no phytonutrients, and no fiber. The lack of fiber in the diet leads to more constipation and a greater risk of colon problems. The average American consumes only 7 to 11 g of fiber a day, when the recommendation is at least 40 g of fiber a day. In those cultures around the world that consume 90 to 120 g of fiber daily through their diet have virtually no incidences of colon cancer. I recommend that you figure out how much fiber you consume daily and then increase slowly by 5 g per week. If you do this, you will avoid any immediate constipation, as your GI tract will learn how to digest the increase in fiber over time.

In addition, it is crucial that you increase the amount of water you drink in order to make the fiber more effective. Fiber attracts water, which causes it to create bulk that stretches the intestines, which then causes peristalsis— which makes the bowels move. While there's been a lot of debate about how much water to drink daily, the rule I follow is to drink half my body weight in fluid ounces per day. Therefore, if you weigh 150 pounds, then you should be drinking about 75 fl. oz. of water a day. If you do that, you will notice less pain, improved blood pressure, better bowel movements, and overall improved memory and well-being.

Example 4: Arthritis = chronic inflammation of the joints.

But it's my destiny to be the king of pain.
—THE POLICE

Arthritis is the most common cause of disability in the United States, limiting the activities of nearly twenty-one million adults. In the United States, most doctors and patients view arthritis as a disease of aging, but this is wrong.

Through our inflammatory diets and lifestyles, we have created certain medical conditions for ourselves that, as a society and in our culture, have become part of our thinking, too. We expect to get these conditions over time. In most people's minds, arthritis is one of those conditions that are inevitable as we get older.

In actuality, arthritis is just inflammation of the joints that occurs over time; it is not directly due to aging. For example, in countries like Indonesia, the concept of arthritis hardly exists. Remember, *itis* means *inflammation of* whatever word you place before it. Thus, arthritis is inflammation of the joints, and instead of treating our symptoms with NSAIDs, steroids and immunosuppressive agents we should investigate what is triggering our joints to be chronically inflamed.

The Levee Point

> *When the levee breaks*
> —LED ZEPPELIN

I have coined the concept of the "levee point"—the point at which function becomes dysfunction in the body. Similar to the levees that protect against flooding from waterways, each cell and organ has its own "levee point," or the point at which the level of water (in this case inflammation) can only go so high (reaching our cells' and organs' tolerance) before the levee breaks and the water spills over, causing damage (from metabolic dysfunction to pain to organ destruction).

Each cell, organ, and tissue in our body has its own "levee point," at which the burden of chronic inflammation becomes too much to manage. We all remember the disaster that occurred from Hurricane Katrina. The levees in New Orleans were not strong enough or high enough, and when they broke, the water they unleashed into New Orleans caused immense damage and destruction. A similar thing happens in the body when the inflammatory "levee points" are breached.

The other problem with inflammation is that the various fuels—inflammatory foods, stress, injury, and so on—can accumulate in the body, causing the flames of the inflammatory fire to burn higher and faster. It's like adding gasoline to a fire, and then adding diesel, and then adding kerosene. The more fuel you give the fire, the faster it grows. If the fire burns high enough and long enough, the result is a cataclysm of dysfunction and pain. If we consider just the effects of eating typical SAD amounts of pro-inflammatory foods and our individualized food allergens, the inflammatory fires never go out.

I talk to so many patients who tell me they have not fe
many months or even years. Many will couch that by saying som
"Well, at least I don't feel as bad as I used to!" But they never tel   .at
they are feeling normal, let alone better than normal. I tell them that I don't
want people to feel that barely keeping their head above water is normal.
That is not even close to being good enough, although most new patients
of mine seem to feel that way. I want my patients not just above water
but sailing. That is the difference between only feeling good and achieving
optimum health.

If you're ready to get to the bottom of whatever your health concern
may be—or if you simply want to feel good—I recommend that you do
these five things to start:

- Switch to eating a plant-based diet.
- Find ways to exercise and reduce your stress.
- Based on your history of symptoms and health conditions, test for
  food sensitivities (IgE and IgG4) and celiac/gluten/gliadin sensitivity
  (and test for inhalant allergies if you have seasonal allergy symptoms
  or asthma/COPD).
- If you have a history of heavy antibiotic use; if you experience bloating, gas, fatigue, and brain fog after eating sugars (regardless whether
  from fruits or sweets); or if you have a history of yeast infections,
  then I would test for candida.
- If you or your child is struggling with depression or severe behavioral
  problems, then I would test for sensitivities to food additives, colors,
  and chemicals.

If you want to see the full list of laboratory tests I recommend to my
patients, see **Side Notes: Dr. Pai's Recommended Laboratory Testing**.

The Wheat Misunderstanding: Not the Root of All Illness

The ice age is coming, the sun's zooming in,
Engines stop running, the wheat is growing thin.
—THE CLASH

Wheat is on everyone's mind these days. Some people say it's at the root of all illness, while others believe avoiding wheat can at least help improve their health or help them lose weight.

So, is wheat bad? The answer is a "No, but…"

The type of wheat, how it is made, and what it is exposed to make all the difference. Doctors and scientists around the world have discovered a strong correlation among this increasing sensitivity to wheat in the US population, the increase of GMO-wheat varieties, and the industrialized manner in which wheat is processed.

Let's start with what wheat is exposed to. Most wheat (as of the time of this publication) is not GMO but is nevertheless exposed to a harmful chemical called glyphosate—the active ingredient in the broad-spectrum herbicide Roundup from Monsanto. In her interview with Dr. Mercola, Dr. Stephanie Seneff, a senior research scientist at the Massachusetts Institute of Technology (MIT), claims that glyphosate appears to be strongly correlated with the rise in celiac disease and has links to other diseases, including autism.[105] Both Dr. Seneff and her fellow researcher, Dr. Anthony Samsel, have published research on the connection between glyphosate and the development of a wide array of modern diseases.[106] Dr. Seneff believes that glyphosate may in fact act as a transporter for aluminum (a common vaccine adjuvant) into the brain. Glyphosate also appears to transport arsenic into the kidneys. If that weren't bad enough, glyphosate has also been shown to severely damage gut flora and cause chronic diseases rooted in gut dysfunction. The use of glyphosate on wheat crops has risen in tandem with the rise in celiac-disease diagnoses.

Farmers apply glyphosate immediately before the harvest of nonorganic wheat crops in order to reduce the amount of chemical residue and to get a head start on next year's weeds. According to Dr. Seneff, desiccating nonorganic wheat crops with glyphosate just before harvest became popular in the mid-1990s. When you expose wheat to glyphosate, it actually releases more seeds. "It 'goes to seed' as it dies," Dr. Seneff explains. "At its last gasp, it releases the seed."[107] This results in slightly higher crop yield. In addition, glyphosate kills ryegrass, a major weed problem for wheat growers that is resistant to many other herbicides. Glyphosate certainly seems like a win-win for farmers!

Monsanto, however, ignores the fact that ryegrass helps rebalance the soil after the wheat harvest; from that perspective, it is actually a beneficial plant. As a result of trying to increase yield at the last moment, the nonorganic wheat supply is contaminated with glyphosate. While it is claimed there are only trace amounts of residue left on the wheat, glyphosate use is like the proverbial "death by a thousand paper cuts." A large percentage of processed foods are made from wheat—it's in everything from seasonings to snack cakes—helping to explain the veritable explosion of celiac disease and other gut dysfunction since this practice began.

Glyphosate ultimately gives us highly indigestible wheat. Dr. Seneff and Dr. Samsel's research indicates that glyphosate may attach to gliadin as the result of a chemical reaction. The end result is that your body develops an immune reaction to this contaminated wheat.

Glyphosate also chelates trace minerals in the gut such as manganese, iron, cobalt (cobalamin), molybdenum, and copper. Through this disruption to the trace minerals in the gut, the body's "good" bacteria (our probiotics) cannot make use of them appropriately and, thus, cannot work effectively. According to Dr. Seneff, these "good" bacteria have an unusual mechanism to protect themselves from oxidative damage, and this mechanism involves manganese. If the manganese hides inside the glyphosate molecule, it creates dysfunction in the gut and lowers immune function. Ultimately, this dysfunction triggers inflammatory reactions, which in turn negatively affect the pathways that, according to Dr. Seneff, control the production of "sterols: cholesterol, vitamin D, and all sex hormones—estrogen, testosterone, and DHEA. On the other side, you have all the neurotransmitters. This is the dopamine, melatonin, serotonin, and the adrenaline. All of those transport sulfate. They're all derived from this pathway that glyphosate disrupts."[108] Furthermore, as previously mentioned, glyphosate has been very strongly statistically significantly correlated to the rise in twenty-two health conditions since its introduction in the US food supply.[109]

Recently the World Health Organization (WHO) classified glyphosate as a possible carcinogen. Many consumer organizations, scientists, and doctors are advocating and educating people about the health risks of glyphosate. One of them is an organization called FeedTheWorld.info. They provide updated scientific information about glyphosate studies and also discuss the current levels that are deemed safe and acceptable. FeedTheWorld.info can even help you get tested to see what your level is, and they will then use that information (anonymously) to further the scientific and legal battle to work toward banning this chemical. You will be surprised; even if you primarily eat organic and "clean" foods, your levels most likely will be much higher than the acceptable limits. This chemical is now almost ubiquitous in our food and environment. It is one more triggering mechanism to disrupt our immune system and cause increased health problems.

Humans in all cultures, all over the globe, have a very long history of consuming wheat products. So, why is wheat suddenly the enemy? The answer should be obvious: modern agricultural practices—including GMO wheat and, more importantly, the chemicals this wheat is exposed to—have a seriously negative impact on our health.

Instead of advocating avoidance of wheat products as a quick fix (and a quick fad for diet books), we should advocate for organic, non-GMO foods instead. We should be educating our elected officials and demanding that our food be what it used to be—organic, clean, and grown without chemicals. I am hopeful that, over time, the public will demand organic foods or, at least, organic-food standards. Certain states have voted against GMOs and for mandatory labeling when GMOs are added to our foods. Unfortunately, Monsanto is suing those states. They believe it is their right to provide those chemicals to you, and they assert that they are harmless. I disagree completely, and hopefully, after you do more research (including reading this book), you will agree with me.

Another reason for the modern-day wheat problem is rooted in the way we cook our wheat. Michael Pollan is one of my favorite authors and investigative food journalists. In his book *Cooked*,[110] he talks about *how* we eat our wheat and *why* it's causing us so many problems. The most glaring example of how eating wheat has changed for the worse can be found in the very cornerstone of most of our diets: bread.

Western cultures used to make bread by mixing multiple strains of yeast with flour and letting it ferment for long periods of time—sometimes an entire day. Thanks to modernization and industrial food processing, we now use fast-acting single-agent yeasts to make bread very quickly—within a few short hours. This turbocharged fermentation does not breakdown the protein and enzyme structures effectively, causing the wheat to react differently in our bodies, especially when we consume a lot of wheat, as in the SAD. Pollan suggests that those with sensitivities to wheat may not react to "real" bread, like a traditional sourdough that requires about twenty hours just to ferment the dough. This demonstrates how the preparation of food can affect our body's reaction to it; our digestive woes are almost never the fault of the food itself!

Over the past few years, books like *Wheat Belly*[111] and *Grain Brain*[112] have jumped on the antigrain bandwagon, claiming that grains are the cause of all our health problems. But that is not necessarily true. For example, most of my patients with wheat sensitivities, gluten/gliadin sensitivities, or celiac disease do not have any flares when they travel to Europe or other countries that have non-GMO wheat. Most Americans consume way too much highly processed, refined, and GMO grains—but the grain is not the problem. As people learn more about traditional grains and traditional preparation methods, I believe this wheat- or grain-free fad will fade.

Gluten Sensitivity and Celiac Disease

Every trip to the grocery store or to a restaurant these days results in a "gluten-free" food or menu-item sighting. While some treat the gluten-free trend as a new diet plan to lose weight, gluten sensitivity is actually a serious issue that has become a health epidemic.

When I was in medical school, celiac disease was considered a rare condition. It was so rare that instructors used to have a saying about it: if you had a celiac-disease patient in your practice, it was rare, but to have two celiac patients in your practice would be like beating the odds to win the lottery.

From 1950 to 1989, the chance of encountering a celiac patient was about 1:100,000—like winning the lottery. Since 1990, the chance of encountering a celiac patient has become 1:100. It's true that we have improved the diagnostics through laboratory testing, and more doctors are listening to their patients' symptoms and learning about food sensitivities. But that still does not account for the alarming increase in occurrence.

The problem is twofold. First, we used to only diagnose celiac disease with pathology—in other words, from a biopsy of the colon taken during a colonoscopy. Now we have a variety of blood tests we can also use to see whether celiac antibodies are present. The convenience of a blood test means we can test more people for celiac disease. But there is still a problem.

Conventional medicine still defines celiac disease based on a pathological diagnosis only, meaning you have to already have enough damage to your colonic tissue that a biopsy and antibody tests would be positive. Herein lies the problem, and it is a great example of the difficulty with the way conventional medicine diagnoses and treats most conditions. We wait until the patient has severe damage to say, "You have celiac disease. Now you have to stop eating gluten because it's causing your body to attack itself." This is standard practice.

Almost every disease occurs on a spectrum over time. Someone doesn't just wake up one day with heart disease or diabetes or even obesity. Diseases almost always progress gradually. For example, no one suddenly wakes up with cholesterol of 250, blood sugar of 300, and fifty pounds overweight. Poor choices in dietary and lifestyle factors—many of which are marketed to us over a lifetime—result in poor health outcomes. If we focused more on prevention than intervention, we would be able to detect and diagnose so many conditions before they became pathological or severe. Conventional medicine waits until you have a heart attack or diabetes, or are morbidly obese, before providing treatment, which is then expensive and does little to resolve the condition, only maintaining, treating, and managing symptoms.

Every day I see patients with severe IBS, Crohn's, ulcerative colitis, and other chronic inflammatory conditions, including joint and muscle pain, fibromyalgia, fatigue, allergies, memory problems, and more. They all have seen their GI doctors, and they bring in blood tests that show that they do not have celiac disease because they do not have antibodies in their colon yet. But those standard tests do not let them know whether they have gluten/gliadin sensitivity or not. In the eyes of most GI doctors, patients with celiac symptoms may not be "broken" enough for a diagnosis of celiac disease (the end condition), but they could have a spectrum of disorders such as gluten/gliadin sensitivity or inflammation triggers coming from ingestion of gluten/gliadin.

Fortunately, there are lab companies that test not only for the usual celiac antibodies (tTA, endomysial, and reticulin) but also for other inflammatory triggers, such as gluten and gliadin sensitivities, that cause IgA (GI-tract inflammation) and IgG (systemic or all-over inflammation). When I order these tests for my patients **(see Side Notes: Dr. Pai's Recommended Laboratory Testing)**, I hope that they come back negative. But if they are

positive, I tell the patient that he or she has a gluten/gliadin sensitivity,
means that he or she has inflammatory reactions to the ingestion of glu_..i/
gliadin (most heavily found in wheat products). Then we can start to change
the diet to lessen symptoms.

In my practice, I have found a very high correlation (almost 80 percent)
between positive gluten/gliadin sensitivity and autoimmune diseases such
as rheumatoid arthritis, lupus, Hashimoto's thyroiditis, and multiple sclerosis. Most of these patients have been told that having an autoimmune
disease means that their body is attacking itself. To my mind, this is a very
misguided idea.

I tell each of my patients that using the word *autoimmune* in conventional medicine is like saying *idiopathic*: we are saying that we don't really
know what's causing the problem. We have named dozens of autoimmune
conditions, yet none of them have a definitive diagnostic test. Hence, it takes
the compilation of several tests pointing to certain symptoms to suggest
an autoimmune diagnosis; more often than not, this battery of tests points
to inflammatory symptoms in specific organ areas (e.g., rheumatoid in the
joints, lupus in the kidneys, MS in the central nervous system, or Hashimoto's
in the thyroid). All of these are inflammatory conditions, just focused on different places within the body.

The body is not meant to attack itself. Under normal circumstances, the
human body is efficient and functions perfectly within a variety of systems.
The body doesn't just wake up one day and say, "I think I'll start attacking
myself." Contrary to what conventional medicine might tell you, nobody's
cells just decide to hurt the body out of the blue. There is always a reason.

Cells don't go rogue randomly; instead, they are victims of "bullying"
from inflammation. But, again, conventional medicine doesn't care if inflammatory "bullying" triggers cellular inflammation; it is only interested in treatment and symptom management. In many instances we doctors haven't
even attempted to look for triggers, since symptom-treatment options are
so readily available. Again, the misguided approach of only managing symptoms has caused millions of patients to suffer needlessly, when they could
instead learn ways to improve their health conditions—even if they do have
an autoimmune condition.

Conventional medicine even takes the patient's own innate healing
response out of the equation, as conventional-medicine practitioners think

that autoimmune disorders are out of the patient's control (and sadly, some doctors blame the patient for the condition). But these practitioners are either ignorant of or in denial of the truth, which is that inflammatory triggers can be discovered, and that in most instances the immune system can be strengthened (an idea in direct opposition to the standard drug-therapy treatment of autoimmune diseases that seeks to suppress the immune system).

Gluten sensitivity and celiac disease are very serious autoimmune conditions, but they are commonly misunderstood for the following reason: most doctors have not been trained in nutrition and do not know much about food in general. How can physicians advise their patients on proper diet if they have only been trained to treat disease? Once celiac or gluten intolerance is diagnosed through pathology, the treatment is very straightforward for most doctors: drugs and avoidance of gluten. End of story.

The biggest problem with having gluten/gliadin sensitivity in relation to it being classified as an autoimmune disorder is that the inflammatory reaction that occurs from gluten exposure is an *extremely* long-lasting insult to the body. Instead of experiencing an immediate IgE (within one hour) reaction or the delayed IgG4 (from a few hours later until about four days later) reaction, the person with gluten/gliadin sensitivity of IgA or IgG can experience a reaction that lasts from one week up to *three months* after exposure! The chronic long-term inflammation that occurs in these sensitive individuals then triggers the body to go into an autoimmune-like state. But it may be just the duration of the gluten exposure that makes it look like the body attacks itself. Your body is held hostage by inflammatory triggers (in this case, gluten), and as long as your body remains a hostage it can only do what those triggers tell it to do.

To see whether you have a wheat/gluten/gliadin allergy, I recommend not just inhalant testing (to rule out other triggers) but food-allergy testing (both IgE and IgG4), a celiac-disease panel that includes gluten/gliadin sensitivity (both IgA and IgG), and candida testing **(see Side Notes: Dr. Pai's Recommended Laboratory Testing)**.

If you are a grain skeptic, you're probably thinking something like this right now: "OK, Dr. Pai, if grains are OK, why do so many people feel better off grains?"

Well, to begin with, by eliminating grains most people are eliminating highly refined carbohydrates from their diets—which is a good thing.

Everyone feels better when they don't eat doughnuts, white flour tortillas, white breads, or foot-long sub sandwiches. That's a no-brainer. On top of that, everyone loses weight by eliminating highly refined carbohydrates and sugar, which is what makes these types of diets popular.

Although removing highly refined carbohydrates from our diets is important, replacing them with other inflammatory and cholesterol-rich foods will, in the long run, cause other problems, like heart disease. New "revolutions" in diets—Atkins, paleo, ketogenic, South Beach, Mediterranean, primal—offer short-term benefits, not long-term sustainability or even overall health benefits that help reduce the risk of developing disease.

When my people ask me what I think about the latest fad, low-carb, high-protein-diet books, my first question regards the author's background. Is the author a trained in nutrition? A physician? Even though people who adopt these diets might be experiencing improvement in certain aspects of their health—like weight loss and even less systemic inflammation (if they are wheat or gluten/gliadin sensitive)—their success for me only raises more questions, questions for the authors of these diets—especially if they are physicians.

For instance, do they still prescribe statins and blood-pressure medications to the patients on their diet? (Hint 1: they usually do.) Do their patients still get routine cardiac testing like echocardiograms, EKGs, stress tests, and angiograms and make money on such testing? (Hint 2: they usually do.) Do they still prescribe Alzheimer's and neurological medications? (Hint 3: they usually do). If the diets they're touting are as good as they proclaim, why do the majority of patients who follow these diets still need prescription drugs and interventional treatments? Some of these physicians have stated on their websites that they don't follow their diets or recipes, but they recommend that others do. Why would they recommend a revolutionary diet to change everyone's health for the better, yet not follow it? Doesn't that seem strange?

I don't mean to be critical, but if everyone remembers similar diets over the past twenty years, such as the Atkins diet, many who followed those diets still went on to have heart attacks, high blood pressure, and other health problems. A dramatic drop in heart disease and other conditions should have occurred following the introduction of these diets, but instead we have only seen the rise of such conditions over the years. Again, I agree with the general recommendation of reducing our consumption of highly refined wheat products and processed carbs and sugars, but I have a big problem with the recommended replacements.

The Paleo Myth: Caveman Thinking Sold to the Masses

"Make tool! Caveman. No fool! Beat rock!
Hunt meat! Caveman. Rock beat!"
—THE CRAMPS

Many people are advocating the Paleo Diet—directly or indirectly—by blaming grains for their health problems. Again, grains are a fantastic scapegoat, as many people do have sensitivities to wheat/gluten/gliadin, and most Americans are eating too many highly refined and processed GMO wheat products, which cause health problems even absent any underlying sensitivity to wheat/gluten/gliadin.

But to replace grains with animal protein is not only bad advice—it's bad science. We want to reduce the amount of pro-inflammatory foods in our diet to improve almost all aspects of our health. Animal proteins, as I've noted in this book over and over, are incredibly pro-inflammatory. Comprehensive short- and long-term clinical trials and prospective large epidemiological studies demonstrate that whole-food, plant-based diets showed better health outcomes in *all* categories—from chronic pain, cancer, and heart disease, to diabetes, blood pressure, and weight loss. So why would anyone advocate that we eat more animal proteins?

The answer is universal: because it's what most Americans want to hear. It's easy. From a publishing standpoint, "easy" sells millions of books, products, and diet programs. A diet that eliminates a single dietary item makes for best sellers, but it doesn't provide people with comprehensive healthy eating-habit and lifestyle recommendations. The short-term benefits of diets like the Paleo Diet include the reduction of blood-sugar spikes, the elimination of sugar cravings, and the calming of inflammatory triggers—benefits that can be felt immediately. Thus people jump on the bandwagon because they feel good right away; they see the elimination of wheat products as the cure for their health problems. But replacing processed grains with pro-inflammatory animal protein is, according to scientific consensus, foolish and unwise in the long term.

Many people and special-interest/lobby groups for the meat and dairy industry are thrilled about the Paleo Diet trend, but the scientific data is not on their side, and quoting meat-industry-sponsored studies should not inspire confidence in consumers. But low-carb diets do sell. The Atkins Nutritional Company made over one billion dollars from its related books and products. Today, the meat industry continues to reap the benefits of bad science and "not-as-bad-as-SAD" diet trends.

It takes effort to make significant changes to your diet. It wasn't easy for me, either, in the beginning. To decrease or to stop eating things that you have been used to eating for many years or decades is hard to do—especially when you're used to foods that are easily available, cheap, and abundant. In addition, many publishers and conventional medical doctors believe that most people can only learn to exclude one item at a time; thus, doctors assume that if they suggest an overly detailed diet plan, their patients will not comply.

I believe that patients are smarter than many doctors give them credit for. Instead of dumbing down information, we physicians should provide our patients with as much detailed information as possible and help explain what they may not understand, thereby allowing our patients to make truly informed decisions for their health.

I have given dozens of lectures about inflammation over the past few years in tandem with educating my patients on an individual basis. There are always those who will reject outright the notion that animal proteins are not good for them and don't need to be consumed. But even for those who won't stop eating animal protein, a reduction in the amount and frequency of consumption, along with an enhancement in the quality of the meat consumed, will help move them toward better health. But this is getting harder and harder to do (see chapter 3).

I have my share of Paleo Diet advocates as patients as well, and they are very determined to eat what the Paleolithic person did. So, let's explore for a moment the actual diet these early humans ate.

Firstly, Paleolithic people did not consume meat on a consistent basis. In fact, meat was scarce. When early humans did manage to get meat from a successful hunt (not just driving up to a window to pick it up), they gorged on it because they needed to consume the kill all at one time. There was no refrigeration, no leftovers, no "fixins." (There were certainly no layered foods with multiple meats like a bacon cheeseburger.) They shared with the rest of their group and then went on hunting and gathering again. Animals, when available, were just one of many items that the Paleolithic person ate.

The diets of those animals, however, were completely different from what is fed to livestock today. The animals during that time ate grass, not grains. They were wild and very lean, and they were not exposed to hormones, antibiotics, or other chemicals. This is not the type of animal protein that the majority of Americans consume.

The Paleolithic person ate grains, legumes, berries, and seeds. Stone-tool artifacts from thirty thousand years ago (twenty thousand years before the agricultural age) include tools similar to mortars and pestles, used to grind up seeds and grains. Fossilized dental plaque allows us to identify plant microfossils and other evidence of ancient diets. Myriad plant remains have been found in the dental calculus of Paleolithic people, and these include seasonal, real, non-GMO, unprocessed whole grains (e.g., barley), legumes, tubers, seeds, nuts, and berries.[113] Based strictly on necessity, the average Paleolithic person ate more whole grains, fruits, legumes, and vegetables than animal protein—by a wide margin.

The idea that the Paleolithic person was healthier than we are because of their diet is a misconception. During that time period, most children died before the age of fifteen, and adults rarely made it to forty. A study of ancient mummies in *The Lancet* revealed that the average Paleolithic person had alarmingly high rates of atherosclerosis, or hardened arteries; 47 of 137 mummies were suspected of having the disease.[114] This discovery does much to cast doubt on the theory that the Paleolithic person ate an ideal diet.

Don't get me wrong—avoiding highly refined and processed grains, refined sugars, and highly glycemic starchy foods (like refined fried potatoes) is always good advice. But you don't need to follow the Paleo Diet to do so. The Paleo Diet is sold to people as a way to eat more meat instead of carbs to be healthier. If Americans ate the actual diet that the Paleolithic people did, their health would certainly improve upon reducing the consumption of meat and upping the intake of seasonal whole grains, vegetables, legumes, and fruit. Unfortunately, our consumption of bacon double-cheeseburgers, meat lover's pizza, baby back ribs, and so on, means an average American consumes more meat in one day than a Paleolithic person would have consumed for several days.

Paleolithic people also expended most of their time and energy hunting and gathering, often covering dozens of miles daily—on foot. The closest "paleo-like" nomadic culture alive today, the Masai in Africa, travel between twenty and thirty miles daily to hunt for food. Even the most hardcore competitive fitness athletes would have a hard time keeping up with the Masai! For even greater comparison, most Americans walk between two and three miles per day.[115] Although this diet has worked for the Masai, it doesn't appear to confer the same benefits to the average American. To my knowledge, I have not found an American that can eat the same diet and have the same body type as the Masai. Paleo Diet proponents like to cherry-pick the parts they like (bacon) but don't disclose what they don't like to think about. The Masai eat raw organ meats and drink the blood of the animal that they themselves have hunted, and most certainly Paleolithic humans did as well. Strangely, the Paleo Diet does not promote this practice.

Unfortunately, the modern person does not hunt but only gathers. You expend no energy when driving your car up to a fast-food window to get a Baconator. Or even worse, going to restaurants that have the word *corral* in the name, which implies humans eating in a feedlot. Let's be honest: the majority of the population uses the Paleo Diet as an excuse to eat more unhealthy animal proteins.

I do have patients, however, who hunt and eat only what they have caught. This is a true Paleolithic diet. But they also eat vegetables and fruits in large amounts. If most people researched what factory farming is really like, they may not start hunting for their own meat, but they would almost certainly reduce their intake of those foods **(see Side Notes: Books and Movies)**.

Some doctors are now recommending a "paleovegan" diet for their patients. This means they recommend basically a plant-based diet that includes animal proteins if they are grass-fed or sustainably hunted in their natural environment. This option would be acceptable for most people in theory, but it is an exclusionary option that targets the few who can afford to spend more for expensive animal protein or who are skilled enough to hunt their own game (in the wild without a high-powered rifle). That is not the average American. Average Americans do not have access to or do not spend their money on grass-fed meats, particularly every single time they eat animal protein (including all restaurant visits). On top of that, the introduction of GMO grass means that even grass-fed meats are no longer a better option for consumers **(see chapter 3: The Grass Is Not Greener on the GMO Side)**.

If you eat grass-fed animal protein, it's a significant improvement over factory-farmed meat. It has lower omega-6 levels, less cholesterol, and fewer calories. A six-ounce grass-fed beef tenderloin may have nearly one hundred fewer calories than the same cut from factory-farmed, grain-fed cattle. "If you eat a typical amount of beef per year," says Jo Robinson, author of *Pasture Perfect*, a book about the benefits of pasture-raised animals, "which in the United States is about 67 pounds, switching to grass-fed beef will save you 16,642 calories a year."[116] It would also, if you paid supermarket prices and dined on tenderloin, cost you about three hundred dollars more. On average, it costs five to nine dollars per pound for organic, grass-fed/grass-finished beef, compared to three to five dollars per pound, on average, for factory-farmed, corn-fed beef.

Despite the growth of its popularity among consumers (due mainly to Paleo Diet marketing and conscious consumers demanding more sustainable farming practices), the demand for grass-fed beef is relatively insignificant, amounting to *less than 3 percent* of all US beef sales. That's a mere drop in the bucket for that industry, too small to represent a sea change in the way Americans consume beef. Thus the argument and marketing that suggests most Paleo Diet adherents are eating clean food misstates the reality of the situation. Plus, soon Monsanto, through their Scotts division, will introduce GMO grass, and even grass-fed animal protein may no longer be a "clean food" source for that 3 percent of beef sales.

When I advocate healthy eating to my patients, I want the diet I recommend to be something that everyone can have access to and can afford. Reducing or avoiding animal protein altogether is one of the simplest ways to improve one's health through diet. It costs very little to do, and it has the biggest impact on all the important health markers: it decreases inflammation, cholesterol, and other unwanted hormones and reduces the amount of unnecessary antibiotics and chemicals in our diet. Simply structuring your diet around a more plant-based philosophy also benefits the workers in

animal-processing factories (who are often expo̲
which is heavily impacted by vast amounts of anin̲.
cal byproducts of modern animal production **(see c̲**
Myth and Side Notes: Books and Movies). For those w̲
more about how their diet is triggering inflammation, in additī
sensitivity testing, one can easily test high sensitive c-reactive prɔ̲
(more specific for cardiac inflammation) and cytokines (IL-2, IL-6, IL-̲
IL-17, TNF-α, IFN-γ). Cytokines are immune signal molecules which aid cell
to cell communication and stimulate cells to move toward sites of inflammation. Imbalances in these markers point to specific inflammatory states and
also influence other aspects of our health such as hormones, neurotransmitters and our overall immune function.

What Do I Do with the Results of Laboratory Testing for Sensitivities?

> *Got the whole thing down by numbers.*
> *All those numbers!*
> *Give me guidance!*
> —GENESIS

After all this discussion of the different types of allergens, different allergy
therapies, and the plethora of dietary misinformation, the simple truth is that
allergy testing is the most effective way to fine-tune your diet for ideal health.

If testing reveals food allergies, then the easiest and most cost-effective option is just to avoid eating the triggering foods as much as possible.
Based on the severity of your symptoms and the type of your allergic reactions—either IgE (immediate) or IgG4 (delayed)—you can choose when or
if you want to consume the foods you're sensitive to (assuming, of course,
your sensitivities are not sufficient to trigger anaphylactic shock, in which
case you must take more extreme precautions). The more you avoid foods
you're sensitive to, the better you will feel, as the inflammation that these
foods trigger slowly subsides over time. (You will also notice flare-ups and
the exacerbation or worsening of your symptoms when you then consume
these foods.)

whatever reason, you have to eat the foods you have sensitivities gy testing allows you to choose the food that gives you the least ptoms. Here are my recommendations if you must eat foods that you're nsitive to:

When it comes to IgE foods, I recommend strict avoidance in general. With delayed IgG4 reactions, after complete avoidance for one month you can reintroduce some of those foods by rotating them back into the diet (for instance, rotating the foods into your diet every four days—we provide a rotational diet plan for our patients). After a few months of this controlled exposure, your body will become more tolerant of foods to which you have IgG4 sensitivities.

Even in the face of anaphylaxis, it's almost impossible to completely avoid all food allergens. When it comes to non-life-threatening food sensitivities, I tell my patients to follow the 90:10 rule: avoid 90 percent of the foods that you're sensitive to; always remain conscious of what you eat, but leave a 10 percent "window" for travel days, holidays, and special occasions when you might have to eat those foods because of physical or social restrictions. It is possible to preempt allergy symptoms by following a simple protocol that I give to my patients for that 10 percent of the time when they can't help but consume triggering foods **(see Side Notes: Preemptive Protocol for Food Allergies)**. In addition to avoidance, I offer Allergy-Drops Therapy and SAAT treatment for desensitizing and improving tolerance through controlled exposure to allergens (as described earlier in the chapter).

ADHD/Behavior Problems in Children and Psychiatric Problems in Adults

In the sixteen years that I have been specializing in integrative medicine and investigating inflammatory triggers in patients, I have found that the condition that has the strongest correlation to food allergies—especially in children—is the diagnosis (or, should I say, misdiagnosis) of Attention Deficit Hyperactive Disorder (ADHD) and other behavioral problems.

Almost every child diagnosed with ADHD who I have evaluated has come back positive for food allergies or sensitivities. The more severe the behavioral problem, the more allergies and food sensitivities he or she has.

I have seen too many extreme cases where young children, between the ages of seven and ten years old, have been prescribed dozens of antipsychotics, antidepressants, and antianxiety medications without any noticeable improvement of their symptoms over time—only side effects. I've seen some children with behavioral symptoms that were so bad that they had to be admitted to psychiatric inpatient institutions. Their parents came to see me feeling defeated after all conventional treatments seemed to have failed. My suggestions are never earth-shattering. In almost all behavioral-issue cases, I suggest simple blood work to rule out any food sensitivities or allergies before looking at adjusting their conventional treatments.

Without fail, every single child I've seen with severe behavioral problems has had severe food sensitivities—with both very high immediate and delayed reactions. Fortunately, many of these sensitivities were limited to just a few foods. When those foods were removed from the child's diet, the symptoms would almost universally start to improve within seventy-two hours.

I clearly remember once case in which a child in an inpatient psychiatric facility had been on over thirty different medications by the time the child was eight years old. The child's parents were wonderful people—hardworking, loving, and attentive—nothing amiss at home whatsoever. Their other child was happy and healthy; nothing could explain why one child had such behavioral problems and the other didn't. While he was in the psychiatric facility, his behavior was monstrous and extremely violent. His parents didn't understand why any of this was happening, as they had been nothing but nurturing.

When we had this child tested for food sensitivities, the results were off the charts for three foods in particular—foods that the child was being fed even in the hospital. Once the parents removed those foods from his diet, their child started to calm down—in just seventy-two hours. Two weeks after eliminating these foods entirely, the child was moved from an inpatient to an outpatient facility. Two months later, he was in public school.

I saw the child a few times afterward in my office without any issues. He was very pleasant, coloring with crayons and playing with toys. I did see him once after accidental exposure to a prohibited food, and within minutes he became extremely violent and lashed out. It was like turning a switch from *off* to *on*.

You're probably wondering, how does food cause such horrid, out-of-control behavior? These children do not have any areas of brain trauma, pathology, or overuse. So, what is the problem? If you've been reading this book continuously, you know what the answer is: inflammation. In this case, it's inflammation in the brain caused by food allergies.

Going back to the analogy of the roof leak, if rain doesn't find the weakest point in the roof and leak out slowly, then it can collect quickly and collapse the whole roof. Inflammation usually finds its way to a child's brain, which is very sensitive. But sometimes too much inflammation overloads the developing brain and causes severe reactions. Therefore, in my medical opinion, inflammation is at the root of most behavioral and psychiatric conditions, and emerging research is bearing this out. Research is revealing that many cases of depression are caused by an allergic reaction and inflammation.[117] By focusing on treating the inflammation symptoms of depression versus the neurological ones, new clinical trials are demonstrating that adding anti-inflammatory medicines and natural anti-inflammatories such as omega-3s and curcumin may have similar effects. It is great to see how science comes full circle with simple concepts of nutrition, physiology, immunology, and what traditional medicines have been demonstrating over thousands of years.

Approaching ADHD and other behavioral problems not as diseases but as dysfunctions of the brain due to inflammatory triggers has changed the way I look at treatment options for my patients. I see the same types of inflammatory food reactions in children with chronic eczema, asthma, and unexplained symptoms and medical work up that has found no pathology or cause. And, not surprisingly, I see the same correlation of dietary triggers with adult psychiatric conditions such as bipolar disorder, depression, and a host of anxiety disorders.

Food sensitivities trigger inflammation in the brain, affecting the baseline of the person's personality. Thus, just as one can experience flare-ups of any disease triggered by inflammation, behavioral flare-ups can occur in those with psychiatric disorders. In sensitive people, inflammation can cause a quiet, shy type to become more depressive, the anxious person to panic, and some people to experience flare-ups of both, depending on their food exposures and the amounts they have ingested—especially around holidays and celebrations, where food choices are limited.

Most of the patients who come to me for their children's behavioral issues or their own psychiatric conditions see me because they (or their children) have not responded as expected to standard psychiatric medications. But when they follow the steps outlined in this book to reduce overall inflammation in their bodies, they experience significant improvements of not only their psychiatric symptoms but also their overall health.

CHAPTER 5

STEP 3: Detoxification—Clearing the Toxins

> *My body's sweatin' toxins,*
> *Of my own demise.*
> —BILLY IDOL

One of the most important and underrated aspects of maintaining optimum health is incorporating a regular practice of detoxification. All traditional medicines and cultures worldwide incorporate this concept into their overall approach to good health. Unfortunately, in the United States most people equate detoxification with juice cleanses or going on expensive spa retreats. But detoxification is simply the process of supporting the body's own ability to remove toxins and helping the body become stronger by doing so.

Fasting, an ancient version of detoxification, is part of most religious practices and is touted as a means to clear the mind and purify the body. Ayurvedic medicine, the four-thousand-year-old traditional medicine of India, is one of the origins of the concept of detoxification. Its Ayurvedic name is *pancha-karma*, which means (roughly) the five actions for cleansing and rejuvenating the body. At Sanjevani, we specialize in providing individualized panchakarma detoxification programs that range from three to five days or longer if needed.

Panchakarma gently detoxifies the body of accumulated toxins (*ama*) in order to prepare it for healing and rejuvenation. Panchakarma includes a series of massages and treatments utilizing pure organic sesame and coconut oils infused with custom-formulated herbs to treat your body/mind imbalance (dosha) and symptoms of disease, along with daily bastis (oil and herb enemas), dietary recommendations (Ayurvedic foods specific to your dosha), yoga, and meditation. It is a time to dedicate oneself to quiet relaxation and introspection so the body can do its work during the cleansing period.

The pure oils and herbs used by Sanjevani's therapists penetrate deep into the cellular level, cleansing and nourishing the entire being. Daily massages and treatments include *abhyanga* and *vishesh* (two-therapist massage), *shirodhara* (stream of oil poured onto the forehead and scalp), herbal wraps (herbal soaked sheets that take three days to prepare), *swedna* (medicated steam), and sound healing (with singing bowls and tuning forks). Along with the cleansing, one receives Ayurvedic education about lifestyle changes to assist in the rejuvenation of mind, body, and spirit and to allow one to embark upon this life journey with a new awareness of the physical, mental, and emotional being in relationship to the environment.

Panchakarma includes an Ayurvedic consultation in which a plan of treatment, specifically tailored to one's constitution, is formulated. It is recommended that one undergo panchakarma treatments for at least five days at the change of each season to assist in the elimination of accumulated toxins. Sanjevani will supply herbs for preparation one week in advance and give you specific dietary and lifestyle instructions to allow the body to rejuvenate following your panchakarma treatments. At Sanjevani our panchakarma programs are unlike any other in the United States. From our clinical experience, we incorporate other aspects of integrative medicine to enhance and improve your outcome. Customizing each therapy based on your health condition, dosha, laboratory (both conventional, functional, and allergy testing), along with energy and sound therapies, each program is individualized and delivered as one may have never experience before.

In addition to panchakarma programs, doing simple juice fasts or eating a plant-based diet can help the body detoxify. The use of natural detoxification foods such as organic chlorella (grown in tanks, not from the ocean or from Japan) and spirulina (grown in tanks) can help the body eliminate toxins—especially heavy metals. These foods are also extremely beneficial after chemotherapy. One can safely use these "greens" instead of chelating agents _h as DMSA, which are expensive and difficult to come by and require medical supervision.

I encourage the use of fresh, organic (why add to the toxins you need to remove?), plant-based foods for detoxification. Specific plants that help the body flush itself of toxins are parsley for the kidneys and cilantro for the liver. You can eat or, even better, juice these plants to get greater amounts of their beneficial compounds.

All fruits and veggies help provide not only the fiber needed to bind and eliminate toxins in the colon but also the phytonutrients and antioxidants that help rejuvenate the body after the removal of toxins. For those on the go or those who have difficulty accessing fresh organic foods, I recommend using our organic, vegan and vegetarian, plant-based shakes that contain all the protein, fiber, phytonutrients, vitamins, adaptogens, and antioxidants needed to help balance the major bodily systems: digestive (stomach and intestines), circulatory, respiratory, urinary, glandular (endocrine), nervous, structural (muscles and bones), immune, and emotional/mental **(see Side Notes: Plant-Based Health Shakes)**.

At Sanjevani we carry a variety of plant-based health shakes targeted for different health conditions, so you can easily find one that is right for you. Although they are not replacements for fresh foods, these shakes can be used as meal replacements when one cannot prepare full meals, or is in a debilitated state, or has a low appetite, or simply to improve metabolism. I personally use these shakes in addition to my healthy breakfast as part of my morning regimen.

To complete a detoxification program and improve recovery and rejuvenation, I recommend fulvic-acid and humic-acid products. Due to conventional petrochemical farming methods, we have lowered these important compounds in the foods that we grow. There are many books written and much research completed on these compounds, so I will just mention that these natural bioavailable organic compounds that come from the earth have wonderful healing properties; most importantly, they contain dozens of trace minerals and amino acids. They are true powerhouse compounds, increasing cellular energy function, assimilation, metabolism, and electrochemical balance and enhancing nutrient absorption and immune support. I have worked closely with nationally recognized experts in the field of fulvic and humic acids, such as my colleague Dr. Dan Nuzum, all of whom have assisted me to ensure these powerhouses have true clinical benefits. These experts have helped me find fulvic and humic acids derived from the most potent and clean sources so that they are the most effective for detoxification protocols.

Finally, I always recommend that a detoxification protocol include liver support to help the liver improve its functions (this is especially good for those who have elevated liver-function tests). The liver is your body's main filter, so ensuring it can filter and process everything that goes into your body is essential to any detoxification program. Ingredients such as milk thistle, NAC, alpha-lipoic acid, and selenium, found in clinically effective doses in *Sanjevani Liver Formula Forte*, help keep the liver healthy and improve its ability to remove toxins from the body (**see Side Notes: Detoxification Support Protocols**).

CHAPTER 6

STEP 4: Avoid Smoking

> *I smoke my cigarette with style.*
> —GUNS N' ROSES

n order to stay healthy and decrease overall disease risk, one must quit and avoid smoking. By now everyone knows the dangers and risks of smoking, but too many Americans and people worldwide persist in this dangerous habit. Because the dangers of smoking are well known to Americans thanks to well-funded educational efforts, tobacco companies have created new markets in foreign countries and have introduced new delivery systems to keep their share of the market.

The most recent data on smoking rates was reported in *The Health Consequences of Smoking—50 Years of Progress: A Report of the Surgeon General, 2014.*[118] This official report showed that, in the United States alone, the cost of smoking is about $289 billion per year for taxpayers. This is four times the federal budget for education! With all the cuts to federal programs that help hardworking Americans, imagine what we could do if we simply encouraged our friends and family not to smoke? Although every adult has the individual right to smoke if he or she chooses, as a society we have the right not to be stuck with the health-care bills of those who do.

If the economics doesn't convince you to quit or avoid this nasty habit, then think about how many lives are lost. Over the past fifty years, twenty million Americans have died from smoking—that is more than all the deaths from all the wars in that time combined. To put that into even greater perspective, that is like killing everyone in New York City, Los Angeles, Chicago, Houston, Philadelphia, and Phoenix—all from cigarette smoking.

Every year, about five hundred thousand people in the United States will die prematurely from smoking. Not only is that a horrible fact, but at a cost of four to fourteen dollars per pack, cigarette consumption wastes money better spent on healthy, organic foods and other healthier lifestyle behaviors. If you currently smoke and don't have enough money to pay your rent, buy a new car, or even take that hard-earned vacation, just calculate how much money you spend on cigarettes each year—that is money you are just throwing away (or that is literally going up in smoke). Not to mention the health-care costs you're accruing, both indirectly and directly, through lost hours at work and the impending long-term health costs associated with smoking (e.g., for diseases such as emphysema, COPD, heart disease, and lung/mouth/throat cancer).

The good news is that overall smoking in the United States has been declining for years. In 1980, 41 percent of males in the United States smoked; that has decreased to 31 percent in 2012. In 1965, 42 percent of all adult Americans smoked, versus only 18 percent today.[119] Such dramatic reductions have a direct savings impact on our health-care dollars. When New York City banned smoking in common workspaces and public places like restaurants in 2004, in one year after the ban, there were 3,800 fewer hospitalizations from heart attacks, and the city saved over fifty-six million dollars—that's in one city in just one year![120]

Overall, we are headed in the right direction. But tobacco companies do not give up that easily. When they were being pushed out of big US markets like New York City, they switched their focus and entered foreign markets in a big way. Cigarette smoking in other countries has grown rapidly over the past decade. For example, China now has an estimated 350 million smokers—that's more smokers than the entire population of the United States!

One of the ways that "big tobacco" is getting around the decrease in cigarette consumption is via e-cigarettes. From a public-health standpoint, e-cigarettes are better because there is no secondhand smoke exposure, only water vapor. E-cigarettes are becoming more and more popular, and people are viewing them as a safe cigarette, but I would be very cautious. E-cigarettes are the product of an industry that feels no shame in killing twenty million Americans and hiding the data on the known health risks and addictive qualities of tobacco for decades. They are simply using a newer technology to keep people addicted to nicotine—now without the smell.

While e-cigarettes may contain carcinogens, some studies suggest that smokers inhale more deeply when using them and therefore are exposed to higher levels of nicotine per puff. In addition, while we don't have the data (though I am sure the industry does), the direct inhalation of vaporized nicotine with flavor enhancers is absorbed more quickly into the system. Thus, even though the e-cigarette does not contain over three thousand other deadly chemicals, as does a regular cigarette, it is still highly addictive—if not more so than traditional cigarettes. Maybe the tobacco industry calculated that it wants not to kill you off with addiction but to keep you alive longer to continue the addiction. This would certainly be more profitable for them, with the added bonus of changing their public image to that of a responsible industry, harnessing technology to make products that appear less harmful than they once were.

The e-cigarette industry is growing and becoming more profitable thanks to nicotine e-liquids, which require no farming or related labor. With the invention of e-cigarettes, companies are attracting celebrity spokespeople again. In some companies, the celebrity spokespeople are actually stockholders. Thus every time people use an e-cigarette, they are making the celebrity spokesperson even more money, one breath at a time.

E-cigarettes are sometimes billed as a way to wean a smoker off traditional cigarettes. But given the increased amounts of nicotine in e-cigarettes, this is most definitely not the case. For those who smoke and want to quit, I recommend setting a goal of a quit date and having other supportive measures, such as counseling, hypnotherapy, yoga, meditation, acupuncture for smoking detox, or even EMDR therapy. A microfrequency device called Alpha-Stim has had a promising amount of success in treating people who have a nicotine addiction. One of my colleagues, Dr. William Eidelman, has treated over a thousand patients using this noninvasive device and has reported about 98 percent success in helping his patients with their nicotine cravings. I use the device in my practice and have observed benefits including lowered anxiety and depression and reduced insomnia almost instantly after a session. Although the FDA has approved Alpha-Stim for use in those conditions, one can also use it "off-label" clinically to reduce nicotine cravings **(see Side Notes: Therapies to Help with Anxiety, Depression, and Insomnia)**. It is very simple to use. I simply place its ear clips on a patient's earlobes and press a button on the device; it then runs through a patented program to create more alpha waves in the brain. Producing an alpha-wave state provides a calming effect almost instantly. Most smokers will lose their nicotine cravings within *two minutes* of wearing the device (which they wear for twenty minutes to one hour). Once the cravings come back (depending on the individual, that can take twelve hours or more), the patient will notice that the cravings don't feel as powerful. Over a few weeks, the person eventually stops feeling these cravings altogether and quits smoking completely. Although the physical cravings will be eliminated, the person who smokes still has to overcome the psychological cravings of a habit that they have performed for such a long time. This is where supportive therapies can be helpful in maintaining smoking cessation.

There is not one single treatment that has been found to be the most successful in helping people quit smoking, but one should try a variety of options (like the ones mentioned above) and see what works. I prefer nontoxic, nicotine-free, nonpharmacologic substitutes for cigarettes. Support from friends and family is also crucially important in the process, but in the end it is up to the smoker to take the first step. As with any addiction, the addict must decide to make a change for the better.

For more information about Alpha-Stim, or to purchase one, please visit **www.sanjevani.net**.

CHAPTER 7

STEP 5: Avoid NSAIDs—The Unknown Dangers

I balance my Excedrin
And Anacins in stacks.
I'm a pain reliever junkie;
I got a Bayer on my back.
—ALICE COOPER

NSAIDs, or nonsteroidal anti-inflammatory drugs, are the most widely used class of drugs in the United States today. There are over thirty different types of NSAIDs, with over eighty million prescriptions written and over thirty billion OTC (over-the-counter) products purchased every single year in the United States alone.

This means that almost *one-third* of all Americans take a prescription NSAID. When we include OTC NSAID use, it is equivalent to every man, woman, and child in the United States taking an NSAID daily for over three months! Even for pennies on the dollar, the NSAID market is incredibly lucrative.

Most of us have taken NSAIDs, but maybe we don't know what class of drug we were or are taking. Let me give you a few examples of common NSAIDs:

- Ibuprofen (Motrin, Advil, Caldolor)
- Naproxen and naproxen sodium (Aleve, Naprosyn, Midol, Pamprin, Anaprox)

- Aspirin (Bayer, Anacin, Bufferin, St. Joseph)
- Diclofenac (Voltaren, Voltarol, Cataflam)

As the class name suggests, nonsteroidal anti-inflammatory drugs (NSAIDs) reduce inflammation but are not related to steroids, which also reduce inflammation. NSAIDs work by reducing the production of prostaglandins, chemicals that promote inflammation, pain, and fever. Prostaglandins also protect the lining of the stomach and intestines from the damaging effects of acids (including stomach acid) and promote blood clotting by activating blood platelets. Prostaglandins also affect kidney function.

The enzymes that produce prostaglandins are called cyclooxygenase (COX). There are two types of COX enzymes, COX-1 and COX-2. Both enzymes produce prostaglandins that promote inflammation, pain, and fever; however, only COX-1 produces prostaglandins that activate platelets and protect the stomach and intestinal lining.

NSAIDs block COX enzymes and reduce the production of prostaglandins, which is how they reduce inflammation, pain, and fever. Since they reduce the prostaglandins that protect the stomach and promote blood clotting along with pain and inflammation, NSAIDs can cause ulcers in the stomach and intestines without warning and increase the risk of internal bleeding. In fact the new cardiology guidelines are showing that NSAIDS such as aspirin should not be used for primary prevention of cardiovascular events, since the harm is now outweighing the good.[121]

Unfortunately, even with such data, medical practitioners downplay the dangers of NSAIDs, as do the pharmaceutical companies that make these popular OTC drugs. Over the last twenty years or so, dozens of published clinical research studies have demonstrated the dangers of NSAID use.[122] Most of this research, however, was completed and published in Europe and the rest of the world, and, thus, the results did not get the attention of the medical establishment in the United States. This is largely due to grievances expressed by pharmaceutical companies and lobbyist groups who influence the regulatory systems that are supposed to protect us. Sadly, our scientific journals aren't much better; they are almost all funded by their advertisers—pharmaceutical companies.

What exactly are the dangers of NSAIDs that these pharmaceutical companies want to downplay? If you regularly use NSAIDs to treat your arthritis, for example, you are in for quite an unpleasant surprise.

The downplayed international research reveals that NSAIDs have been shown to do the following:[123]

- Accelerate the progression of osteoarthritis
- Decrease joint-space width
- Increase joint forces/loads
- Increase risk of joint replacement
- Inhibit proteoglycan synthesis (the proteins in connective tissue)
- Inhibit synthesis of cellular matrix components (molecules that provide structural and biochemical support to the surrounding cells)
- Inhibit chondrocyte proliferation (the cells that form cartilage)
- Inhibit collagen synthesis (the structural protein found in connective tissue)
- Inhibit glycosaminoglycan synthesis (molecules that form substances that act as a lubricant and shock absorber)

The scientific literature makes it abundantly clear that NSAIDs—from in vitro and in vivo studies, in both animals and humans—have a significant *negative* effect on cartilage matrix, which causes an *acceleration of the deterioration* of articular cartilage in osteoarthritic joints. The preponderance of evidence shows that NSAIDs have *no beneficial effect on articular cartilage* and *accelerate* the very disease for which they are most used and prescribed!

This is why those of you who have taken NSAIDs for years or decades still have joint pain. Although NSAIDs temporarily help with pain, they actually degenerate your joints; therefore, arthritis sufferers keep taking NSAIDs because the pain persists.

The immediate pain relief offered by NSAIDs leads most people to not question why they have taken something for so long and, most crucially, why their problem hasn't been resolved. So many patients of mine will tell me that they started using an NSAID like ibuprofen to treat their arthritis pain. They clearly remember only taking one or two pills a day and then, over time, needing to take more and more to the point that they may take one to two pills every few hours *plus* another NSAID like naproxen sodium (i.e., Aleve). Some of these people have been taking NSAIDs for over twenty years, without a doctor once warning them about the damage this long-term use is causing in their joints.

My soapbox speech about NSAIDs revolves around their inappropriate use and the deceptive marketing pushing their overuse in the United States, which began in the early 1980s. If you remember the NSAID commercials from back then, they generally showed a person who was over sixty-five taking an Advil or Motrin for joint pain caused by playing golf or lifting their grandchildren. Over time, the people in the commercials became younger and younger. Now when you see an NSAID commercial, many of the people shown are under the age of twenty-one. Some are even teens—riding bikes, holding backpacks, etc. The change was so gradual that no one seems to have noticed or asked, "Why are young teens taking Advil?"

Aleve is well known for advertising the fact that you need to take just two Aleve, versus many ibuprofen pills, for "all day long, all day strong" relief. The problem is that although the pain relief from Aleve may last longer than that from ibuprofen (Advil, Motrin, etc.), it still causes the same side effects! Even more concerning to me is that most MDs, health-care providers, pharmacists, and patients do not know that NSAIDs—both prescription (e.g., Celebrex) and OTC (e.g., Advil, Motrin, Aleve, Midol, and Pamprin)—all carry what is called a "boxed warning" or "black-box warning."

What Are the Side Effects of NSAIDs?

And the label said, "Take two for the pain."
—MÖTLEY CRÜE

I will get to the black-box warning in just a moment. First, there are a few other important things you should know about NSAIDs.

Every drug on the market today has a monograph; this is a set of important information about the drug that the drug company provides to the FDA. The monograph shows pictures of how it is supplied and tells the proper dosages, indications and conditions the product is used for, drug interactions, adverse reactions, safety monitoring, and manufacturing/pricing. Every drug, whether prescribed or OTC, has what are called "common reactions." These are side effects that commonly occur when the product is taken.

Common Reactions (Side Effects) of NSAIDs

The *common reactions* for NSAIDs, in general, follow:

1. Dyspepsia
2. Nausea
3. Abdominal pain
4. Constipation
5. Headache
6. Dizziness
7. Drowsiness
8. Rash
9. Elevated ALT, AST (liver enzymes)
10. Fluid retention
11. Tinnitus
12. Ecchymosis (bruising)
13. Dyspnea (shortness of breath)
14. Photosensitivity (sensitivity to light)

This list of common reactions means that someone who takes an NSAID will often experience one or more of these side effects. None of these common reactions are immediately life threatening, but they can become problematic, as they can cause the person experiencing them to go to the doctor for more medications to treat the side effects. For example, if an NSAID causes heartburn, a doctor might prescribe a proton-pump inhibitor (acid blocker) such as Prilosec or Nexium, creating the beginning of a "drug cocktail" situation.

Most worrying to me as a physician is that NSAIDs commonly cause mild elevations in serum aminotransferase levels (AST liver enzymes); this occurs in up to 18 percent of patients taking NSAIDs over a prolonged period.[124] Many physicians downplay this elevation because it is considered mild. Most of us were taught that the liver enzymes (AST, ALT, and Alk Phos) had to be severely elevated to cause problems. But most MDs were not trained to understand what liver-enzyme testing actually measures.

From a functional standpoint, liver enzymes only elevate when about 60 percent of the liver is having some difficulty performing its normal metabolic breakdown of all foods, medicines, supplements, and so on, after digestion. Thus a mild elevation is not dangerous but will cause someone to be temporarily unable to break down toxins. This mild elevation causes some medications (and supplements) to metabolize either more quickly or more slowly than expected. This in turn causes medications, like those for blood pressure or blood sugar, to have a stronger or weaker effect. If the patient (and often the physician) does not know about this side effect of mild liver-enzyme elevation, the resulting change in blood-pressure or blood-sugar numbers may cause the doctor to make unnecessary changes to the dosage of the relevant medications.

Doctors are accustomed to warning their patients about consuming alcohol, for example, while on certain medications; they advise that a glass of wine or beer may feel either stronger or weaker than usual when taken in tandem with many other medications, but they seldom mention NSAIDs. More importantly, mildly elevated liver enzymes can affect medications used for prevention, such as oral contraceptive pills. So, if you are taking birth-control pills and if your liver enzymes are ever elevated, I recommend using a second form of birth control until those enzymes return back to normal.

One does not have to take NSAIDs for long periods of time to experience one or more of the common side effects. One double-blind trial found that six out of thirty-two healthy volunteers (or 19 percent) developed a gastric ulcer that was visible on endoscopic examination after only one week's treatment with naproxen (at a commonly prescribed dose of 500 mg twice daily—the same amount as five nonprescription Aleve).[125] Even worse, NSAID use can cause erosions and ulcerations in the small intestine (which is not visualized on normal endoscopy) causing chronic iron-deficiency anemia and protein loss due to increasing gut permeability.[126]

Mild side effects from NSAID use are altogether too common. But these mild side effects are not the main problem with NSAIDs. The main problem with NSAIDs is what are called "serious reactions."

Serious Reactions (Side Effects) of NSAIDs

Serious reactions are those types of adverse reactions that can be life threatening or cause severe damage to one's health. The *serious reactions* for NSAIDs, in general, follow:

1. GI bleeding
2. GI perforation/ulcer
3. MI (myocardial infarction: heart attack)
4. Stroke
5. Thromboembolism
6. Hypertension
7. Congestive heart failure
8. Renal papillary necrosis
9. Nephrotoxicity
10. Hepatotoxicity
11. Anaphylaxis/anaphylactoid reaction
12. Bronchospasm
13. Exfoliative dermatitis
14. Stevens-Johnson syndrome
15. Toxic epidermal necrolysis (Lyell's syndrome)
16. Thrombocytopenia (reduction of platelets in the blood)
17. Agranulocytosis (dangerously low white-blood-cell count)
18. Aplastic anemia
19. Anemia, hemolytic
20. Neutropenia
21. Leukopenia
22. Angioedema

These are side effects that you *definitely* do not want. But these aren't even the biggest problems with NSAIDs. The biggest problem with NSAIDs is that they carry black-box warnings.

The Black-Box Warning—Your Worst Nightmare

It's a dead man's party.
—OINGO BOINGO

After reading about all the mild and serious NSAID side effects, you're probably wondering how it could possibly get any worse.

A black-box warning **(see fig. 25)** is a warning that manufacturers have to place on the insert and inside information about a drug once serious reactions serious enough to put users into a *black box* become common. Yes, a black-box warning is the FDA's attempt to let you know that you can end up in a coffin or casket if you are unlucky enough to suffer one of a medication's serious reactions.

Now, not every serious reaction becomes a black-box reaction, but the serious reactions that happen frequently enough to require a black-box warning are far more likely to put you in a black box **(see fig. 26)**.

> **Cardiovascular Risk**
> *May increase risk of serious and potentially fatal cardiovascular thrombotic events, MI (heart attack), and stroke; risk may increase with duration of use; possible increased risk with cardiovascular disease or cardiovascular disease risk factors; contraindicated for CABG peri-operative pain.*
>
> **GI Risk**
> *Increased risk of serious GI adverse events including bleeding, ulcer, and stomach or intestine perforation, which can be fatal; may occur at any time during use and without warning symptoms; elderly patients at greater risk for serious GI events.*

Figure 25: The black-box warnings for NSAIDs

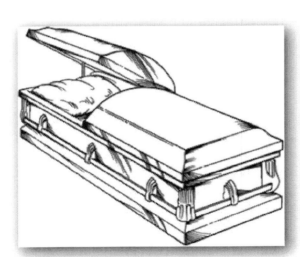

Figure 26: The black box

Again, this all means that tens of millions of people today are at risk of heart attacks, strokes, and GI bleeds from America's love affair with NSAIDs. And we are unlikely to fall out of love with NSAIDs anytime soon. As long as most people in the United States follow some variation of the pro-inflammatory standard American diet, the average person will want to take NSAIDs, putting him or her at an even greater risk of heart attacks and strokes. Even more frightening is the fact that the risk is still there, even if someone doesn't have elevated cholesterol/lipids (heart disease), if that person has heart-disease risk factors such as obesity, high blood pressure, and diabetes.

Consider for a moment how common the risk of stroke and heart attack is in America today. Americans suffer approximately 735,000 heart attacks per year; that amounts to almost two people having a heart attack per minute.[127] It is nearly impossible to find someone in the United States who is not at risk of taking one too many NSAIDs and winding up in the black box. In fact, at time of publication of this book, the FDA issued a new safety announcement to strengthen the black-box warning. New data from the FDA has shown that NSAIDs increase heart attack and strokes up to 50 percent![128] The danger of NSAIDs has been a theme of mine for years. I have been educating the public (and physicians) at national conferences and seminars, on radio shows, as well as with each of my patients. The dangers of NSAIDs is one of the main reasons I wrote this book, and now the data is so overwhelming that even the FDA cannot hide from the truth.

Over the years, many physicians and patients who did not believe me would justify their continued recommendation or use of NSAIDs. They would note that the black-box warning stated that these drugs "may" cause increased risk, and therefore it was a possibility, not a direct problem. Now with the new, updated black-box warning soon to take effect, the FDA will require the drug manufactures to remove the word "may" and now state that the medication will "cause an increased risk" of serious heart attacks and strokes. The black-box warning will also include the following language: "The risk of heart attack or stroke can occur as early as the first weeks of using an NSAID. The risk may increase with longer use of the NSAID. In general, patients with heart disease or risk factors for it have a greater likelihood of heart attack or stroke following NSAID use." More disturbingly, "patients treated with NSAIDs following a first heart attack were more likely to die in the first year after the heart attack compared to patients who were not treated with NSAIDs after their first heart attack." Finally, there is also an "increased risk of heart failure with NSAID use."[129]

In addition to heart attacks and strokes, the average NSAID user is at high risk for life-threatening GI bleeding. Again, the warning states, "bleeding ulcer, stomach or intestine perforation, which can be fatal at any time, can occur *without* warning symptoms." Can you believe this? How many people already have GI problems and are taking antacids and acid blockers such as Zantac, Pepcid, Prilosec, and Nexium? If they add NSAIDs to the mix (and they almost certainly are), they are putting themselves at an even greater risk of a fatal GI bleed.

In addition, think about all the people who get ulcers just from high amounts of stress. What about everyone who drinks alcohol in excess (occasionally or regularly) or who smokes? What about everyone who takes any number of other medications that cause stomach irritation? What about those people with food allergies who deal with constant stomach or intestinal issues? Or people with IBS, ulcerative colitis, or Crohn's disease? Or people having chemotherapy? People are being set up for serious health consequences from something that is marketed as being very benign. NSAIDs are in everyone's medicine cabinets, office drawers, lockers, purses, and backpacks, and millions take them on a daily basis. This false sense of security means that you might never see a black-box side effect until—at best—you wake up in the hospital, or at worst, you never wake up again.

If this all seems sensationalistic because you've been taking NSAIDs for years and have never experienced anything but pain relief, please believe me; black-box events are terrifyingly underreported. You might be wondering, in that case, "If these drugs don't help my joint pain in the long run and are putting me at an elevated risk of a heart attack, stroke, or fatal GI bleed, why are NSAIDs still on the market?"

The answer is that the companies that make these drugs have no incentive to take them off the market. Once a drug gets a black-box warning, this information is simply listed (or alluded to) on every insert, printout from the pharmacy, and web page (usually buried deep down), and it is included in small print on the bottom of the screen during every prescription-NSAID television commercial (e.g., Celebrex). The black-box warning has been provided to you whether you realize it or not, and therefore, drug companies are free of legal liability.

For example, on every Celebrex commercial, you will see and hear the black-box warning in full. Yet most people don't notice it, as they are misguided by the wonderful images of people walking, hiking, and being pain-free, accompanied by upbeat music in the background. Pay attention next time you see an NSAID commercial; listen closely to the black-box warnings and hear all about the side effects you are legally agreeing to experience.

The Black-Box Warning—The Unknown, Unconsented Agreement

> *You just can't get agreement*
> *In this present tense.*
> *We all talk a different language,*
> *Talking in defense.*
> —MIKE AND THE MECHANICS

Once the black-box warning has been placed upon a product, you, by opening the product bottle and swallowing the pills, or even by picking up the prescription at the pharmacy, have given consent to the "terms and conditions herein." Yes—whether you knew it or not—by opening the bottle or package *you have accepted that these black-box warnings of serious and fatal side effects can occur.*

An analogy to this is the "terms and conditions" form you agree to when you're updating software for your smartphone or your computer. You see a pop-up that asks, "Do you want to upgrade?" Of course you do, so you click the box that says, "I agree to the Terms and Conditions." Most of us, and I'm guilty of this myself, agree on a daily basis to "terms and conditions" we haven't read. Have you ever read a T&C agreement? These agreements free software, computer, and phone companies from any liability if your data is lost or stolen, if your information is sold to third-party vendors, if your personal information is collected, and if you encounter any number of other invasion-of-privacy-type situations. What choice do we have, really? In order for us to upgrade our software, we must agree to the "terms and conditions," or we will be left behind.

As bad as an invasion of privacy is, no one has had a heart attack, stroke, or GI bleed after upgrading his or her software (at least not as a direct result). However, hundreds of thousands of people each year have heart attacks, strokes, or GI bleeds after agreeing to black-box warnings on drugs, never knowing that they were at risk. To my mind, these sorts of blanket, fine-print black-box warnings are un-American and grossly unethical.

How can there be *no* legal liability upon a manufacturer if you have a stroke from taking their product? Why are products with such severe side effects sold over-the-counter? You cannot call "1-800-BAD DRUG" if you end up having any of the serious side effects, because you have accepted that those risks can occur just by opening the bottle or package.

So why does almost every retail outlet and pharmacy in the country still sell these products? The answer is what it always is: money and greed. Almost two-thirds of the US population takes an NSAID at least once a week, and fully one-third takes an NSAID on a daily basis. Remember, there are seventy million NSAID prescriptions filled in the United States every year; minimum estimates show that over thirty billion OTC NSAID medicines are purchased every year as well.[130] In 2013 Americans bought more than 275 million boxes of over-the-counter NSAIDs, racking up $1.7 billion in sales, according to retail tracker IRI.[131] Visit any pharmacy today and you will see dozens of companies selling NSAIDs, from brand names to generics. Since NSAIDs are incredibly popular, and there is no legal liability associated with their use, lots of companies sell their own versions. NSAID sales benefit pharmacies, too, as pharmacies themselves make money selling them to you. If you're unlucky enough to get a common or serious side effect from taking the NSAID, doctors, emergency rooms, hospitals, medical- and surgical-equipment companies, and insurance companies make money trying to save your life. There is plenty of money to be made by everyone involved. But if true health care were the goal of these pharmaceutical companies, pharmacies, and conventional health care, they would have warned you not to take NSAIDs in the first place.

Most of the patients I see for an initial integrative-medicine consultation tell me that they take ibuprofen on a daily basis. Almost everyone in the United States has a bottle of NSAIDs in his or her locker at school, at the gym, in a desk drawer, purse, briefcase, medicine cabinet, or even glove compartment in the car. People go to warehouse stores and purchase huge bottles of two thousand pills or "twin packs" of four thousand tablets. I even have soccer moms and dads who give every kid who leaves their minivan one ibuprofen before the game and one after the game. Many active adults and children are taking four to eight ibuprofen tablets daily; that's two tablets every few hours.

Before my integrative-medical training, I too took an NSAID if I had a headache or back pain. Like most people, I thought, "Those side effects won't affect me," or "Side effects only happen to those people who take too many pills." I thought, "I only take them rarely," or "It hasn't bothered me so far." And I was well aware of the black-box warnings. I think we all (including doctors) inherently believe that we are exceptions to the rule, as no one wants to think something terrible could happen out of the blue. It's in our nature to think we will beat the odds, or that such terrifying side effects happen only to other people.

I haven't taken an NSAID in fourteen years. I stopped taking them once even conservative medical journals started publishing statistics about the shocking number of deaths that occur from taking NSAIDs. I was not expecting data that was so overwhelming and compelling, and I am eternally grateful that one journal in particular was confident enough to publish researchers' findings. I immediately made a lifestyle change that has protected me from this common, unnecessary risk, which most Americans are exposed to every day. It also led me to develop Bosmeric-SR.

So, how compelling is the data? Is it really so bad that it compelled me to formulate a replacement product? You bet it is. After learning what I did, you may (and should) change how you think about NSAIDs.

Here is the data that will make you think twice about taking another NSAID—ever:

Conservative estimates published in *The American Journal of Medicine, The New England Journal of Medicine, Journal of the American Medical Association, Therapeutics and Clinical Risk Management,* and *The Journal of Rheumatology* all have stated that the average number of people hospitalized for complications from NSAID use *as properly prescribed* is over one hundred thousand per year—with *about twenty thousand deaths every year* (see fig. 27).[132]

This means that when health-care providers prescribe an NSAID such as Advil, Motrin, Aleve, or Celebrex and the patients take it appropriately, one

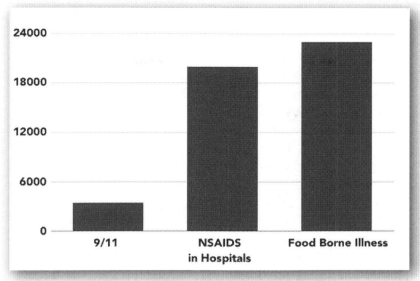

Figure 27: Estimated deaths per year from NSAIDs in US hospitals

hundred thousand of these people end up in the hospital from complications each year. Each hospital admission is estimated to cost between $15,000 and $20,000.[133] (The study was conducted to assess the origins of uncontrolled health-care costs.) And that's if the patient is fortunate enough not to end up as one of the twenty thousand who never leave the hospital alive.

What affects me deeply as a doctor is the fact that these are conservative estimates and *do not include inappropriate use* (taking more than recommended or prescribed dosages) *or OTC administrations*. That's right—the one hundred thousand hospitalizations and twenty thousand deaths annually do not include the thirty billion OTC NSAIDs that are purchased at pharmacies, grocery stores, or big-box stores.

To put these numbers in perspective, Sept 11, 2001, was a tragic day in our nation's history. Over 3,500 people died in the terrorist attacks that day. That means the annual number of deaths related to prescribed NSAIDS is almost seven times that of the fatalities on 9/11. In other words, it's like fourteen World Trade Centers falling year after year, senselessly killing innocent Americans. And, again, that doesn't include the deaths from OTC use or intentional overdoses. Let's have a look at those numbers.

The most recent data from 1984 to 2009 show that approximately 300,000 people have died from GI complications due to NSAIDs, with almost 1.7 million hospitalizations, at a cost of $38.8 billion.[134] To put these total statistics into perspective, the number of people killed from NSAID GI bleeding is *greater than* the number of Americans who died during the Revolutionary War, the War of 1812, the Mexican-American War, the Spanish-American War, World War I, the Korean War, the Vietnam War, the first Persian Gulf War, and the conflicts in Iraq and Afghanistan—combined (287,371 versus 300,000).[135] The total number of people hospitalized from 1984 to 2009 due to NSAID bleeding (1.7 million people) is higher than the American casualties from all American wars combined (1.4 million people).[136]

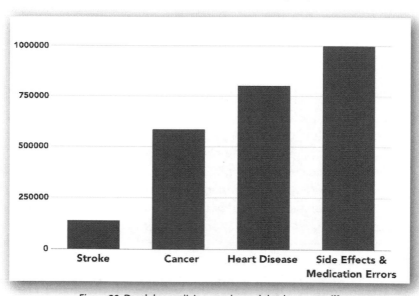

Figure 28: Death by medicine—estimated deaths per year[135]

Even worse, now the number-one cause of death in the United States is adverse drug reactions and medical errors **(see fig. 28)**. Yes, you read that correctly. More people die from the drugs that we are using to treat them (or more precisely to manage their disease) than the diseases themselves!

These adverse drug reactions and medical errors kill more people yearly than heart disease (number two), cancer (number three), and stroke (number four). You don't hear about this data because the cause of death is not a disease. Most people know that heart disease is the number-one cause of death (from a disease). But don't be misled by worrying only about heart disease, cancer, and stroke. Your bigger risk comes from some of the approaches and treatments of our current medical system, which in my opinion has aspects and behaviors like those of a disease.

This is a hard truth to swallow, but millions of Americans swallow it every day without thinking about it.

In addition to the side effects listed in the black-box warnings, NSAIDs also do the following:[138]

1. Increase cardiovascular problems, like heart attacks, by 40 percent to 60 percent;
2. Increase the risk of heart failure by 60 percent;
3. Increase the risk of miscarriage by 80 percent;
4. Increase the risk of hearing loss up to 20 percent;
5. Increase the risk allergic reactions in people with asthma by 10 percent to 30 percent.

Remember the NSAID called Vioxx (rofecoxib)? In 2004, it was pulled off the market because over sixty thousand people were killed from cardiac events; in addition, at least eighty-eight thousand, and possibly as many as 139,000 Americans, experienced a nonfatal heart attack as a result of taking Vioxx. In 2005, another similar drug, Bextra (valdecoxib), was pulled off the market. In 2007, Prexige (lumiracoxib) was also removed. Can you see a pattern here? Maybe NSAIDs cause more harm than reported?

Celebrex (celecoxib) was spared from this regulatory carnage because it put a black-box warning on its label while these other drugs were being taken off the market. With this warning on the label, however, it was freed from liability in the United States (even though it has been pulled off the market in other countries). The makers of Celebrex got a very lucrative green light, and today many other drug companies continue to sell NSAID drugs like Celebrex because *you the consumer are the only one to blame legally* if something goes wrong when you're taking them.

While it is clearly easy for me to write about the many dangers of NSAIDs, there is an alternative. It's the result of years of research conducted by some of the most venerable physicians in the world, and it is a far better option to help with pain and inflammation. I mentioned it earlier, and you're about to learn all about it in the next chapter. It's called Bosmeric-SR.

CHAPTER 8

STEP 6: Decrease Inflammation through the Use of Bosmeric-SR

For a miracle, a miracle drug
—U2

From allergies to asthma, from fibromyalgia to arthritis, from colitis to cancer—most if not all disease, research now suggests, begins and worsens with inflammation.

In addition to eating an organic, non-GMO, plant-based diet and testing for specific individual food allergies, one of the most important parts of preventing, treating, and reversing diseases can be the daily use of Bosmeric-SR.

What Is Bosmeric-SR?

Bosmeric-SR is the superior natural anti-inflammatory dietary supplement for pain and inflammation support.* It contains four specific natural ingredients that have been clinically tested and patented, using precise potencies that are not only important by themselves but also have a *synergistic effect when combined in a unique delivery system.*

What Are the Benefits of Bosmeric-SR?

Bosmeric-SR provides superior pain and inflammation support* for the following:

- Arthritis
- PMS, menstrual irregularities, and fibroids
- Headaches and migraines
- Joint and muscle pain
- Fibromyalgia and chronic pain
- Ulcerative colitis and Crohn's disease
- Psoriasis and acne
- Allergies, asthma, COPD, emphysema
- Heart disease
- Diabetes and related neuropathy
- Obesity
- Liver dysfunction from toxic insults
- Memory and cognition problems
- Alzheimer's disease, Parkinson's disease, and other neurodegenerative diseases
- Autoimmune diseases (e.g., rheumatoid arthritis, multiple sclerosis, and lupus)
- Various cancers (e.g., brain, breast, colon, thyroid, prostate, and lung)

The ingredients of Bosmeric-SR support inflammatory physiological response mechanisms that are vitally important to the health of the entire body, and they have been shown to play a critical role in supporting cardiovascular, pulmonary, immune, neurological, gastrointestinal, joint, and connective-tissue systems—and more. Not only is Bosmeric-SR *clinically tested and very effective,* there are *no kidney, liver, or GI side effects.* **(For more details on the side effects of NSAIDs, see chapter 7.)**

How Does Bosmeric-SR Work?

More than you know
—EDDIE VEDDER

The ingredients in Bosmeric-SR have been shown to safely and effectively *reduce inflammation*. Unlike NSAIDs that block only one inflammation pathway—like cyclooxygenase (COX)—Bosmeric-SR helps reduce *at least ninety-seven different biological inflammatory mechanisms or pathways*. Inflammation is now regarded as a root cause of several diseases and chronic health conditions; hence, it is important to inhibit inflammation. Inhibition of inflammation at its origin can prove a significant strategy to counter the increasing occurrence of several chronic diseases.

Targeting inflammation at multiple pathways before problems start can dramatically reduce symptoms, prevent further damage, and in some cases, reverse the disease or dysfunction altogether. This comprehensive approach provides a balanced and more effective outcome. Using Bosmeric-SR is a better alternative than trying to put out a fire using a single fire hose (the single-target approach of pharmaceuticals); Bosmeric-SR provides an entire sprinkler system to extinguish the flames.

Just like our military has different weapons to use—from assault rifles to machine guns, rocket launchers, missiles, and even lasers—our immune system (remember, our soldier cells) has hundreds of different types of inflammatory signals that it can deploy when triggered by reactions, foods, and other things that cause inflammation in the body.

The ninety-seven biological inflammatory pathways that Bosmeric-SR either lessens or *inhibits* include the following: nuclear factor kappa B (NF-kB), COX-2, 5-LOX, C-reactive protein (CRP), interleukin-6, macrophage inflammatory protein, tumor necrosis factor alpha (TNF-a), IGF-1, HER-2, inflammatory matrix metalloproteinase, human leukocyte elastase (HLE), several types of protein kinases, adhesion molecules, and genes involved in inflammation. In addition to reducing and inhibiting factors that aggravate health conditions, Bosmeric-SR also activates important protective factors such as Nrf2.

Factors such as NF-kB, a protein complex, have now been discovered to be one of the main switches in the immune system, which then triggers multiple pathways of inflammation. This systemic inflammation leads to almost every chronic disease and every type of cancer.[139] My good friend and colleague Dr. Bharat Aggarwal—a world-renowned researcher and professor at the Department of Experimental Therapeutics, Division of Cancer Medicine, The University of Texas MD Anderson Cancer Center in Houston—has published dozens of studies with regards to the anticancer and anti-inflammatory effects of the Curcumin C3 Complex, a major ingredient in Bosmeric-SR, as well as of boswellia, ginger, and black pepper. In particular, his research focuses on the natural agents that inhibit NF-kB **(see www.bosmeric-sr.com/research)**. The ingredients in Bosmeric-SR block NF-kB naturally and effectively.[140]

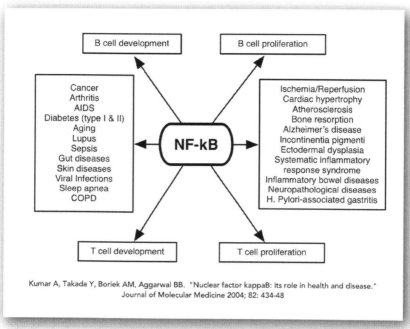

Kumar A, Takada Y, Boriek AM, Aggarwal BB. "Nuclear factor kappaB: its role in health and disease." Journal of Molecular Medicine 2004; 82: 434-48

Figure 29: NF-kB activation has been linked to most major diseases[139]

The infographic above **(fig. 29)** illustrates that compounds that block NF-kB can positively affect a staggering variety of disease. With its NF-kB blocking capabilities, Bosmeric-SR enables people to utilize one natural product with almost limitless benefits. With its unique natural ingredients, it can help people to inhibit the inflammation at its root source, before it becomes chronic and degenerative and even pathological.*

Inflammation is a complex process involving a series of actions and reactions and a broad range of biologically active substances (e.g., bradykinins, histamines, prostaglandins, thromboxanes, hydroxy-fatty acids, leukotrienes, lysosomal enzymes, and lymphokines) triggered by the body's immunological response to tissue damage. Through the arachidonic acid pathway leukotrienes, important mediators in inflammatory and allergic processes are produced by the key enzyme 5-lipoxygenase (5-LOX).

Prostaglandins and thromboxanes are also important mediators in inflammatory and allergic processes, and these are also produced from arachidonic acid by the key enzyme cyclooxygenase (COX-2). **(See fig. 10.)** Arachidonic acid is an essential fatty acid synthesized in the body.

Bosmeric-SR *inhibits both 5-LOX and COX-2 pathways* in a manner similar to NSAIDs, but *without the dangerous side effects described in chapter 7.** **(See fig. 30.)**

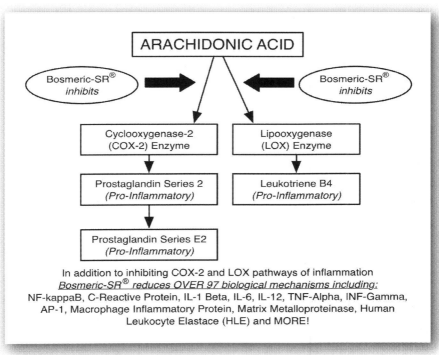

Figure 30: Pathways by which Bosmeric-SR blocks inflammation

What Makes Bosmeric-SR So Effective and Different from Other Natural Anti-inflammatories?

Bosmeric-SR is a sustained-release bilayered vegetarian caplet that synergistically combines the highest doses of Curcumin C3 Complex, Boswellin PS, ginger extract (with 20 percent gingerols), and BioPerine available today. Genesis of Bosmeric-SR comes from Ayurveda and its use of the relevant ingredients for centuries to manage several health conditions and diseases, especially inflammatory (*pitta*) conditions. Bosmeric-SR actually takes this historically successful Ayurvedic concept to the next level by combining these ingredients in a highly standardized and potent form. Further, to give long-lasting support against inflammation, I created Bosmeric-SR using a highly specialized delivery system that provides an immediate onset of action within twenty minutes and a sustained-release effect for eight hours.

While you may have taken these ingredients individually or together with other ingredients, poor selection of herbs at origin, subpar potencies and purity, and substandard manufacturing control often lead to poor efficacy and mistrust among the average consumer. This is why I endeavored to make Bosmeric-SR the best example of true integrative medicine, using the ancient knowledge of Ayurveda delivered via modern pharmaceutical technology to ensure enhanced benefits, effectiveness, and safety.

You may have tried many products on the market that contain turmeric, boswellia, ginger, and black pepper. You may have had some or no benefit at all. Most people don't realize that there is a major difference in how herbs are grown and manufactured. There are vast differences in the potencies and purities, meaning that many people taking supplements won't experience *real clinical benefits*. That's just not acceptable.

If you have experienced benefits from curcumin/turmeric supplements, I will show you how the better, more potent form of those spices and herbs in Bosmeric-SR can improve your response. If you've taken curcumin/turmeric supplements and wondered what all the fuss was about, I will show you examples of the ways in which your product failed you (or, more accurately, why the manufacturer of those products failed in delivering a truly clinically effective product).

After my training in India, I started to recommend turmeric, boswellia, ginger, and black pepper to my patients at Sanjevani very successfully. Unfortunately, I soon found out that most of my patients could not take each of these ingredients separately, multiple times daily, in large enough doses. Taste was a major issue, and so compliance started to wane.

My continued study and research of Ayurvedic medicine led me to discover a different way, thousands of years old. I learned that the most successful Ayurvedic medicines were not single agents taken separately but formulas. The herbs I was recommending to my patients not only were beneficial individually but also had synergistic and improved effects when used in combination with each other. This made the formulas not only stronger but also more balanced and less prone to causing side effects. Again, conventional Western medicine does not teach this approach or even bring it into our common thinking. Our training in pharmacology teaches us to use drugs that only target one specific reaction. We only think of one agent equaling one outcome; we never consider the power of therapeutic synergy.

The beauty and ingenuity of Ayurvedic medicine is that it involves an understanding of the complexities and the symphony of interactions and synergies among multiple ingredients, which improve overall efficacy. With this understanding, I felt drawn to investigate and research the best forms of Ayurvedic ingredients to address the root cause of most illness—inflammation.

My research led me to develop a unique way to use technology while respecting traditional medicinal formulations. Bosmeric-SR was the result, and it is unlike anything that is currently available in the market: a thoroughly modern, ancient formulation that is incredibly powerful.

Curcumin C3 Complex

Let's start with the first ingredient of Bosmeric-SR, Curcumin C3 Complex—turmeric.

Turmeric is widely used in India as a spice and has been around for over four thousand years. It is a cornerstone of Ayurvedic medicine and other traditional medicines from around the world. Turmeric is not spicy, as some people may think, but is used to add a rich flavor to foods. It is the common ingredient in many curries. Grown as a root crop, it can be used as a root directly (as it often is in cooking) or converted to a powder for use as a spice. For example, turmeric seasons yellow curry at Thai restaurants and a variety of curry dishes at Indian restaurants. Commonly known as the "yellow-colored spice," it is even used as a natural coloring agent in foods in the United States, for instance in French's mustard and other products that have a yellow color.

Although mustard does have some turmeric in it, it is not a good source for obtaining the clinical benefits. I have attended quite a few conferences over the past few years, and I have heard doctors recommending that their patients eat a packet of mustard daily (i.e., the amount of mustard found in packets taken from ballpark hot-dog stands). Whenever I hear this recommendation, I cringe. These doctors clearly lack a rudimentary understanding of the importance of turmeric potency and, more importantly, the importance of the purity of turmeric and its compounds when it comes to actual health benefits. I think these doctors mean well, but perhaps marketing from food companies has fooled them into believing that just because something contains a beneficial ingredient, it must provide tangible health benefits. When large food manufacturers use turmeric as a colorant, they do not prioritize the source, grade, and type (family or genus) of turmeric root. For that reason, these foods usually contain the lowest grade turmeric possible, which then provides lower potencies of the important constituents such as curcumin. Again, most companies are not looking for health benefits but simply using the turmeric to make the mustard turn yellow. When using turmeric as a food (or dietary supplement), one should take into consideration important factors such as whether it is synthetic, GMO, or grown with the use of pesticides and herbicides. Further, turmeric is available in many grades, ranging from very good to very poor. To get the benefits of turmeric, one must choose the right cultivar.

Turmeric is a very powerful adaptogenic and anti-inflammatory compound when grown and processed responsibly. Its many health benefits come from a powerhouse compound in its root: curcumin.

Curcumin—A Vital Component of Turmeric

Now I wake up dreaming saffron, turmeric, and brass.
—R. E. M.

The most vital therapeutic component in turmeric is curcumin. Vogel isolated curcumin in 1842, and then Milobedzke identified the structure of curcumin in 1910. Lampe further synthesized it in 1913, and Srinivasan discovered that it was a mixture of curcuminoids in 1953.[142] Although curcumin was described over a century ago, the last two decades have seen an explosion of research into the compound and its numerous health benefits. As of the first edition of this book, there are over eight thousand published studies on turmeric and curcumin, making it one of the most researched natural ingredients. Curcumin has been shown to have over six hundred potential health benefits despite making up only 2 percent to 5 percent of the turmeric root on average.

Curcumin: Activities and Actions

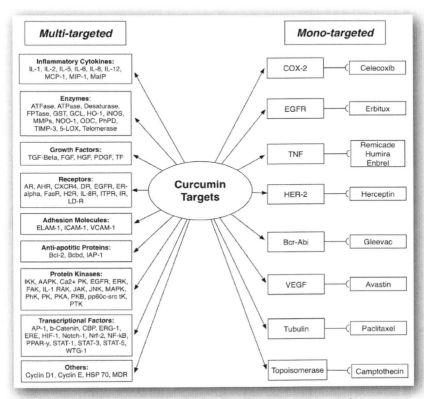

Figure 31: Curcumin actions—multitargeted and monotargeted,
similar to prescribed medications (modified diagram)

As you can see from the above diagram **(see fig. 31)**, curcumin provides both a multitargeted and monotargeted approach to its therapeutic actions.[143] *Multitargeted* means that curcumin works on hundreds of biochemical processes. For example, it works on transcriptional factors, protein kinases, adhesion molecules, enzymes, and inflammatory cytokines through its multifunctional actions and effects. *Monotargeted* means that, like conventional pharmaceuticals, curcumin works specifically on single-targeted pathways. Additionally, curcumin works by inhibiting the same pathways as NSAIDs—in addition to over one hundred other inflammatory pathways—without the unwanted effects.

For those who are interested in the scientific specifics, curcumin has been shown to reduce inflammation via NF-kB, COX-2, 5-LOX, C-reactive protein, IL-1 beta, IL-6, IL-12, TNF-alpha, IFN-gamma, AP-1, macrophage inflammatory protein, matrix metalloproteinase, human leukocyte elastase (HLE), several types of protein kinases, adhesion molecules, and genes involved with inflammation—to name a few. As mentioned before, in addition to reducing and inhibiting factors that aggravate health conditions, curcumin also activates important protective factors such as Nrf2.

Other protective factors include curcumin's demonstrated ability to boost antitumor immunity through different mechanisms. These include: increased population of CD8+ and CD4+ T cells, along with increase in Th1 cytokines like IFNγ, which mediate tumor cell apoptosis. Curcumin can block Treg cell development, thereby decreasing immunosuppressive cytokines like IL-10 and TGFβ. Curcumin also reduces tumor-induced T-cell apoptosis. All these actions help to invalidate the overall immunosuppressive environment created by a tumor (which is how the tumor avoids being recognized by the immune system) and lead to tumor regression. Thus curcumin has the ability to provide a favorable response by supporting the immune system and restoring immune system-mediated elimination of tumors.[144]

The foregoing explanation is heavy on scientific terminology. In simple terms, curcumin has been shown to exhibit the following properties:[145]

- Antioxidant
- Anti-inflammatory
- Antiviral
- Antibacterial
- Antifungal
- Anticancer

The above effects are mediated through the regulation of various transcription factors, growth factors, inflammatory cytokines, protein kinases, and other enzymes. For those who have severe chronic inflammatory health conditions—such as rheumatoid and psoriatic arthritis, Crohn's disease, ulcerative colitis, and even some cancers—you probably have been treated with pharmaceutical immunosuppressive agents and anticancer agents, offering some benefits along with heavy side effects and a large list of black-box warnings **(see chapter 7, Black-Box Warnings— The Unknown, Unconsented Agreement)**. Curcumin has been shown to work similarly to these powerful medications, but without unwanted and unpleasant side effects.

Curcumin: A Natural Pharmaceutical without Side Effects?[146]

Don't regret it, but I still live with the side effects.
—MARIAH CAREY

Curcumin exhibits activities similar to an astonishing number of major pharmaceutical anti-inflammatory drugs and chemotherapy drugs, including (but far from limited to) the following: COX-2 inhibitors (Celebrex), TNF blockers (Humira, Remicade, and Enbrel), vascular endothelial cell growth-factor blockers (Avastin), human epidermal growth-factor receptor blockers (Erbitux, Erlotinib, and Gefitinib), HER2 blockers (Herceptin), topoisomerase inhibitors (Camptothecin), tubulin inhibitors (paclitaxel, Taxol), and BCR-ABL1 tyrosine kinase inhibitors (Gleevec)—*without side effects.* In fact, there are no reports of death or serious injury from the consumption of turmeric or curcumin—just millions of tasty meals!

(As an aside: the ingredients in Bosmeric-SR are derived from herbs, foods, and spices. However, some people may have sensitivities to any of the Bosmeric-SR ingredients. Although reactions are rare, I always recommend food-allergy testing before starting any new dietary supplement.)

So promising is the therapeutic potential of curcumin that a recent turmeric study published in *Cancer Letters* is paving the way for a revolution in the way that we understand and treat cancer, titled "Targeting Cancer Stem Cells by Curcumin and Clinical Applications."[147] Researchers in the United States demonstrated via many cell and animal studies that curcumin has the ability to target cancer stem cells (CSCs), getting to the root cause of tumor formation and malignancy.[148]

CSCs are the deadliest cell types within a tumor or blood cancer, since stem cells have the ability to give rise to all the cell types found within a particular cancer. CSCs are capable of dividing (by mitosis) to form either two stem cells (increasing the size of the stem population) or one daughter cell that goes on to differentiate into a variety of cell types and one daughter cell that retains stem-cell properties. This means that CSCs are tumorigenic (tumor forming) and tumor sustaining. Therefore, it makes good medical sense to focus cancer therapy on treating the disease at this level. CSCs are also increasingly recognized to be the cause of relapse and metastasis following conventional cancer treatment.

Turmeric and curcumin extract have been extensively studied for their ability to kill various cancer-cell lines. Research identifies a number of ways in which curcumin provides an ideal CSC-targeting therapy, including the following:[149]

> **Regulation of the CSC self-renewal pathway:** Curcumin appears to directly and indirectly influence at least three self-renewal pathways within cancer stem cells, namely Wnt/b-catenin, sonic hedgehog 89 (SHH), and Notch. The authors list twelve different cancer-cell lines that curcumin appears to affect positively.

> **Modulation of microRNA:** MicroRNAs are short noncoding RNA sequences that regulate approximately 33 percent of the protein-coding genes in the human genome. They bind to target messenger RNAs (mRNAs), leading to their degradation or inactivation. Curcumin has been found to alter the expression of microRNAs in cancer stem cells in a way that would suggest a strong suppression of tumor formation.

In addition to the dozens of anticancer activities that curcumin has demonstrated, it also acts as a chemotherapy and radiation-therapy sensitizer. This means that it helps sensitize the tumors to cancer therapies, making those treatments more effective. In other words, making toxic therapies more targeted. Curcumin can sensitize tumors to many different chemotherapeutic agents, including doxorubicin, 5-FU, paclitaxel, vincristine, melphalan, butyrate, cisplatin, celecoxib, vinorelbine, gemcitabine, oxaliplatin, etoposide, sulfinosine, thalidomide, and bortezomib.

Chemosensitization has been observed in cancers of the breast, colon, pancreas, GI tract, liver, blood, lung, prostate, bladder, cervix, ovary, head, neck, and brain, as well as in multiple myeloma, leukemia, and lymphoma.

Similar studies have also revealed that curcumin can increase the sensitivity to gamma radiation of a variety of tumors, including glioma, neuroblastoma, cervical carcinoma, epidermal carcinoma, prostate cancer, and colon cancer. How curcumin acts as a chemosensitizer and radiosensitizer has also been studied extensively[150]. For example, it downregulates various growth-regulatory pathways and specific genetic targets, including genes for NF-kB, STAT3, COX-2, Akt, antiapoptotic proteins, growth-factor receptors, and multidrug-resistance proteins.[151]

Furthermore, curcumin also helps protect healthy tissues from the toxic side effects of chemotherapy and radiation therapy. Curcumin has been shown to protect healthy organs and tissues such as the liver, kidney, oral mucosa, and heart from chemotherapy- and radiotherapy-induced toxicity. The protective effects of curcumin appear to be mediated in a variety of ways: through activating Nrf2 and inducing the expression of antioxidant enzymes (e.g., heme oxygenase-1, glutathione peroxidase, modulatory subunit of gamma-glutamyl-cysteine ligase, NAD(P)H:quinone oxidoreductase 1, and increase glutathione—a product of the modulatory subunit of gamma-glutamyl-cysteine ligase), directly quenching free radicals, and inhibiting p300 HAT activity—to name a few.[152]

To summarize all that dense scientific language, curcumin exhibits some of the most amazing anticancer properties, such as the following, which apply to most cancers:

- Inhibits TNF-alpha, NF-kB, and hundreds of other mechanisms that stimulate inflammation[153]
  - As little as 150 mg of curcumin twice daily, standardized to three curcuminoids orally, can significantly decrease TNF-alpha[154]
- Prevents multidrug-resistant cancers[155]
- Destroys cancer stem cells (CSC)[156]
- Protects tissues and organs from chemotherapy- and radiation-induced damage (reducing overall toxicity from these treatments)[157]
- Works synergistically with chemotherapy and radiation therapy to make those therapies more targeted and, therefore, more effective.[158]

In addition to inhibiting and influencing the biological mechanisms of inflammation as described earlier, curcumin has been shown to improve endothelial function and reduce vascular inflammation (which increases blood flow and prevents plaque buildup in the arteries), downregulate adipokines (including resistin and leptin, factors involved in obesity) and monocyte chemotactic protein-1, and upregulate Nrf2 (key factors involved in brain-inflammatory processes and brain-degeneration issues that manifest in disorders such as epilepsy, Alzheimer's, traumatic brain injury, and other neurodegenerative conditions).

So what does all this mean in terms of preventing and treating disease? It means curcumin may be the most powerful natural therapeutic substance for a wide array of acute and chronic health conditions.

Conditions Helped by Curcumin*

- Osteoarthritis
- Autoimmune arthritis (rheumatoid)
- Ulcerative colitis and Crohn's disease
- Cancer (breast, prostate, brain, colon, bone, and liver), via immune-modulating, angiogenesis, tumorigenic properties
- Allergies and asthma
- Diabetes and diabetic neuropathy
- Cardiovascular diseases
- Obesity
- Fibromyalgia and other chronic-pain syndromes
- Neurodegenerative diseases (Alzheimer's disease, Parkinson's, traumatic brain injury, epilepsy, etc.)
- Acne, psoriasis, and eczema
- Liver diseases (toxic insults and dysfunction)

What Form of Curcumin Is Best for Me?

You get the best of what I got.
—BAD ENGLISH

Now that you know some of the amazing benefits of curcumin, and you've seen that there is a lot of low-quality curcumin on the market, how can you tell what is best?

Bosmeric-SR contains the form of curcumin called Curcumin C3 Complex, which is the gold standard for curcumin, used successfully in high-quality supplements for over twenty-five years. It is the *patented form of curcumin* that contains *standardized 95 percent curcuminoids* and is supported by *forty-five human clinical studies (and counting)* at major universities, hospitals, and health-care institutions worldwide, making Curcumin C3 Complex the *most clinically studied* brand of curcumin on the market today.

Full disclosure: I work closely with the company Sabinsa that owns the patent on Curcumin C3 Complex; they closely monitor the farms at which the raw turmeric grows, and they initiated clinical research that has become the standard by which all other curcumin is measured. I can assure my readers that no one is more of an expert about turmeric and curcuminoids than the team that developed Curcumin C3 Complex. Sabinsa is not only the most knowledgeable and experienced with curcumin and turmeric, they helped the US Pharmacopeial Convention (USP) prepare their recently published monographs on curcuminoids and turmeric, developing validated analytical methods for these compounds. Additionally, they supplied the reference standards for individual curcuminoids to the USP.[159] Thus the whole industry follows the standards set by Sabinsa on curcuminoids quality.

Curcumin C3 Complex is not only the most effective form of curcumin *and* the most clinically studied but also contains the three major constituents (curcuminoids) in *specific ratios, guaranteed*:

- Curcumin (70–80 percent)
- Bidemothoxy curcumin (2.5–6.5 percent)
- Demethoxy curcumin (15–25 percent)

These three curcuminoids are guaranteed to be *in the same ratios in every batch*, which is almost unheard of in the natural-product world. Most importantly, these curcuminoid ratios are also *the precise ratios that have undergone the most clinical studies*. This guaranteed uniformity ensures consistency of health benefits and enables physicians to more accurately recommend and administer these incredibly beneficial compounds.

What about Generic Curcumin Extract Standardized to 95 Percent Curcuminoids?

If you're familiar with curcumin supplements, then you're familiar with the ways in which companies try to assure consumers that they're getting what they're paying for. Most companies use generic "standardized 95 percent curcuminoids," but that standardization doesn't guarantee that the curcuminoid ratios are exactly in the proportions that have been clinically studied. Thus generic standardization limits the effectiveness and purity of most curcumin supplements. Generic curcumin has no potency guarantee and is not validated by third-party testing; most supplements fall short of efficacy and safety measures.

Supplement manufacturers from China and India, driving the marketplace to provide the cheapest product possible, generally purchase generic curcumin products. In this competitive international marketplace, corners are cut to further drive down costs; the most basic cuts are to safety (not testing enough or at all) and efficacy (not verifying clinical effectiveness). Most companies (including MLM companies, health-practitioner channels, and retailers) will purchase generic curcuminoids not knowing (or caring) which type of turmeric they come from, how the turmeric is grown (whether pesticides, herbicides, GMO, or synthetics were used), whether harmful solvents were used for the extraction process, whether the product was irradiated, or whether or not the curcuminoids are effective. All that matters is the bottom line and having a "buzz worthy" ingredient. Thus by providing a substandard material and citing the clinical studies done on Curcumin C3 Complex as also applicable to their curcumin, these generic suppliers are misleading the consumers.

Remember, the FDA classifies a dietary supplement as "not intended to treat, prevent, or cure disease." This limitation actually works in unscrupulous supplement companies' favor. Since the FDA has defined what a supplement *can't* do, supplement manufacturers can take advantage of this disclaimer by obtaining the cheapest (even completely ineffective) product because *they are not being held to any standard of efficacy, potency, or purity.* In essence, they don't have to provide products that actually work anywhere close to how they are marketed.

Bosmeric-SR contains only Curcumin C3 Complex—the curcumin supported by the most safety data. This safety data has been reviewed and acknowledged by the FDA for GRAS (generally recognized as safe) status, a process that includes a comprehensive review of safety and toxicology data. Most other curcumin products on the market cannot make that claim. Because Curcumin C3 Complex is made using a patented and proprietary process, the safety data for Curcumin C3 Complex is not applicable to other curcumin products. In fact, many other curcumin-supplement companies derive their indirect and direct health claims and advertising from research studies using Curcumin C3 Complex and not their own products! (More on that in the next section.) And you may see other curcumin products advertise that their curcumin is touted to be safe, but Bosmeric-SR *is the only one that is guaranteed safe.*

The use of turmeric and curcumin supplements has skyrocketed because of the enormous amounts of research published on a near-weekly basis (again, there are over eight thousand studies as of the first publishing of this book). Curcumin is one of the top five best-selling herbal ingredients every year. Because of this high demand, many companies and products state that they use curcumin, but, in actuality, their curcumin compounds are not as potent, as effective, or even as safe as Bosmeric-SR.

All That Glitters Is Not Gold: All That Is Yellow Is Not Curcumin C3 Complex

> *Fools remain, but nothing gold can stay,*
> *All that glitters seems to blow away.*
> —Night Ranger

As I touched on in the previous section, because of the competition in the marketplace and the drive for higher profit margins, you might have thought you tried Curcumin C3 Complex in the past. Over the past few years, companies have been caught claiming Curcumin C3 Complex on their label when in fact they were selling generic curcumin, synthetic curcumin, or turmeric extract. More nefariously, some companies have added a small amount of Curcumin C3 Complex to their product but illegally cut the product with generic curcumin, synthetic curcumin, or turmeric powder to make the margins on the product better. This year synthetic curcumin was discovered being sold as turmeric extract with forged certificates of analysis. A major company selling curcumin extract in India for export to the United States was adulterating their product with synthetic curcumin (43 percent). What makes it worse is that the company was not revealing the synthetic contents. This leads one to a few obvious questions. What was it synthesized from? What chemicals were used? What process did they use to make it? And the most important question: is it safe for consumption by humans? Synthetically made materials may have distinctively different pharmacological activities compared to natural products. If a company is selling synthetic curcumin and not identifying that some or all of the product was synthetically derived, that lack of transparency is not only misleading consumers who think they are taking a product derived from turmeric root, but it has the potential to hurt people. Therefore, in order to avoid questionable contract manufacturers, I prefer to go directly to the source of Curcumin C3 Complex, ensuring each batch is consistent and guaranteed every time.

In a time when it seems everyone is trying to make a fast buck on supplements, transparent quality control and safety protocols have never been more important. Curcumin C3 Complex (as well as Bosmeric-SR) is manufactured in an FDA-inspected facility compliant with CGMP (the FDA's standard for "current good manufacturing processes"). Its manufacturer maintains quality through the sourcing of raw material; they have direct control and access throughout the sourcing and manufacturing process. They use only analytical and biological testing labs audited and certified by the National Accreditation Board for Testing and Calibration Laboratories (NABL). Bosmeric-SR is manufactured in state-of-the-art facilities assessed by NSF International and certified to be in compliance with GMP.[160] Again, although all manufacturing facilities should be up to these standards, because of the staffing limitations of the FDA and other regulatory agencies (since there are hundreds of contract manufacturers opening all over the country on a regular basis), not all companies actually comply with current FDA regulations.

Whether you decide to use Bosmeric-SR or not, it is important that you know the guidelines and the regulations that *all* supplements should abide by. The more informed we are, the higher standards these companies will have to hold themselves to if they want to stay in business.

What about the Newer Forms of Curcumin That Claim to Be Better Absorbed?

What I see is unreal.
—ALICE IN CHAINS

Many companies claim to be selling newer forms of curcumin that they advertise as "better absorbed." I'm always interested in investigating new products—especially if they seem to have an advantage over what I am currently recommending. Over the past few years, I have been investigating the claims of companies that market "new and improved," "better absorbed," and "more bioavailable" products. The industry uses these new buzzwords to help sell products, but as you might imagine, they aren't necessarily providing the results they're promising. I am not saying that some products do not have additional benefits or even improve on the benefits of a previous formulation. But when I started looking into actual formulations and actual data for "better absorbed" curcumin, what I found was shocking.

Bioavailability: A Path and Not a Destination

Destination out of sight
—SCORPIONS

The supplement industry has placed a disproportionate emphasis on the role of bioavailability of their formulations, but bioavailability is not the sole criterion for judging the therapeutic effect of curcumin. Bioavailability is the amount of a substance (in this case curcumin) that is absorbed and made available at the site of physiological activity. Therefore increasing bioavailability is important, but making sure that the substances which are measured also have health benefits is critical.

Vast amounts of research, along with the expert opinions of those who specialize in the field of curcuminoids, have continually maintained that bio-availability is only a "path" and not the "destination." Enhanced bioavailability cannot be used as an alternative to or as a substitute for clinical studies. Now, I *am* interested in increasing bioavailability with all my products **(see Black Pepper—Not Just the Other Shaker on the Table)**, and I also favor those companies that have invested in making their products more bioavailable. But these companies must have also initiated, supported, and invested their resources in several curcumin-based clinical trials. Science trumps buzzwords, always.

Formulations that contain *curcumin-phosphatidyl choline, curcumin-lecithin*, and *micronized and micelle-curcumin* mixtures deliver curcumin as a small fraction of the actual mass (most offer less than 20 percent curcuminoids; one even provides only 7 percent). Although the studies on these products show some benefits (as they should, since they are providing *some* curcumin), their claims of "29 to 60 *times*" to even "185 *times* more absorbed" contain flat-out skewed data. When curcuminoids are absorbed in the body, they are converted to many byproducts or metabolites such as glucuronides. Studies of these newer formulations are measuring not the actual curcuminoids but these *other metabolites*. They are using the increase in the metabolites to show increased absorption, but they are not actually providing those metabolites directly. For example, the above formulations do not inhibit the biotransformation of curcuminoids, which is the limiting factor for improving bioavailability. Instead, these formulations just load the body with more of the inactive glucuronide metabolites of curcuminoids. Additionally, many of these metabolites have been recently discovered to have little to no anti-inflammatory effects![161]

Companies routinely misrepresent data and skew it to exaggerate the comparisons between formulations—especially in relation to other products. In fact, pharmaceutical companies may be the biggest offenders in this area. According to a handful of medical studies on the pharmaceutical industry, most of the comparison graphs and data that pharmaceutical sales reps and advertisements presented to doctors were not accurate.[162]

If this happens within the pharmaceutical industry—which the FDA regulates—you can imagine what happens when there is no regulation or oversight for such marketing from dietary-supplement companies. Exaggerated graphs and data are shown every day in supplement advertising and by sales reps. Store clerks, doctors, and the general public have probably seen a chart that shows "increased absorption" or "better bioavailability." Often these charts are comparing apples to oranges. As one example, I was presented with studies on curcumin that showed increased absorption rates, but those higher rates were for curcumin in a liquid versus a tablet form, and the company giving the presentation *sold only tablets*. This is a common trick in which sales representatives extrapolate data from one form or type of supplement and try to use it to their advantage; most products, when taken as a liquid, deliver better absorption than as a solid. In the case of this tablet company, however, they were attempting to misguide me with inaccurate data that made their product look better than it was.

Another newer form of curcumin uses something called "colloidal dispersion technology" and states that it has "enhanced absorption and bioavailability up to twenty-seven times." A sales rep from the nutraceuticals company marketing this product arrived at my office and tried to tell me that this new curcumin was superior to anything else on the market. He had a colorful graph showing that it was "twenty-seven times" more absorbable than "regular" curcumin.

He did not know that I was familiar with the study used for the infographic. In that study, the authors tested their newer form of curcumin (which contained far less curcumin than most brands) against a turmeric product, but they (purposely) never stated the actual quantity of curcuminoids that the comparison product contained—only that theirs dissolved better in water. Thus, the rep was using an invalid comparison, which is sadly all too common.

Aside from that, however, this salesman didn't mention that his product contained far fewer curcuminoids, and he declined to disclose the product's sources. On top of that, a supplement that disperses better in water does not necessarily correlate to improved efficacy or absorption in the blood. What does this mean to the consumer? It means that dietary-supplement companies that sell these sorts of well-marketed "more bioavailable" products can make bigger claims and bigger profit margins while using lower potency or lower amounts of curcuminoids.

Another wrinkle in the bioavailability competition is the rise of lipid- or nano-encapsulated ingredients. These processes take standard ingredients and encapsulate them in tiny absorbable particles, making them smaller and more dispersible. Nanoparticles may be beneficial, although they certainly have their detractors, but with curcumin I tend to use what is tried and true. To date, no nanoparticle curcumin has been studied against Curcumin C3 Complex—just generic, nonstandardized curcumin powder or extracts without disclosed potencies. Generic forms never test against patented forms. Again, be wary of unsourced supplement studies and read very carefully between the lines—especially when it comes to an extremely popular compound like curcumin.

When assessing the bioavailability of curcumin in the body, ignoring the role of curcumin's metabolites reveals a lack of knowledge and expertise. Curcumin breaks down into certain metabolites, which are mainly tetrahydrocurcumin, curcumin glucuronides, and sulfates. While the positive effects of tetrahydrocurcumin have been recognized, most bioavailability studies have failed to quantify the bioconversion of curcumin into this efficacious metabolite, tetrahydrocurcumin.[163] This means that most studies are not giving the full therapeutic picture. The bioefficacy of glucuronides and sulfate metabolites, which is what the newer forms of curcumin formulations are claiming are better absorbed, has not been well established. They even have been shown to be less active and have weak activity.[164] Furthermore, they have no anti-inflammatory effects, nor do they have any effect on mitotic catastrophe, an important step in preventing proliferation of some cancerous cells.[165]

My colleague Dr. Bharat Aggarwal announced at a cancer conference that his research demonstrated that "curcumin glucuronides show very little antiproliferative activity against human cancer-cell lines and have no inhibitory effect on NF-kB, thus lacking the anti-inflammatory activity of curcuminoids."[166] Although many products sold in health-food stores, on the Internet, through MLM companies, and through doctors' networks may claim better absorption, they are measuring curcumin metabolites—especially the glucuronides—and thus are missing the stronger intended anti-inflammatory effect. In the real world, such absorption claims have nothing to do with efficacy; they're simply the stuff of cleverly written research articles, with graphs that seem to illustrate meaningful differences, and very convincing marketing campaigns. Again, instead of searching for the "new and improved," I tend to go with what has been tried and true—and backed by research.

I agree with a recent statement provided by Dr. Muhammed Majeed, the patent owner and research scientist behind Curcumin C3 Complex. Dr. Majeed stated that, "emphasis on increasing bioavailability alone is by no means a substitute for properly designed and conducted clinical trials that examine what happens to a curcumin product in the body. We don't believe making the assumption that increasing initial bioavailability is valid without doing the work to make sure the resulting substance does what it is supposed to do."[167]

Since many products are being introduced into the market almost monthly, and it would be impossible to go through *all* the comparisons here, I have provided comparisons on the most popular curcumin products being sold as of the publishing of this book. Products compared include BCM-95, Meriva, Longvida, NovaSol, and many others. For details please see **Side Notes: Figure 32: Comparison Curcumin C3 Complex in Bosmeric-SR* vs. others**, as well as our website for general details at **www.bosmeric-sr.com.**

Turmeric Cultivation and Processing: What Is Best?

Since so many supplement companies focus on marketing "better absorption," maybe we should ask them, Better absorption of what, exactly? What type of curcumin are they using, and how is it cultivated and processed? You might make a smoothie with a high-quality blender such as a Vitamix, but that doesn't mean that the smoothie is good for you—especially if it contains conventional, nonorganic, and GMO foods. What makes a smoothie better for you is not just the quality of the blender but, more importantly, the quality of the ingredients.

Like all good supplements, let's first start at the farm. Unlike most turmeric supplements sold in the United States, *Bosmeric-SR is non-GMO, halal, kosher, wheat free, gluten-free, and soy-free.* Most turmeric and generic curcuminoids come from unregulated turmeric grown in China, India and other countries and commonly contain wheat, corn, soy, or gum fillers. Turmeric is a root crop, and almost all turmeric that is grown worldwide has been treated with common chemicals such as pesticides, insecticides, and herbicides. Fortunately, Bosmeric-SR does not contain these harmful ingredients, as they are not used in the cultivation of our turmeric. Our turmeric is cultivated to meet the current guidelines for organic certification. The farms we work with are owned and contracted specifically to grow the best type of turmeric root, as determined by "blueprint fingerprinting" the best crop, measuring the ideal compounds in the turmeric root, and then using those roots to continue to harvest newer crops. The process is similar to that used with heirloom seeds. By using this method, we ensure the potency and purity of the turmeric root that provides our curcuminoids and other important turmeric constituents. Though the Curcumin C3 Complex does not carry organic certification, it still matches the quality of organically grown turmeric and provides the best quality of curcumin. Experts strictly monitor the quality of the turmeric to minimize use of any pesticides and to use GAP (good agricultural practices) processes.

Most companies that sell curcumin products have no control of the actual turmeric crop, nor any control over how it is cultivated (e.g., with pesticides, herbicides, radiation, or GMOs). These companies only worry about getting the cheapest raw ingredients from the world market (mainly from China) and then trying to improve upon them with their proprietary processes.

However, when using foods as medicine, starting with the best ingredients makes the biggest difference. The curcumin in Bosmeric-SR is controlled, from crop cultivation at the farms to the highest certified processing facilities, to a patented process of extracting the specific ratio of curcuminoids—guaranteed batch to batch—to the manufacturing of the unique delivery system. All of this ensures a superior product that is consistent, potent, pure, and effective every time.

Taking things a step further, I have ensured that the Curcumin C3 Complex in Bosmeric-SR *is not irradiated*. Here's why this is vitally important.

Many people are not aware that since 9/11, all food ingredients imported into the United States must be irradiated to ensure "safety" and destroy contaminants (bacteria, fungus, etc.). I have researched extensively and traveled to India (where most of the turmeric is grown) and discovered that almost all curcumin—especially curcumin grown in China, which is the second largest producer—is irradiated prior to being sent to the United States. My experience in India was truly disheartening. During my search for the best type of turmeric/curcumin, I witnessed many batches of raw product being sent to facilities to get irradiated. At these various facilities (which irradiate products and then provide certification of the completion of such treatment), there was *no difference in the amount of radiation used to sterilize each different product.*

For example, I personally witnessed the irradiation of a variety of herbal turmeric products from the biggest exporters in India (exporters that provide turmeric/curcumin to the major retailers and common brands at the health-food stores). These exporters have their products irradiated at *the same dose that is used to sterilize surgical equipment.* We are all familiar with the harmful effects of extreme doses of radiation, and sterilizing the herbal ingredients at that extreme level dramatically decreases the effectiveness of the antioxidants, phytonutrients, and other important aspects.

Curcumin C3 Complex is also nonirradiated to preserve the therapeutic benefits that are stripped out by massive doses of "protective" radiation. It does cost more to obtain certifications and to follow extremely strict importation procedures to ensure that there are no contaminants (bacteria, fungus, etc.) without irradiating anything. Naturally, it takes extra time and extra steps of quality control, but it is worth it to provide the true benefits of these incredibly powerful natural ingredients. Most of my patients who have tried other turmeric supplements said they did not work as well as they expected, but almost all reported that when they took Bosmeric-SR, they noticed an immediate and ongoing difference.

Not only does Bosmeric-SR have ensured potency and efficacy because it uses Curcumin C3 Complex, but it also has guaranteed safety from contaminants like heavy metals. Heavy metals? How do they wind up in any supplement? When supplement manufacturers request turmeric, the bulk spice is shipped to the United States in large containers. Over the past few years—especially in 2008, 2011, and again in 2013—independent consumer groups discovered that 33 *percent of turmeric and curcumin supplements failed quality testing, and many popular brands contained lead and other contaminants.*[168] Turmeric was being shipped in lead containers (mostly from India and China), and the containers' linings were leaching lead into the turmeric. Makes you wonder about other foods, such as grains, shipped in those containers!

During the time of greatest lead contamination, many patients who came to see me were taking turmeric supplements for their joint pain. They told me they were taking it because they had read all the health benefits, but they felt that they were actually getting worse. No surprise: they were taking products from companies whose turmeric/curcumin products failed safety tests for lead contamination. Even worse, the patients had high levels of lead when we screened them using blood testing. This is a tragically obvious example of why purity is so important.

You will almost always get what you pay for. Sometimes a bargain costs you far more in the end. Remember, by the FDA's own definition, "Dietary supplements are *not* intended to prevent, treat, reverse, or cure any disease." Far too many companies follow that rule, but not to avoid getting in trouble for making sensationalistic health claims; instead they use the FDA's disclaimer to absolve them of providing high-quality, effective, or safe products.

Furthermore, it is important to make sure that no harmful, toxic solvents are used in the process of extracting real curcumin from turmeric, as solvent residues do remain on extracted products and can cause harm. No harmful solvents are used in the extraction of the Curcumin C3 Complex used in Bosmeric-SR. Again, this processing is an investment in the health of anyone taking Bosmeric-SR; it *costs* slightly more to make a cleaner and safer product than to use cheap, poisonous chemicals, but it's an investment worth making for so many reasons.

In addition to checking purity and quality of source, one must make sure that they're getting real curcuminoids from real turmeric. Companies in China and India can make synthetic curcuminoids in the laboratory, creating something like a pharmaceutical compound. This is why you see turmeric/curcumin products priced as low as two to five dollars for a bottle on the Internet. These cheap products are usually synthetically derived; you are taking an isolated molecular compound, and therefore, you are not receiving the full benefits of the curcuminoids—as well as the other active turmeric compounds.

Cheaper products mean that more harmful chemicals have been used in the production process, and, thus, they expose you to greater risk of side effects and allergic reactions. Next time you see a cheap generic turmeric product, see if the word "natural" is listed in the ingredients. I can say with near 100 percent certainty that you will see only the words *turmeric* or *curcumin* or *turmeric extract* (or *powder*) or *curcumin extract* (or *powder*). All the supplements with their ingredients listed this way will be priced at or below five dollars per bottle. On top of that, some branded turmeric or curcumin products are actually synthetics. Some supplement companies sell products honestly thinking they are using real turmeric when they are actually purchasing synthetic curcumin or turmeric and don't even know it! The deception can seem insidious, but it's not over yet.

When investigating your dietary supplements, always look for NSF (National Sanitation Foundation) and CGMP (current good manufacturing practice) certifications and a guarantee that the supplements have been formulated and packaged in registered ISO 22000 facilities only. These certifications establish strict guidelines that make sure the manufacturer follows ethical practices that all boil down to ensuring that the label matches the contents of the bottle. These certifications ensure compliance by requiring audits that verify that the company is meeting the highest standards of manufacturing and handling of products at all times.

I prefer to obtain a finished product directly from the company that owns the patents and ingredients instead of buying from third-party vendors—especially when it comes to turmeric, because of all the pitfalls I described above. Since the FDA does not regulate dietary supplements but only offers guidelines (which are not enforced until after an adverse report or event), many companies cheat their customers and increase their bottom line by blending patented ingredients with generic ones. In essence, this means that they can state on their labels they are using the patented ingredients—like Curcumin C3 Complex—when in fact the product might contain only 5 percent to 10 percent Curcumin C3 Complex. The rest could be generic turmeric powder or even synthetic curcumin extracts. This practice is so widespread as to be epidemic. Consumer groups decry it, but federal agencies do not have the resources to investigate every supplement manufacturer.

Since I work closely with the manufacturers of the ingredients I use in my products, I know the raw cost of the product—that is, the actual price of the product before it is sold to wholesalers and then to retailers. Even nutrition companies that sell exclusively to health-care providers and on the Internet join the many online discount vitamin companies (I like to call them the "big-box vitamin shops" or "discount warehouses" of supplements) that sell Curcumin C3 Complex at prices lower than the actual raw cost of the product! No matter how much volume discount a company receives, the price of *any* product at retail should never be lower than the raw cost. Products sold below raw cost guarantee that the branded ingredient is being cut or diluted with generic or synthetic ingredients, or it contains other ingredients altogether. If you look at a patented ingredient and find a competitor with a price that is greatly lower or even half the price, you're virtually guaranteed that the cheap product would not meet its label claims of potency or purity if tested.

Therefore, when looking for turmeric/curcumin—and, really, any other natural products—make sure they are:

- Tested for heavy metals (there is a high risk of lead contamination in cheap supplements)
- Produced in an NSF- and CGMP-certified facility
- Manufactured in an ISO 22000–certified facility
- Guaranteed for potency and purity, with documentation and third-party test results
- Using patented ingredients (like Curcumin C3 Complex, for example) to ensure quality, potency, and purity
- Certified GRAS (generally regarded as safe) by FDA

How Much Curcumin C3 Complex Should One Take?

Now that you better understand the potential pitfalls of generic curcumin, I would like to talk about the product I know best and tell you how you can use it best to achieve your health and wellness goals.

Most of the clinical studies on the use of curcuminoids suggest a daily dose from 1 g (1,000 mg) to 3 g (3,000 mg), in divided doses for a better response (e.g., 1,000 mg three times a day). I recommend the divided doses because when curcumin is absorbed into the body, it has a short "peak" and then falls off over time. Therefore, multiple doses provide a better response throughout the day. The more chronic or severe the health condition, the higher the dose that the person would require. Some studies suggest upward of 8 g (8,000 mg) or more for severe, life-threatening diseases or end-stage cancers.[169]

When I first started recommending turmeric—and especially Curcumin C3 Complex—my patients were taking multiple pills three times daily, as there were no other options. That was one of the driving forces behind the development of **Bosmeric-SR**. I made sure we improved the efficacy of curcuminoids (through a combination of synergistic ingredients) and the potency of curcumin itself through a unique delivery system that requires just *one to two caplets, twice daily with food.* (Those with severe health conditions, such as cancer, can take two caplets up to three times daily with food for twenty-four hours of full support.)

Bosmeric-SR comes in an easy-to-swallow bilayered vegetarian caplet that has an immediate action—meaning it is designed to start working within twenty minutes (like a "fast tab") but also incorporates sustained release for over eight hours of support. This specific type of sustained release provides the clinical benefits of 3 g (or more) of curcuminoids with the intake of just 1 g.

What about Taking Curcumin Products during Chemotherapy, Radiation, or Imaging Such as CT and PET Scans?

In the past, most oncologists and internal medicine physicians advised their patients not to take anything herbal while undergoing their chemotherapy and radiation treatments. Thankfully, this is now considered to be out-of-date advice.

Most recent studies (in vivo studies on various cancers) have shown that animals and human patients that took the combination of conventional treatment along with curcumin did better than those taking conventional treatment alone. Curcumin has been shown to have both chemo-protective and radio-protective benefits.[170] In other words, it helps protect the healthy cells from the damaging effects of chemotherapy and radiation. Thus, curcumin has a threefold effect:

1. Curcumin reduces the toxic side effect of damage to healthy cells.
2. Curcumin decreases inflammation and other dangerous cancer signals that aggravate cells **(see fig. 31)**.
3. Curcumin sensitizes cancer cells to chemotherapy and radiation, which makes these toxic therapies more targeted (helping to attack the cancer, while leaving healthy, unaffected cells and tissues unharmed).[171]

Curcumin is only one means that might be able to improve someone's treatment outcomes. Bosmeric-SR and all of its synergistic compounds (detailed below) may be an important part of an overall protocol for those suffering from cancer. The ingredients in Bosmeric-SR have not only healing aspects but also protective or preventative aspects. For that reason, I recommend all my patients take Bosmeric-SR for added radiation protection when they get CT and PET scans, and other imaging as well, including full-body scans at the airport.

I know some may find my opinion on airport scanners a bit overcautious, but I always recommend that those traveling through airport security request a pat down instead of going through the full-body scanner as much as possible. A number of reports from as far back as 1995 have shown increased risk of exposure to radiation (this comes from backscatter machines) and now of radio frequencies (the current scanners at most airports that spin around you) and the more frightful terahertz scanners (similar to microwaves) that are yet to come. The closer one is to those machines and the longer the exposure, the higher the risks of cancer and other concerns like fertility problems.[172] With this logic in mind, the TSA officers are at highest risk, since they work around these machine all day, as are the flight attendants, pilots, and flyers who go through them frequently. If I can easily avoid anything that can increase my risk of health problems, such as by getting a pat down instead of going through a machine, then why would I not?

I request a pat down every time I travel, and TSA officers get upset with me, as it is more work for them. They usually ask me why I am requesting it, and I tell them that as an MD who sees a lot of cancer patients, I choose not to increase my risk through unnecessary exposure.

One of my cancer patients is an older gentleman who worked for five years as a TSA agent. He told me that during his training, he had to practice going in and out of the body scanner about two hundred times! He also worked around full-body scanners for full shifts—forty hours a week for five years. He came to see me after his diagnosis of leukemia. Coincidence? Not according to a study that showed that military personal exposed to radiofrequency and microwave radiation had eight times the risk of lymphoma and leukemia of those who were not exposed.[173]

On a recent trip, I did my usual opting out of the body scanner, and again a TSA officer asked me why. Once I told him my reason, he smiled and replied, "Oh, you read the report!"

How unfortunate that we knowingly put people in an occupational-hazard area for our own protection; what about theirs? Why not fully educate the TSA about their risks or, better yet, encourage them to do pat downs as a way to give them a break from their long-term exposure? Or, even better, why don't we pat down everyone and treat everyone equally while developing better screening methods that are safe for the public and for those who are providing protective screening measures?

Let me be clear: you won't get cancer from going through a full-body scanner a few times. But any radiation exposure, no matter the source, can and does contribute to your overall radiation-exposure load over your lifetime. We get enough inflammatory triggers and hits to our DNA daily; why add more?

Consider this: the full-body scanner has to emit just enough radiation to provide a full-body image (in less than three seconds). Those who travel often are accumulating an unnecessary lifelong exposure risk. When you consider that the United States is the only country that uses body scanners—and not just metal detectors and full pat downs for everyone (which is what has been occurring in most places for the last twenty years)—even though data suggests that body scanners increase the risk of cancer, you have to wonder. Are body scanners yet another case of profits before people? It would seem so.

I recently attended a cancer conference where one of the specialists provided information that pilots and flight attendants were at the highest risk of getting cancers because of long-term exposure from the natural radiation from the sun at thirty thousand feet. A trans-Atlantic flight is equivalent to one chest x-ray's worth of radiation exposure. That's actually not too much radiation, but if you are a pilot or flight attendant, your exposure greatly increases as part of the occupation. This risk is so great that when a governmental report documented the correlation between the higher risk of cancers—such as leukemia and lymphomas—in pilots, airplane manufacturers started to place a thin lining of lead in cockpits to shield them from this subtle but dangerous lifelong exposure (and more importantly, to protect themselves from legal liability). Interestingly, they only added this protective lining to the cockpits—not the entire plane—because pilots are under a different type of legal contract than flight attendants. Because flight attendants (and passengers) do not carry that same liability, plane manufacturers kept their costs to a minimum and only protected those people who are their greatest liability (pilots). Therefore, I recommend that all flight attendants or passengers take Bosmeric-SR to help prevent the stress and damage from natural radiation exposure during air travel.

Boswellia: Activities and Actions

It all began with the three wise men
Followed a star took them to Bethlehem
And made it heard throughout the land
Born was the leader of man
All going down to see the Lord Jesus
—QUEEN

Boswellia serrata is a species of tree that primarily grows in India (and also grows in the Arabian Peninsula and northeastern Africa). It produces a resin commonly known as frankincense. Biblical references to frankincense—including it being one of the gifts that the magi brought to baby Jesus—have made it popular worldwide in recent years. But it is an almost "magi-cal" compound that has been used for thousands of years in India, China, and Greece for treatment of inflammatory conditions.

Here is a short list of the documented activities and actions of boswellia:[174]

- Anti-inflammatory
- Antiarthritic
- Antirheumatic
- Antidiabetic
- Antihyperlipidemic (prevents elevated blood lipids)
- Antiasthmatic
- Anticancer
- Analgesic (pain-relieving)
- Hepatic-protective (liver protection)
- Colon-protective
- Immune-modulatory (positively affects or strengthens the immune system)

The magi brought gifts of frankincense, myrrh, and gold; interestingly, these three items can be further identified as three powerful herbs:

- "Frankincense" is boswellia.
- "Myrrh" is almost certainly the guggul plant (*Commiphora wightii*).

- "Gold" is thought to be turmeric, as it was the "golden spice" and was traded more than gold during the height of the spice trade.

Today we understand the three wise men were bringing Ayurvedic medicines to baby Jesus!

Frankincense was very popular worldwide for thousands of years. During the sixteenth century in France, frankincense was used in battlefield medicine for the treatment of acute pain and swelling. Although practitioners of Ayurvedic medicine have also used *Boswellia serrata* for thousands of years to treat arthritis and asthma, a more recent scientific consensus appears to show that frankincense positively impacts inflammation throughout the body and is effective for a number of conditions, including osteoarthritis and rheumatoid arthritis,[175] inflammatory bowel disease (colitis),[176] colon polyps,[177] and lung diseases such as allergies and asthma.[178]

Frankincense is even the subject of increasing research on its anticancer and anti-inflammatory effects on traumatic brain injury and brain tumors.[179]

Frankincense is not only historically important as internal medicine, but it has been used throughout various religious communities for centuries as incense. You might have experienced frankincense at church or seen it on a televised religious broadcast. Typically, a priest or other clergy member will walk down the main aisle in the church holding a ceremonial censer of smoky incense, which burns throughout the ceremony. Research into why frankincense has been the preferred incense used in religious practices indicates it may be due to its documented mildly psychoactive properties, which relieve a variety of stressful emotional states like anxiety and depression. Research appears to support its positive effects and its purported ability to draw people toward contemplation, meditation, and prayer. Frankincense stimulates the areas of the brain utilized in states of focus, relaxation, and calm. Therefore, the choice of frankincense might be purposeful, putting us in a calmer state, enabling us to get in touch with our inner being, and fostering a feeling of safety.[180] It is quite amazing how *Boswellia serrata* reduces not only the inflammation of the body but also that of the mind.

Thanks to the emergence of natural boswellia products, there are now more than four hundred published studies on boswellia, with an average of one to two studies published weekly.

Which Boswellia Extract Is Best for Me?

You might have tried supplements with boswellia before with some or limited success. This is because, as is also the case with curcumin, most boswellia is not standardized. Consumers often get boswellia extract from bark or root powder when the actual anti-inflammatory properties come from the gum resin. Thus, the part of the boswellia tree that manufacturers use makes all the clinical difference.

Without standardization of certain components (boswellic acids, AKBBA, polysaccharides, etc.), the effectiveness of a boswellia supplement can vary from batch to batch, bottle to bottle, manufacturer to manufacturer, season to season, and species to species. Beware of products on the market that are using other parts of the boswellia plant—like the leaves and bark—since these plants are grown more for their use as an incense and not as an efficacious, potent, and pure supplement. But they can still be listed as "boswellia" on supplement bottles!

Research has now shown that certain primary components of boswellia are responsible for its health benefits. Therefore, in order to get true therapeutic value, you must ensure that you are obtaining those components. Various types of boswellia have been shown to have more or greater benefits than others, with *Boswellia serrata* leading the research.[181]

Let me help educate you on what to look for when it comes to a boswellia product.

First, look to see if it is standardized to a certain amount of *boswellic acids*. Boswellic acids exhibit anti-inflammatory, analgesic, and antiarthritic activities through a unique 5-lipoxygenase (5-LOX) and human leukocyte elastase (HLE) inhibition mechanism. These acids are crucial to creating an effective boswellia product **(see fig. 29)**.

Boswellic acids also inhibit the activation of NF-kB and, consequently, downregulate TNF-alpha and decrease the pro-inflammatory cytokines IL-1, IL-2, IL-4, IL-6, IFN-gamma, and LTB4.[182] This means that boswellia helps the lower various inflammatory markers involved in many diseases. Boswellia has recently gained significant attention due its effect on chronic inflammatory diseases and its anticancer properties.

If a boswellia product is not standardized to contain boswellic acids, then you are not getting the full benefit from it. I would not take a boswellia product that contains *no* boswellic acids. In general, clinical studies have found that products standardized to contain from 30 percent to 85 percent boswellic acids are the most effective on their own. (But the results are even better when combined with other boswellia components. See below.)

Second, look for how much AKBBA (acetyl-11-keto-beta-boswellic acid) is in the product. This should also be standardized to a certain percentage (between 5 percent and 30 percent AKBBA). This component appears to be just as important in improving effectiveness as boswellic acids alone. Products standardized to have AKBBA and boswellic acids are much more effective than *Boswellia serrata* (extract or powder) alone.

Third, look for PS (Polysal—polysaccharide). A newly discovered part of boswellia has been named a Polysal (PS) fraction. In Bosmeric-SR, this Polysal fraction is called Boswellin PS. It is the new benchmark for boswellia supplements as it contains all three major components of the compound (Polysal, AKBBA, and boswellic acids).

Without all three of these components, you simply aren't getting what your boswellia product is promising.

Boswellia serrata—Boswellin PS: The New Gold Standard

Boswellin PS is the new gold standard for boswellia. In addition to its documented anti-inflammatory effects, this combination of the three critical compounds at specific potencies has been shown to be more readily and more quickly absorbed. Boswellin PS contains the key polysaccharide fraction Polysal that improves therapeutic benefits and increases the absorption and efficacy of both the boswellic acids and AKBBA.[183] Studies have been conducted to see how much of each of these main components one needs to maximize the anti-inflammatory benefits of boswellia.

In developing Bosmeric-SR, we intended to create full-spectrum anti-inflammatory activity that has an immediate onset of action (water soluble) and a sustained-release effect that lasts over eight hours. Boswellin PS gives us a clinically significant synergistic effect from a patented compound. Boswellin PS contains only clinically tested, specific dosages of Polysal, boswellic acids, and AKBBA, providing for maximum clinical benefits every time.

Once an ingredient has shown promise, most companies will try to cram the highest dose possible into their supplements. For example, some companies use only AKBBA at 90 percent concentration, with no boswellic acids or Polysal. This type of "more is better" approach, which I consider to be the general pharmaceutical approach, does not necessarily translate into better results. Scientific data has shown that synergistic compounds—not a "scorched earth" approach that bombards the body with high doses—appear to have the most beneficial effects.

Careful scientific investigation into each of the three important synergistic components of boswellia has detailed the specific ratios that provide the greatest anti-inflammatory effects. Bosmeric-SR uses these ratios. When it comes to a boswellia product, high concentrations of these three ingredients matter less than specific potencies in the right combination. Bosmeric-SR provides just that.

How Much Boswellin PS Should I Take?

If you take a product that is standardized to have at least 65 percent boswellic acids and 10 percent AKBBA, then I recommend 500 mg twice daily with food. But if you take Bosmeric-SR, which contains the patented components of boswellia in the most effective ratios (Boswellin PS), then you need to take only 200–400 mg (that's one to two caplets of Bosmeric-SR) twice daily with food. Again, with the synergistic and enhancing benefits of curcuminoids (combined additionally with ginger and black pepper), Bosmeric-SR is more effective than even boswellia products that may offer higher concentrations of AKBBA or boswellic acids alone.

Please see **Side Notes: Figure 33: Boswellin PS in Bosmeric-SR vs. others** for a comparison of boswellia products and see our website for general details at **www.bosmeric-sr.com**.

Ginger and Gingerols

Bring me the fragrance of ginger.
—BING CROSBY

We all know about and have eaten some ginger during our lifetimes. It's a sweet, aromatic root with a pungent and hot taste. Some people enjoy drinking it as a tea, some eat it with sushi, and others enjoy it as candy. Ginger the rhizome (otherwise known as the underground stem of the plant *Zingiber officinale*) is a common food ingredient that has been used for thousands of years in Ayurvedic and traditional Chinese medicine to treat a wide variety of conditions. Practitioners most commonly use ginger to treat conditions related to digestion: nausea, vomiting, upset stomach, diarrhea, and motion sickness. To this day, many people grow up sipping ginger ale when sick with a stomach bug. Clinical studies have shown ginger to be helpful for nausea during pregnancy, and it is one of the safest natural therapies for this type of condition. In fact, it is the only natural product—which is actually a food—that even conventional medicine recommends and has given an "approved use" stamp for nausea in pregnancy, as all other medications have side effects that are harmful to mother and baby.

Ginger contains nutrients that have good *spasmolytic* properties, which is just a way to say that ginger micronutrients soothe and relax the intestines. Doctors commonly recommend ginger to patients who have undergone intestinal surgery, as it also confers great protection against infections. Ginger helps aid many anti-inflammatory problems that occur in smooth muscles or even in the skeletal muscles.

People use ginger not only for GI troubles but also for arthritis, the common cold and flu, painful menstruation symptoms, headaches, and even various cancers. As of the writing of this book, there are over 2,400 studies on the various benefits of ginger published in the scientific literature.

Ginger: Activities and Actions

Ginger has been shown to have the following properties:[184]

- Immunomodulatory (strengthens the immune system)
- Antitumorigenic (prevents tumors development)
- Anti-inflammatory
- Antiarthritic
- Antihyperglycemic (prevents elevated blood glucose)
- Antihyperlipidemic (prevents elevated blood lipids)
- Antiemetic actions (prevents nausea and vomiting)
- Chemopreventive actions (helps prevent cancer growth when consumed frequently)

Some of the most studied actions of ginger are its analgesic and anti-inflammatory effects through the inhibition of NF-kB, COX-2, and 5-LOX (the major pathways and switches of inflammation mentioned previously). Ginger also has been shown to protect against cancers and to demonstrate a chemo-protective effect, meaning it protects the body from the side effects of chemotherapy. Some characteristics of ginger's actions include the following:[185]

- Induction of apoptosis (programmed cell death) of cancer cells
- Inhibits IkBa kinase activation (upregulates apoptosis)
- Upregulation of BAX (a proapoptosis gene)
- Downregulation of Bcl-2 proteins (cancer associated)
- Downregulation of prosurvival genes (anti-apoptotic) Bcl-xl, Mcl-1, and Survivin
- Downregulation of cell-cycle-regulating proteins, including cyclin D1 and cyclin-dependent kinase 4 (CDK4) (cancer associated)
- Increased expression of CDK inhibitor, p21 (anticancer associated)
- Inhibition of c-Myc, hTERT (cancer associated)
- Abolishes RANKL-induced NF-kB activation
- Inhibits osteoclastogenesis (type of bone cell that breaks down bone tissue to remodel and repair)
- Suppresses human breast-cancer-induced bone loss

If you or a loved one has been stricken with cancer, then you probably know the importance of all of these functions. Thus, it's easy to see that ginger can play an important role in regulating not only inflammation but also various signals that affect cancer cells.

Ginger and its constituents have been shown to inhibit the following cancers:[186]

- Breast cancer
- Colon and rectal cancer
- Leukemia
- Liver cancer
- Lung cancer
- Melanoma
- Pancreatic cancer

- Prostate cancer
- Skin cancer
- Stomach cancer

To demonstrate just how important ginger can be to helping eliminate cancers, let's look at one example: ovarian cancer.

In ovarian cancer, there are usually some indicators of the inflammation, such as vascular endothelial growth factor (VEGF), interleukin-8, and prostaglandin E2 (PEG2). Ginger extracts have been shown to greatly decrease these inflammatory markers in ovarian-cancer patients.[187] Thus not only can it be taken as a tea or food to help warm someone who may feel cold or have nausea (especially those being treated with chemotherapy), but ginger also has a beneficial effect for those with serious health conditions like ovarian cancer.

Another interesting aspect of ginger is its hypoglycemic effect against enzymes linked to type 2 diabetes. Anyone who has diabetes or even mild insulin resistance can enjoy this added benefit of ginger; it is not harmful to those who are taking diabetes medication. Instead, it may improve overall glucose control. In addition, keeping blood glucose in the lower/normal range is optimal for those with cancer, even if they do not have diabetes (I will discuss this in more depth later).

To sum up, ginger is a strong antioxidant that can help with metabolic syndrome, diabetes, cardiovascular disease, dementia, and inflammatory conditions such as arthritis, osteoporosis, and even cancers. Thus, in addition to taking Bosmeric-SR, one should try to include organic ginger in the diet as much as possible. Try adding it to foods like salsa, smoothies, or stir-fry. Ginger is a staple in most Thai and Indian curries and sauces, which are both fun and easy to make at home to liven up the flavors of any meal. You can also cut off half an inch of organic ginger root and blend it in a juicer along with other veggies and fruits to give your juice a kick of spiciness. For those with weak digestion, **see Side Notes for Ginger Elixir Recipe** to jump-start your digestive system before meals.

What about Ginger Supplements—Which Is Best for Me?

Research shows that gingerols are some of the most important bioactive anti-inflammatory components in ginger. Most people have taken ginger products, but they may have experienced limited benefits because the supplement contained plain ginger powder. Most dietary supplements on the market contain ginger powder, which is virtually devoid of the beneficial compounds found naturally in ginger.

Ginger extract should be standardized to contain from 10 percent to 20 percent gingerols; the higher the percentage of gingerols, the stronger the health benefits (and the more pungent it is). Bosmeric-SR contains the highest amount of gingerols available today, standardized at 20 percent. A product that says it contains "ginger powder" or "ginger root" and that is not standardized to have gingerols in it truly is not worth taking. You are much better off buying organic ginger root and consuming it as a food, making it into a tea or using some of it in your cooking.

If you take a ginger dietary supplement, make sure it has at least 10 percent standardized gingerols and take 100 mg twice daily with food (most products recommend taking ginger with food). Bosmeric-SR gives you 200 mg of 20 percent gingerols twice daily, with a sustained release that offers lasting effects over eight hours—virtually your entire working day.

Since all four ingredients in Bosmeric-SR act upon cancer pathways,[188] the formulation may help those who have cancer. Its anti-inflammatory and stomach-calming effects are wonderful for those undergoing chemotherapy, as nausea is a common side effect. Taking Bosmeric-SR may not only reduce feelings of nausea safely but also help the condition and protect the noncancerous cells at the same time. For everyone else, Bosmeric-SR may be a wonderful way to help reduce systemic inflammation in the body and prevent future chronic diseases and cancers from occurring in the first place.

See Side Notes: Figure 34: Ginger comparisons in Bosmeric-SR vs. others, as well as our website for general details at **www.bosmeric-sr.com**.

Black Pepper—Not Just the Other Shaker on the Table

Shake it, shake it, shake it.
—MICHAEL FRANTI & SPEARHEAD

Almost everyone has eaten black pepper. It is a common ingredient in many recipes, and most every table in homes and in restaurants worldwide holds a shaker.

Historically, black pepper was used as a spice and as a medicine. The underlying reason it became so ubiquitous is rooted in science. Black pepper enhances bioavailability. In other words, black pepper helps improve the absorption of whatever one takes with it, improving the digestive process and the absorption of foods in tandem.

Black pepper is used not only in foods but also in Ayurvedic medicine. It has been a staple in formulations to improve the absorption of natural medicines for thousands of years.

BioPerine is a patented and standardized extract of black pepper (*Piper nigrum*). Piperine, an alkaloid contained in black pepper, causes its pungent bitterness; BioPerine has been patented and standardized to contain exactly 95 percent piperine. When BioPerine is added to Curcumin C3 Complex, it has been shown to increase the absorption and length of time for penetration in organs such as blood, bone, heart, liver, spleen, kidney, and muscle more than just with Curcumin C3 Complex alone.[189] This is why Ayurvedic medicine traditionally places black pepper with curcumin in medicines and also why we cook our spices together in our foods. Bioperine also has been shown to increase other vitamins and nutrients dramatically **(see fig. 35)**.

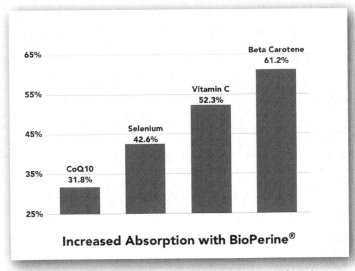

Figure 37: BioPerine increases bioavailability of vitamins and nutrients

BioPerine has the ideal bioavailability-enhancing potency needed from black pepper, and it has been clinically demonstrated to aid in the absorption of many supplements. Piperine has been shown to improve the absorption of curcumin, boswellia, and ginger from 30 percent to 60 percent. That is a *big* difference. Not only are you getting the most potent and clinically effective forms of curcumin, boswellia, and ginger in Bosmeric-SR, you are getting 30 percent to 60 percent increased absorption—sustained over eight hours.

BioPerine: Activities and Actions[190]

There are currently over five hundred modern cell, animal, and human studies that describe the following actions and properties of black pepper (piperine), contained in BioPerine.

- Anti-inflammatory (e.g., COX-2)
- Antioxidant (i.e., lipid peroxidation)
- Antiasthmatic/anti-COPD
- Immunomodulatory
- Chemopreventive (prevents cancer cells from growing)
- Controls progression of tumor growth
- Anticancer (i.e., decreases NF-kB, STAT-3, and MMP-9)
- Assists in cognitive brain functioning
- Boosts nutrient absorption and bioavailability of herbal and conventional drugs
- Improves gastrointestinal functionality
- Antimicrobial
- Antiulcer (gastro-protective)
- Antidepressant
- Antiamoebic

BioPerine helps to boost the anti-inflammatory, antioxidant, anticancer, and gastro-protective properties of the Curcumin C3 Complex, Boswellin PS, and ginger extract combo while enhancing the overall absorption of the formula.

How Much BioPerine Should I Take in a Supplement?

For those who take BioPerine in a dietary supplement, the clinical dose for enhanced absorption of curcumin is 5 mg per 250–500 mg of curcumin (the same dose applies to boswellia and ginger). Many companies tend to put less than 5 mg of BioPerine in their supplements, just enough that they can include it on the label and market the increase in absorption. But, more often than not, these amounts aren't even close to the clinical dose needed for improved absorption. If you see a product with less than 5 mg of BioPerine, question the other ingredients in the product as well. Again, this is where the industry uses hard data for marketing purposes, employing a bait-and-switch tactic, whereby they make consumers aware of the benefits of BioPerine but then shortchange them by providing so small a dose that it delivers virtually no clinical benefits. This bait-and-switch tactic again illustrates the frequency with which companies prioritize profits above efficacy, safety, and purity.

If a product contains "black-pepper extract" only, then beware of this as well. You're probably not getting a product standardized to contain 95 percent piperine (the clinically effective concentration), and therefore, you will not get the results that the company claims (directly or indirectly).

See Side Notes: Figure 38: BioPerine comparisons in Bosmeric-SR vs. others, or for more details visit our website, **www.bosmeric-sr.com**.

Can Black Pepper Be Dangerous?

Over the past few years, this question has come up, not only from consumers or from people who have had problems but also from other supplement companies that sell natural anti-inflammatory products and do not want to use the patented form of piperine (i.e., BioPerine) or use black pepper at all (again, to keep their profits higher). In fact, some of these companies have their director of education/marketing state that the increased absorption provided by black pepper could potentially increase interactions with prescription medication and cause liver problems. Let me assure you that this is just a scare tactic.

First, black pepper has been used safely for thousands of years without any side effects or harm. I have been practicing medicine for nearly twenty years, and I have never heard of any fellow doctor or health regulatory agency warn the public to be careful of taking medication with meals that may contain black pepper. You probably had some black pepper the last time you ate lunch or dinner. Black pepper has never been banned from a restaurant table anywhere in the world!

In fact, it's quite the opposite. Millions of people worldwide take their medications daily with food that has black pepper in it. In some cultures and dishes, there may be dozens of times more black pepper than you would get in any dietary supplement.

Try not to become a victim of fear mongering and scare tactics. Companies use educational, marketing, or sales people to disseminate this misinformation on purpose—to drum up sales for whatever they are selling or to discourage customers from purchasing a competitor's product. Nothing more. No actual MD or anyone trained in nutrition would ever tell you to avoid black pepper unless you have an allergy to it. Most respectable supplement companies understand these scare tactics, but unfortunately many wholesalers, retailers, and health-care providers don't. Don't buy into the hype. More importantly, you might want to question companies that go to such lengths to create such misinformation.

What Is the Recommended Dosage of Bosmeric-SR?

Now that we have discussed all the various ingredients in Bosmeric-SR, you may be wondering where to begin. I have formulated its composition to make this very easy.

Take two caplets twice daily with food for the clinical dosage. This is what I recommend for those with moderate to severe inflammatory pain or related conditions. I also recommend that most of my patients take this amount for at least two to three weeks or until their discomfort is improved. Then they can reduce to one caplet twice daily with food for maintenance. If patients cannot reduce their dose to one caplet twice daily, then this tells me that they have more inflammation in their body and that they must follow the **Ten-Step Approach to Optimum Health and Longevity** fully, as outlined in this book.

Those who need cancer-supportive treatments or are having a severe flare up of their condition may choose to take two caplets three times daily with food to get full twenty-four-hour benefits until their symptoms and conditions resolve.

Why Is the Price So Different from Other Products with Similar Ingredients?

Bosmeric-SR is the strongest natural anti-inflammatory dietary supplement for pain and inflammation support currently available.* Read that again.

In order to make a statement as bold as that, I needed to ensure that the product not only works but also works better than everything else. That is why I only use the patented and standardized forms of all ingredients (when possible) and the exact potencies that have been shown to have the best clinical outcomes. All of that, coupled with the unique instant-yet-sustained delivery system, is what makes Bosmeric-SR so different and so effective: it actually works, and it works very well.

Bosmeric-SR provides another benefit. Since it works for so many inflammatory conditions—including allergies, asthma, arthritis, colitis, cancers, and more—you should be able (with guidance from your health-care provider) to eliminate repetitious products that you are taking to treat these conditions symptomatically. For example, for most of my patients who are taking numerous dietary supplements, on average, *Bosmeric-SR will replace between four and twelve different products*—that includes supplements, OTC, *and* prescription medications. This provides immediate cost savings to the patient and an efficacy boost that immediately helps with a wide swath of health conditions.

Once you take the above into consideration—or even look at the cost of separately obtaining the ingredients at the same potencies and purity of Bosmeric-SR—the cost savings are *huge*. Again, for detailed comparisons to other products on the market, please visit our website (**www.bosmeric-sr.com**). Although some of these products may seem less expensive than Bosmeric-SR, they are actually more expensive, since most of them provide smaller amounts (a typical bottle might contain only a fifteen to twenty day supply), have reduced potency, or contain only one ingredient (not multiple synergistic and patented ingredients).

For example, here is how some (unnamed) competing brands compare:

- One brand sells a bottle of forty-five capsules for $56; at a recommended serving size of three capsules, this gets you a fifteen-day supply.
- Another brand sells a bottle of sixty capsules for $59; at a recommended serving size of two capsules a day, this gets you a thirty-day supply.
- A third brand sells a bottle of sixty capsules for $27; at a recommended serving size of four capsules a day, this gets you a fifteen-day supply.

On top of that, these other "pure" supplements do not provide immediate onset of action (i.e., make you feel better right away) and then sustained release over eight hours (i.e., keep you feeling better for longer). I encourage all readers to take a closer look at what quality supplements are really worth to them in terms of money spent and health improved.

What about Other Similar Turmeric and Boswellia Combinations?

One of the most successful (in terms of sales) products on the market contains a combination of another patented form of curcumin and boswellia. It seems to be slightly less expensive and seems to have two ingredients similar to those in Bosmeric-SR. Is there a difference? Absolutely.

For those interested, I will explain these differences on the Sanjevani website, but I do want to at least explain a trick ingredient that these products contain, which has been used in other brands to fool consumers.

Below us the ingredient label of one of the most popular dietary supplements on the market today:

3 capsules per serving.
Proprietary Complex: **2,181 mg**

DLPA (DL-phenylalanine), Boswellia (*Boswellia serrata*) Gum Resin Extract (BosPure) standardized to contain >70 Percent Total Organic and Boswellic Acids with AKBBA >10 Percent, with less than 5 Percent beta-boswellic acids, Curcumin (*Curcuma longa*) Rhizome Extract

(BCM-95) standardized for curcuminoid complex (curcumin, deme-thoxycurcumin and bisdemethoxycurcumin), Nattokinase.

Let's start with the ingredient that is used in so many of these "combination anti-inflammatory" products: *DLPA* or *DL-phenylalanine*. DLPA is an amino acid that does not decrease inflammation but makes the brain or its nerve receptors perceive that there is no pain. It has an immediate onset of action once ingested, so the user may feel that his or her pain is lessened, but in essence the pain hasn't gone away—only the user's *perception* of the pain has. This is a similar effect to someone taking a narcotic medication. Narcotics help take the mind out the body, but they do not act as anti-inflammatories. Thus, when the narcotic wears off, the pain is still there, requiring the person to take more medication.

DLPA is an inexpensive amino acid that manufacturers use as a pain-relieving ingredient, but let me stress this again: it is *not* an anti-inflammatory. Thus, companies that use this as the first ingredient in a formula (or in the top two or three ingredients) are watering down their product to give the consumer the *perception* that their pain is better without ever treating the underlying cause of that pain by reducing inflammation.

Now, in the above product, you can see that they do add curcumin and boswellia (at lower potencies and within narrower spectrums), but, more importantly, they do not list the amounts of each of those ingredients that are actually in the product. Remember, when a product lists a "proprietary blend" on the label, the first ingredient has the largest amount in the product. Using the above example, out of 2,181 mg of total product, how much is DLPA? I guarantee you that it is most of the product, meaning the product contains less curcumin, boswellia, and other ingredients.

The other trick with "proprietary blends" is that, since the individual ingredients are not listed *per capsule* or *per tablet*, the manufacturer can adjust those doses as they see fit whenever any of the ingredients becomes cheaper. They can also change the actual doses of each ingredient to make different SKUs or bottles or products.

For example, you might see a product with various price points and different bottle sizes that don't necessarily correlate with a price difference. That often means the manufacturer is lowering the amounts of the ingredients to make the product cheaper. So, for example, a manufacturer can increase DLPA—which is cheaper than curcumin, boswellia, and many other ingredients—in the same product and then sell it at a different price point.

In addition, be sure to check how many servings you need to take at one time and how many servings the bottle contains. The above example product is sold with seven, twenty, or forty servings per bottle. Therefore, many people will look at the price per bottle and tell me a product costs less...but then when they need enough for a month, it actually costs them more (and is less effective).

Many consumers believe that a one-month-supply bottle is standard, but in the dietary-supplement industry, that is not true. Most companies are moving toward smaller amounts to encourage people to purchase the product more often so they can advertise a lower price point.

When patients who come to see me have used or are using these sorts of products, and I recommend trying Bosmeric-SR instead, they notice huge and significant differences. I will say it again without hesitation: that is because Bosmeric-SR is one of the strongest natural anti-inflammatory dietary supplements available. Those other products sell well because patients get that "perceived" feeling of less pain, but once the DLPA wears off, they need more. And they will always need more because the supplement never really successfully tackles their underlying inflammation (and, therefore, their recurring pain). The formulation of these products compares poorly to the effectiveness and efficiency of Bosmeric-SR.

While the last couple of chapters may have seemed like an infomercial for this product, I hope it is now evident why I feel so passionately about Bosmeric-SR. The specific combination and potencies of Curcumin C3 Complex, Boswellin PS, and ginger extract in Bosmeric-SR with BioPerine to enhance absorbability is not by accident. This formulation has been purposely chosen, and its origin in the thousands of years of historical use in Ayurvedic medicine. In brief, this supplement has been designed to do the most good for the most people.

CHAPTER 9

STEP 7: Increase Immune-System Functioning

You like to think that you're immune to the stuff.
—ROBERT PALMER

The seventh step to obtain optimum health is to increase and maintain a strong immune system.

As I mentioned at the beginning of this book, our body has certain cells (which I like to call soldier cells) that aid our immune system. These soldier cells constitute the body's defenses and protect us against foreign invaders (infections such as viruses, bacteria, yeasts, and parasites). Within these defenses are branches, like the Army Corps of Engineers, that build and maintain systems and infrastructure (walls, levees, and fences) to help keep the immune system running and, in cases of direct attack, help repel invaders. Our immune system comprises the total strength of all of these forces, which together defend our bodies from invasion and help repair both damage from attack and the normal wear and tear that our systems suffer over time.

In addition to **steps 1 through 6**—which are vital to keeping your immune system strong—there are a few other items that power up your immune system's functioning. You can easily incorporate these into a daily regimen or keep them in reserve for when needed for acute or severe illness.

Vitamin D3

Sunshine on my shoulders makes me happy.
—JOHN DENVER

First, let's start with a supplement that you are probably familiar with: vitamin D3. By now almost everyone in the United States has heard of the benefits of vitamin D3, and many are taking it. I can't say enough good things about D3. More than 3,500 studies have examined this vitamin, and overall they have shown the following:

The lower the levels of vitamin D3 in the body, the worse and more degenerative any health condition will be. That's any condition from A to Z, from Alzheimer's to asthma, dermatitis to depression, and colitis to cancer. The higher your levels of vitamin D3, the better you feel and the fewer symptoms you have. I recommend everyone get his or her vitamin D3 level checked via a simple blood test, which most insurance companies cover.

The startling truth is that most people in the United States are deficient in vitamin D3, and most people think their vitamin D3 levels are higher than they actually are.

The vitamin D3 range (measured in nanograms per millilter of blood) follows:

- 0–10 ng/ml = Deficient
- 10–20 ng/ml = Insufficient
- 20–30 ng/ml = Hypovitaminosis D
- 30 ng/ml and above = Normal

Most doctors who have been following the scientific literature understand not only that everyone needs to be above 30 ng/ml (they are measuring mainly for bone health), but also that optimum immune function benefits occur between 50 ng/ml and 100 ng/ml. The data further suggests that when tests show *vitamin D blood levels are between 50 ng/ml and 100 ng/ml, there is reduction in chronic-disease occurrence,*[191] *including an 80 percent reduction in diabetes occurrence*[192] *and 77 percent reduction in all cancers.*[193]

These benefits make vitamin D3 supplementation one of the biggest public-health measures that our country can undertake at a minimal cost. Most other countries' health agencies are now trying to increase their citizens' vitamin D levels so they can lower the risk of chronic diseases and illnesses in their populations. That lowered risk will allow them to spend less money than the United States does on health care.

But misperceptions about vitamin D3 are both numerous and commonplace, including the following:

- **Most people think that their vitamin D3 levels are OK if they live in the Southwest or in sunny areas.** This is not necessarily true. Although there may be more sunshine in those areas, we only get vitamin D3 from direct sunlight on the skin. This is why everyone in general has lower levels in the United States. We all work indoors, go to school indoors, and ride in cars, buses, or subways; we rarely get large amounts of direct sunlight. In fact, when we do get direct sunlight, many of us use high-SPF (sun protection factor) sunblock, which decreases the risk of skin cancer but also decreases our absorption of vitamin D3 from the sun (this decreased absorption has been shown to increase our risk of all other cancers).

- **The darker one's skin color, the higher their vitamin D3 levels.** This is absolutely incorrect. There was a misperception (which still exists) in medicine that we only needed to check for vitamin D3 levels in the stereotypical fair-skinned people with red freckles who easily burn in the sun and, thus, spend most of their time indoors. The truth is, what we know about D3 levels holds equally for those with darker skin color. Unfortunately, many African Americans, East Indians, Mexicans, Latinos, and other people of color are not tested as often, since this misperception still pervades many doctors' thinking. When we look at overall vitamin D levels, the populations that have the lowest across the board are African Americans and East Indians! The skin pigment in darker-skinned people prevents their skin from burning and decreases their risk of skin cancer, but darker skin also limits how much vitamin D3 can be converted and absorbed. Therefore, everyone, regardless of race and gender, should be tested for vitamin D3 levels and supplement with recommended doses to get to a target range (in tandem with appropriate monitoring by doctors). Again, this simple test and supplementation would help decrease future chronic disease and improve everyone's current health conditions.

For those people with vitamin D deficiencies or who simply are not in the optimum range, I recommend a daily average dose of 5,000 IU per day with one's largest meals. I offer my patients a tiny vegetarian capsule (no fillers) or a liquid that provides 1,000 IU per drop. Vitamin D3 is a fat-soluble vitamin, meaning it is better absorbed (up to 60 percent better) when taken with a healthy fat, such as organic ghee, coconut oil, avocados, olive oil, or nut butters.

Prevention is key to lifelong health, and vitamin D3 helps precisely that. Interestingly enough, one can also use vitamin D3 for acute health problems. When patients are coming down with a cold or flu, bronchitis, sinusitis, or some other minor illness, I recommend that, at the instant they start to feel achy or have a sore throat or a fever, they start taking higher doses of vitamin D3 for three to five days. For example, I recommend that most of my patients take 20,000 IU or 30,000 IU daily for three to five days and then return to the 5,000 IU or their regular daily dose once the cold or flu has subsided enough. This increase in vitamin D3 helps upregulate their immune system and causes soldier cells to become more active and help assist the body's own innate abilities to heal itself. Some integrative doctors today give their patients 100,000 IU of vitamin D3 per day for three days instead of a Z-Pak antibiotic for upper-respiratory infections. Although this is very effective, I still would see a doctor for evaluation of your infection, and I may hold on the antibiotics for a while to see if the D3 takes care of the cold, flu, or infection symptoms (which is usually the case).

D3 upregulates the immune system so effectively that pharmaceutical companies are currently undertaking clinical trials to make vitamin D3 a prescription drug as an adjunctive treatment for cancer patients. Yes, you read that right: in the future, vitamin D3 may become a prescription drug.

The problem with most of the recent studies is that the pharmaceutical companies are using vitamin D analogs (chemical compounds with similar properties) in order to obtain patent protection, which will allow them to charge outrageous prices if vitamin D gets approved as a cancer drug (revenues are projected to be in the thousands of dollars per treatment if it is used for cancer). So far, these vitamin D3 analogs do not work as well as the vitamin D3 that is most easily obtained—but not patentable, unless someone figures out a way to patent sunlight.

Hopefully, all of this will convince you of the importance of vitamin D3—when even drug companies see the potential benefits (and potential profits). A substance that can deliver a greater than 75 percent reduction in the risk of developing future health problems, including cancer, *and* it can improve your current health? And all you have to do is take enough vitamin D3 to keep your levels in an optimum range? How easy is that?

As always, it is not how *much* of a supplement you take that makes the difference, but whether or not you are in the optimum target range between 50 and 100 ng/ml. Once you get to the target goal, whichever dose you have been taking should become your daily dose to keep you in that range. I recommend testing every six months. Vitamin D testing costs very little to add to routine screening labs, like for lipid and blood-glucose levels.

I do see some patients who have received vitamin D by prescription from their doctors. The problem that I have encountered with prescription D is that when a physician writes a prescription for vitamin D3, the pharmacy can actually fill vitamin D2. (I wrote a prescription for myself and later checked to see if this was true—it was.)

The problem is that vitamin D2 is an inferior form of D. It is not as bioavailable and does not absorb as well as the D3 form. Therefore, when I checked the D levels in my patients who have been taking prescription D, most were absorbing far less than the high doses prescribed—even in people taking 50,000 IU in a single dose every week! As an aside: A one-time "mega dose" can be helpful for those who have trouble remembering to take daily pills, but I have found over the years that it is best to take a consistent daily dose rather than creating a peak and then a fall over the next few days until the next dose. It appears that the immune system likes to remain at a constant level of strength and support.

Another aside: If someone has digestive issues (as serious as IBS) and is taking an acid blocker, when that person takes a "mega dose" of vitamin D once a week, I find that he or she almost always has lower D levels. If the GI system is already having a malabsorption problem, the patient won't get the full absorption or the full benefits of vitamin D3.

Finally, make sure that whatever vitamin D3 you take does not contain fillers or unnecessary ingredients. It should only contain a vegetarian capsule, vitamin D3, L-leucine, and silicon dioxide (to stabilize it). Avoid D3 supplements that have multiple inappropriate ingredients such a SLS, colors, and other fillers. The same goes for vitamin D3 in a liquid form.

Beta Glucans

Now that you understand the overall immune-supportive benefits of Vitamin D3, I want to teach you how to specifically stimulate your soldier cells to be more active. This is through the use of *Sanjevani Beta Glucan 300*. This all-natural formula uses specifically beta 1,3D glucan, which is scientifically proven to support, balance, and strengthen the immune system. More than ten thousand published studies demonstrate beta glucans biological benefits to health and immune system activity. Beta glucans are natural compounds that increase macrophage activity. Macrophages are part of the immune system that help trap and consume foreign substances that do not belong in the body, such as viruses, bacteria, and cancer cells. Motivated by this significant field of research, several dozen companies over the past decade have emerged that make beta glucans from a variety of sources, all claiming to be of superior quality. They all have impressive marketing materials and show benefits in their marketing studies.

I was using these products with success to treat my own patients when I asked myself, Is there a better form of better glucans, in terms of efficacy? To find an answer, I took it upon myself to investigate which form provided the best quality, potency, and purity of beta glucans. This investigation led me to Dr. Vaclav Vetvicka, one of the leading scientists in the field of beta glucans research. I learned from him what the actual scientific data demonstrates is the best source.[194] I then sought to find the owner of the patent (immunologist AJ Lanigan) on the best source and created **Sanjevani Beta Glucan 300**.

Sanjevani Beta Glucan 300 is produced with a minimum of 83 percent Beta-1,3D Glucan content, with no harmful contaminants. In comparative studies of competitor products in the beta glucans market, our source outperformed all others. It has been tested side-by-side with all of the best-known and most widely available immune supplements and modulators, and it has outperformed all of them.[195] This superior performance includes better phagocytosis of neutrophils, stimulation of Interleukin-2, stimulation of antibody response, increase of superoxide production and increase in IFN-γ (interferon gamma). Most other beta glucan products are less potent compounds, so much less potent that an 8-fold, 16-fold, 32-fold, 64-fold, 128-fold, and even 160-fold dose would be required to obtain the benefits contained in a single dose or even a fractional dose of Sanjevani Glucan 300. The material in Sanjevani Beta Glucan 300 is *biologically active* at 1/8th the dose or even 1/16th the dose recommended for a 100 mg capsule, and we provide only a 500 mg dose. In other words, it would take thirty to fifty times the dosage of another product to elicit an immune response even close to Sanjevani Beta Glucan 300's effects. The purity, biological activity, and the potency of Sanjevani Beta Glucan 300 surpass all others. (**See Side Notes: Sanjevani Immune-Support Protocols, Sanjevani Glucan 300 for more details.**)

I recommend two capsules daily on an empty stomach (eating nothing for thirty minutes) for general health maintenance. For those with chronic health conditions or cancer, one capsule should be taken for every 50 lb. of weight (i.e. for a 150 lb. person, three capsules daily on empty stomach). It takes about two weeks for Sanjevani Beta Glucan 300 to start to modulate the immune cells from the bone marrow. Therefore I recommended for cancer patients or chronic-disease patients to start two weeks prior to chemotherapy, radiation therapy, or surgical procedures. For more information of the benefits and comparisons of Sanjevani Beta Glucan 300 to other beta glucans on the market, please search **Sanjevani Beta Glucan 300** at **sanjevanistore.com.**

I recommend taking certain other natural products in addition to Sanjevani Vitamin D3 and Sanjevani Beta Glucan 300 to keep your immune system strong when someone is sick or entering regions or situations where they may get sick.

Some of my favorite immune-system boosters follow.

1. Sanjevani Vitamin D3 (capsules or drops)
2. Sanjevani Beta Glucan 300
3. Sanjevani Immune Formula

4. Sanjevani Complete Probiotic Formula (pills or powder)
5. Sanjevani Vegetarian Strengthen Shake
6. Sanjevani HistaPlus Formula
7. Megaway Shakes
8. Cannabiseology Shakes
9. CBD (cannabidiol) products
10. Organic India Tulsi Teas
11. Manuka Honey (+15 actives or MGO 400+ or higher, for adding to teas or beverage during flu/cold seasons or when sick)

(See Side Notes: Sanjevani Immune-Support Protocols for more details.)

Physical Vascular Therapy—BEMER*

Improving your circulation will also increase and keep your immune system strong. Blood circulation is the human body's transport system. It supplies the tissues and organs with all the important nutrients and vital oxygen while removing and disposing of resulting waste products. It also helps stimulate the immune system by keeping the white blood cells (the soldier cells of the immune system) flowing and actively working to fight, fix, and repair. About 75 percent of this activity takes place in the smallest blood vessels, where it's called "microcirculation."

Although one can improve general circulation through exercise and yoga (see chapter 11), health conditions cause many people to have trouble with improving their microcirculation. Most people do not exercise enough once they have chronic pain due to injury or conditions like fibromyalgia, obesity, or even chronic fatigue. Although movement would be best for them, because of their pain, discomfort, and immobility, they remain static. Sometimes scar tissue from corrective surgeries for back injuries keeps patients in bed or on the couch. Others, due to injury or debilitation, may have to use wheelchairs. This lack of movement leads to stagnation of the microcirculation and increases pain. This leads to a vicious cycle in which one's mood can worsen over time and lead to depression. Most of us during our lifetime have had an acute back injury that made it difficult to move, but there are many people who, due to degeneration of the lumbar discs from a variety of causes, have that pain chronically.

At Sanjevani we use Physical Vascular Therapy, which is the new classification of a patented waveform of the next generation of pulsed-electromagnetic-therapy (PEMF) devices called *BEMER*. Although PEMF devices are very popular for home use and in doctors' offices and pain clinics, few are supported by published studies, except for a patented device called BEMER, which has been used in Europe for over fifteen years. When we apply Physical Vascular Therapy technology, by having the person lie on the specialized BEMER mat, we see significant improvements in microcirculatory characteristics such as increased capillary perfusion, venular outflow, and oxygen utilization (a 29 percent increase for up to twenty-four hours after a twenty-minute session).[196]

Increasing microcirculation can improve the transport of cellular and humoral factors of the immune system, leading to decreased pain and increased healing responses. Various clinical studies have shown the benefits of improving microcirculation, including improved blood-glucose response and utilization in organ tissue, improved immune response, increased physical-rehabilitation response, improved wound healing, decreased pain and neuropathy, and increased pain-free walking in patients with peripheral arterial disease.[197] It even can help with erectile dysfunction.[198] Furthermore, increasing microcirculation has been shown to significantly lower pain and fatigue and improve sleep and quality of life.[199]

I strongly recommend that integrative or holistic health-care providers use the BEMER physical vascular therapy in their clinics. For patients who have difficulty in finding a clinic that offers it or who prefer to use it more frequently (which is recommended for optimum benefits), I recommend they obtain a BEMER Pro-Set for their personal use. For more information, visit **www.sanjevani.net** and look up **BEMER** or see **Side Notes: BEMER Physical Vascular Therapy**.

I have successfully used the BEMER on my patients who have a variety of conditions, from chronic back pain to fibromyalgia. It even works well with people who have macular degeneration, who after treatment demonstrate an improved ability to read an eye chart. It even has helped one of my patients with retinitis pigmentosa; after each treatment, his visual fields and color perception improve. We have never experienced this in conventional ophthalmology. When circulation (and overall immune functioning) to the eye structures improves, better blood flow and nutrients can penetrate and help improve the overall condition of the eyes. Now, BEMER therapy may not bring back sight for someone born with this type of condition, but any improvement in perception makes a world of difference to someone's quality of life. Since writing a chapter on "Peripheral Neuropathy" in David Rakel's medical reference textbook *Integrative Medicine*,[200] I have successfully treated many patients with this approach. I even treated one of my oldest patients, an eighty-seven-year-old who suffered painful peripheral neuropathy of her feet. I had treated her with neuro-acupuncture for two years, but although I decreased her pain successfully (for three to four weeks with each treatment), I could not significantly improve the level of sensation in her feet. That was not my normal outcome of treatment **(see Side Notes: Neuro-Acupuncture)**. However, after this patient's first treatment with the BEMER, she felt the sensation of the acupuncture needles, which was quite a surprise for both of us. Not only did the combination of the neuro-acupuncture treatments help her, but now with the increased microcirculation in her feet, the supplements that we provide for her neuropathy could penetrate better and provide her better healing responses **(see Side Notes: Peripheral Neuropathy Protocols)**. In Europe they use the BEMER for not only improving the microvascular circulation but also increasing the penetration and efficacy of any prescribed medications. Therefore, when using the BEMER, one may over time (with guidance of their health-care provider) be able to decrease their medications.

In addition to the above conditions, at Sanjevani we use the BEMER to help support cancer patients. Physical Vascular Therapy is very helpful to help facilitate their body's detoxification mechanisms, immune system support, and improve overall function though increased oxygenation of the body. Whether patients undergo conventional oncologic treatment or natural therapies, enhancing small-vessel circulation improves white blood cells' movement throughout the body. This is important to augment the healing response especially in areas of damage from surgery, chemotherapy, or radiation, which causes inflammation, swelling, and tissue damage. BEMER therapy in my patients has been able to help reduce their toxicity from these treatments, make those treatments more effective (patients respond better), and my help patients recover faster.* Even for those patients who are treated with pain medications that cause constipation, the BEMER has been critical to gently improving bowel function. Many integrative and holistic cancer clinics are now applying BEMER Physical Vascular Therapy to areas of concern prior to hyperbaric, hyperthermia, ozone, and IV therapies to improve outcomes.

CHAPTER 10

STEP 8: Maintain Healthy Glucose Levels and Avoid Excess Sugar and Salt

> *Pour some sugar on me.*
> —DEF LEPPARD

If you eat a lot of highly refined sugars, high-fructose corn syrups, and fructose from other sources, you are in for a rude awakening. High levels of sugars—especially fructose—have been *directly* linked in various studies to cardiovascular disease, diabetes, fatty liver, obesity, high blood pressure, mineral imbalance, osteoporosis, and impaired brain function. Even more worrisome is the rise in cancer risk, especially for breast cancer, triggered by the consumption of sugar and highly refined carbohydrates.[201] More than one hundred publications have shown the relationship between sugar and cancer.[202] In my opinion and clinical experience, too much sugar is not good for any chronic disease or any type of cancer.

Although most of the research has focused on the sugar that is added to processed foods or drinks—or sprinkled in coffee or cereal—we must remember that sugar has been added to so many foods that we don't consider sweet. Hundreds of brands of breads, pasta sauces, and salad dressings contain astonishing amounts of sugar. In fact 74 percent of packaged foods contain sugar.[203]

Even though Americans, on average, consume a variety of foods that are abnormally high in sugar, we get most of our excess sugar from sodas.

Therefore, the following sections in this chapter will focus not only on the general consumption of sugar, but primarily on the consumption of sugar via soft drinks. (As a side note, most of the studies on sugar did not include naturally occurring sugar in fruit. I usually recommend that my patients eat their fruit, not drink it, so that they may avoid higher concentrations of sugar.)

I recommend you take the time to review the following brief links and articles if you're as interested in the impact that sugar has on our health as I am:

- "Sugar: Killing Us Sweetly: Staggering Health Consequences of Sugar on Health of Americans," by Dr. Gary Null, on the Centre for Research on Globalization website, GlobalResearch.com, Feb. 4, 2014
- "Soda Contributes to Behavior Problems Among Young Children" by Alexandra Sifferlin, *Time Magazine*, Aug. 16, 2013
- Any article on KicktheCan.info, a website sponsored by the California Center for Public Health Advocacy

I recommend that all readers review these articles and websites for excellent references and specific details on this controversial topic. I have added some additional commentary and data in this chapter to emphasize the various health risks associated with excess consumption of sugar and sweeteners, as well as the importance of maintaining healthy glucose levels for optimum health.

Sugar and Health-Care Costs

In 2013 a Credit Suisse Research Institute report titled "Sugar: Consumption at a Crossroads" detailed the rising cost and ramifications of sugar consumption on the health of Americans. The report revealed that "30%–40% of health-care expenditures in the USA go to help address issues that are closely tied to the excess consumption of sugar."[204] The figures suggest that *our national addiction to sugar runs us an incredible one trillion dollars in health-care costs each year*. The Credit Suisse report highlighted several health conditions—including type 2 diabetes and metabolic syndrome, coronary heart disease, and obesity—that numerous studies and consumption data have linked to excessive sugar intake.[205]

In 2012 the popular newsmagazine show *60 Minutes* aired a report by Dr. Sanjay Gupta titled "Sugar," which addressed the question of whether or not sugar is bad for your health. Dr. Gupta presented new research showing that aside from causing weight gain, sugar can be dangerous to your health by increasing the risks of heart disease and even cancer. Endocrinologist Dr. Robert Lustig gained national attention after a lecture he gave in 2009 titled "Sugar: The Bitter Truth" went viral. Dr. Lustig's research (over twelve published studies) has focused on the connection between sugar consumption and the increase in chronic diseases in the United States. Dr. Lustig's data illustrates that excessive sugar consumption is a major factor in the development of obesity, type 2 diabetes, hypertension, heart disease, and many types of cancer. His research led him to conclude that 75 *percent of all diseases in America today are brought on by the standard American lifestyle and are entirely preventable.*[206] A majority of doctors and scientists in the United States now share his conclusion.

Here are the current guidelines for daily sugar intake:[207]

- Women—no more than 6 teaspoons daily (about 100 calories)
- Men—no more than 9 teaspoons (about 150 calories).

Given that sugar is in nearly every packaged food, how do you know how many teaspoons of sugar you're consuming daily? The simple way is to check out *how much sugar, in grams,* a given product contains. Four grams of sugar is equal to about one teaspoon. Therefore, according to the guidelines above, the daily limit for women is 24 g, and for men it's 36 g.

A recent Gallup poll indicates that nearly half of all Americans consume soft drinks on a daily basis; those who drink soda average about 2.6 glasses per day, or 20.8 oz.—about two cans.[208] If those cans of soda are regular Coke (Pepsi is slightly higher), then that would equal about 67.6 g of sugar every day—that's 242 calories from soda alone.

Just two standard cans of soda put both men and women above the recommended daily intake of sugar. (Two cans of soda give women 2.6 *times* their recommended daily intake of sugar and men 1.8 *times* their recommended daily limit.) However, this amount of soda is just the tip of the sugar iceberg for Americans. It doesn't include Big Gulps, supersized drinks, morning doughnuts or bagels, snack foods like candy bars or trail mix, sweetened blended coffee drinks such as lattes, or the hidden sugar that makes up for the flavor lost in low-fat packaged or prepared foods.

The latest statistics tell us that the average American consumes *130 pounds of sugar each year—or more than one-third of a pound every day.*[209] On average, sugar adds about five hundred calories each day, which adds up to about one pound of body weight per week. Thus, if people do not exercise to burn those excess calories, they will gain weight almost instantly. This excess sugar is one of the major factors contributing to the obesity epidemic in the United States.

If you want to lose weight, the first step isn't exercise; it is to eliminate soft drinks from your diet. Just by doing this one simple thing, most of my patients start seeing immediate weight loss and overall improvements in their health. (Once they start moving toward a more plant-based diet and avoiding their food sensitivities, their health improves even more.)

When it comes to children and adolescents, excess sugar has even more insidious effects. A growing preteen may consume, on average, as much as 50 teaspoons of sugar every day; young males alone may be consuming over 100 teaspoons daily.[210]

A single serving of Baskin Robbins's Chocolate Chip Cookie Dough Sundae can have about 107 g of sugar,[211] without any additional toppings. That doesn't include the pizza, soda, and candies that one would normally consume at a birthday party. We have all experienced the way children and teens get physically and emotionally out of control at birthday parties.

To further demonstrate this point linking sugar and behavior, the latest research indicates that among five-year-olds, those drinking more sugar-sweetened sodas showed increased aggression, withdrawal symptoms, and difficulty paying attention compared to those drinking little to no sugar-sweetened beverages.[212]

This research represents the first time that the effects of sugared beverages have been traced to behavior issues among young children. But these findings mirror similar trends among adolescents; a 2011 study published in the journal *Injury Prevention* found that teens who drank more than five cans of soft drinks every week were significantly more likely to have carried a weapon and acted violently toward peers, family members, and dates.[213]

Another study from Sara Solnick and David Hemenway reported that high consumption of soft drinks was associated with a range of aggressive or mood-related behaviors, from fighting or feeling sad or hopeless to being suicidal.[214]

In a 2013 study published in the *Journal of Pediatrics*, parents reported that 43 percent of the five-year-olds participating in the "Fragile Families and Child Wellbeing Study" drank at least one serving of soda every day, and 4 percent consumed four or more servings daily.[215] This is a staggering number of children consuming a staggering amount of sugar each day. When one considers that an average five-year-old weighs about forty pounds (that's four times less than an average adult male), one serving of soda for a child is far more damaging than one serving of soda for an adult. Worst of all, consuming this amount of sugar consistently from an early age may be setting up our children for one of the most serious health crises of all: addiction.

Sugar and Addiction

I just want to make you go away,
But you taste like sugar.
—MATCHBOX TWENTY

Sugar has been called "the food cocaine" because of its sweet intoxication. That's right; the links between sugar and addiction are actually well documented in a number of studies. Dr. Carlo Colantuoni, an obesity researcher, famously demonstrated that excessive sugar intake causes serious dependence and that abstention from sugar creates withdrawal symptoms; in fact, Dr. Colantuoni and his colleagues showed that withdrawal from sugar is qualitatively similar to withdrawal from morphine or nicotine.[216]

Dr. Colantuoni's study is far from the only research on the topic. Numerous researchers have published similar findings concerning sugar addiction.[217] Using MRI scanners that measure the brain's reactions to sugar, scientists at the Oregon Research Institute established that sugar has an effect on the brain very similar to the effect of highly addictive drugs like cocaine.[218] I recommend watching an informative documentary called *Hungry for Change* that explains in simple terms how we become addicted to sugary foods and why it is so difficult for us to stop eating them.

Sugar and Aging

Pay your surgeon very well to break the spell of aging.
—RED HOT CHILI PEPPERS

Sugar doesn't only adversely affect children and young adults. Emerging research suggests that sugar is one of the most powerful aging substances known.[219] One of the most integral negative effects to consider when discussing the chemistry of aging is the bonding between glucose and collagen, called glycation. Glycation can result in many negative effects on an otherwise healthy body, including stiffening of the joints, muscle weakness, thickening of the arteries, and persistent and acute pain, all the way up to organ failure and death. While we may associate these health issues with normal aging, a reduction in sugar intake may actually create healthier aging by reducing both glycation and the production of free radicals significantly (more on that under "Sugar and Heart Disease").

In her July 2000 article in *Scientific American* entitled "AGE Breakers—Rupturing the body's sugar-protein bonds might turn back the clock," researcher Lisa Melton, PhD, discusses the ways in which diabetes hastens aging. The high blood-sugar levels among diabetics accelerate glycation and results in the formation of advanced glycation end products, or AGEs, which cause damage to the human body and rigidity in human tissues from "years of bread, noodles, and cakes." Even nondiabetics can suffer damage from high blood-sugar levels. It is therefore highly likely that restricting our dietary sugar intake (and, therefore, our caloric intake) may actually do more to slow the aging process than any other antiaging therapy currently available.[220]

Sugar and Appetite Suppression

Appetite for destruction
—AARON NEVILLE

We have all heard about "empty calories" when talking about sugary foods and drinks. Research is bearing this out, proving that a lifetime of sugar intake can actually lower your intake of necessary nutrients by suppressing your appetite.

Researchers have identified that a primary mechanism by which carbohydrates regulate satiety and food intake is through their effect on blood glucose. Anderson et al. found that food intake and subjective appetite are inversely associated with blood-glucose response in the sixty minutes following consumption of carbohydrates.[221] Hence candy and snack-food manufacturers will convince you to eat their snacks to control or calm your appetite—"You're not you when you're hungry." In essence your body is being fooled about what it thinks it is getting. These snacks may provide a temporary fix, but they can cause a long-term problem because they lack any real nutrition.

Sugary foods suppress the appetite and prevent people from obtaining a balanced diet. Important healthy nutrients are not found in sugary foods.[222] In other words, sugary snacks can cause malnutrition; the empty calories they provide are why, even though it seems to run counter to logic, obese people may actually be malnourished. They may be consuming nutrient-deficient calories.

Sugar and Heart Disease

The burning of the heart
—RICHARD MARX

An August 2000 study from researchers at the State University of New York in Buffalo reported that excess sugar in the blood increases the production of free radicals—damaged atoms or molecules with an odd number of electrons that damage healthy cells in their quest to even out their number of electrons. These free radicals have been linked to aging and heart disease. (Free radicals result when oxygen interacts with certain compounds via a process called oxidation; antioxidants—which must be supplied through diet—are thought to interact with free radicals to stop this destructive oxidative damage.)

The study demonstrated that healthy adults who received the equivalent of two cans of cola, or 75 g of pure glucose, experienced a significant increase in free radicals in the blood one hour after the drink and a doubling of free radicals after two hours. From this ingestion there was an increase in an enzyme that promotes free-radical production and a 4 percent decrease in blood levels of vitamin E. This study looked at sugar only, not the artificial colors, phosphoric acids, preservatives, and other chemicals in a typical soda! One of the researchers, Paresh Dandona, concluded, "We believe that in obese people, this cumulatively leads to damage and may cause hardening of the arteries."[223] Numerous other studies have demonstrated this relationship between high blood-sugar levels and an increased risk of heart disease.[224]

Sugar-Sweetened Beverage Consumption Increases the Risk for Both Diabetes and Heart Disease

Sweet, sweet sugar cola
—LOU BEGA

Compared to those who do not drink sugar-sweetened beverages, individuals who drink one to two sugar-sweetened beverages each day have a 26 percent higher risk of developing type 2 diabetes and a 20 percent higher risk of developing metabolic syndrome.[225] Women who drink more than two sugar-sweetened beverages daily have a 35 percent higher risk of heart disease.[226]

Most frighteningly, high levels of fat in the blood, liver, and abdominal region, which increase one's risk for heart disease and diabetes, can develop after very short periods of time consuming sugar-sweetened beverages. After only two weeks, young men and women who drink three cans of soda daily show a 20 percent increase in levels of bad cholesterol and triglycerides in the blood.[227] After just six months, women and men consuming three sodas daily display increased cholesterol, visceral fat, and fatty liver.[228]

A study by Quanhe Yang and colleagues at the Centers for Disease Control and Prevention (CDC) analyzed national health surveys between 1988 and 2010. This comprehensive study included more than thirty thousand American adults with an average age of forty-four years. The authors of these surveys used national death data to calculate risks of death throughout fifteen years of follow-up. Previous studies have linked diets high in sugar with increased risk of nonfatal heart problems and with obesity, which can also lead to heart trouble. But in this study, obesity didn't explain the link between sugary diets and death. *That link was found even in people of average weight who consumed high amounts of added sugar.*[229]

Adults who obtained at least 25percent of their daily calories from added sugar were almost *three times more likely* to die of heart problems than those who consumed the least (who had less than a 10 percent risk). For those who got more than 15 percent of their daily calories from added sugar—or the equivalent of about two cans of sugary soda—the risk was almost 20 percent higher than the safest level. To put it simply, having a sweet roll with your morning coffee, a supersized sugary soda at lunch, and a scoop of ice cream after dinner is enough to put you in the highest-risk category for heart disease, according to the CDC. That means *your chance of dying prematurely from heart problems is nearly three times greater than that of people who eat foods with little added sugar.*

Again, simply eliminating sodas will do your body a huge favor. You will likely lose weight, lower your blood sugar, and lower your cholesterol levels. This is such a simple lifestyle change, yet it is difficult for most Americans to do. If you are someone who drinks soda daily, you are more than likely to be swallowing a statin or diabetes drug along with it in the years to come, when simply avoiding sugary drinks today could decrease or eliminate some of the scariest preventable health risks you may face in your lifetime.

Sugar and Childhood Learning

> *I want candy.*
> —Bow Wow Wow

Dr. Stephen Schoenthaler has conducted diet research on children for almost thirty years. His simple yet profound studies eliminated sugar and junk foods from the lunch programs of one million school children in over eight hundred New York schools during a seven-year period (from 1976 to 1983).

In these studies, academic performance was established first, and then dietary changes were introduced to determine whether diet affected how well the children learned. In a systematic order, high-sucrose foods were gradually reduced or eliminated, after which selected preservatives (BHA and BHT) and synthetic colors and flavors were gradually eliminated, while researched recorded any changes in learning abilities.

The result? A 15.7 percent improvement (from 39.2 percent to 55 percent) in learning ability compared with other schools during the years that did not make changes to the diet. This improvement in learning was further demonstrated by the data that showed that out of 124,000 children who had once been unable to learn grammar and mathematics, 75,000 (or up to 60 percent) could perform these basic tasks at grade-appropriate levels after dietary changes alone.[230] Therefore, you can increase your child's intelligence and abilities just by eliminating sugar from his or her diet. Most of my patients who have taken their children off sugar have reported similar successes.

Removing excess sugar from the students' diets improved their behavior at school, which in turn improved their ability to learn. With the increasing consumption of sugar and lower education rankings over the past decade, all parents who have children with learning or behavioral problems should take a serious look at what they are feeding their kids (and what the school systems are also feeding them). We must wonder how much of a toll sugar is having on our children, their health, and their future ability to compete in the world marketplace. A simple, cost-effective lifestyle change like this should be a national priority, or at least a priority for every family.

Our current educational system is in crisis. The 2012 Program for International Student Assessment (PISA) ranked the United States twenty-seventh in math, twentieth in science, and seventeenth in reading.[231] While everyone is arguing about funding cuts and teaching programs, nobody is talking about the cheapest and easiest solution to help improve students' performance: taking sugary foods and drinks out of schools and providing real, healthy food.

Most people think that we are already doing that by replacing sodas with fruit juices, but that is a common misperception. Let me give you a few examples of vending-machine fruit drinks and their sugar content.

A bottle (16 oz.) of Minute Maid Orange Juice contains 48 g (12 teaspoons) of sugar; a bottle (16 oz.) of Langer's Apple Juice contains 52 g (13 teaspoons) of sugar; and a bottle (20 oz.) of Minute Maid Lemonade contains 67 g (about 17 teaspoons) of sugar. Therefore, fruit juices are no better than sodas when it comes to sugar content—many of them have even more sugar! When one remembers that most of these juice products are from brands owned by soft-drink companies, removing sodas was a relatively painless matter of a simple swap. Fruit juices give the same addictive effects as soda (spikes in blood sugar), though they're cleverly disguised as being healthier. Most of this "juice" that is advertised as being healthy actually states on the label that it "contains less than 5% juice"!

If we could replicate Dr. Schoenthaler's research—research that has been available for over thirty-five years—in schools nationwide right now, how much of a difference could this simple switch make for the youth of the country? As long as large food corporations have a say in what our children consume, we unlikely to ever find out.

Sugar and Childhood Behavior (or, More Accurately, Misbehavior)

Misbehaving
—QUIET RIOT

Sugar has been linked to increased misbehavior in children, yet this remains a controversial fact. With regard to sugar intake in particular, Dr. Schoenthaler again led the way. He worked with the Los Angeles Probation Department Diet-Behavior Program and observed 1,382 incarcerated teenagers at three juvenile detention halls. When eating a low-sucrose diet, these young delinquents showed a 44 percent drop in antisocial behavior on average. The greatest reductions in antisocial behavior, however, were seen in particular groups: repeat offenders (86 percent drop in antisocial behavior), narcotics offenders (72 percent), rape offenders (62 percent), burglars (59 percent), murderers (47 percent), and assault offenders (43 percent).[232]

Additionally, he followed the behavior of 289 juvenile delinquents at three juvenile rehabilitation centers. With the reduced intake of sugar, they exhibited a 54 percent reduction in antisocial behavior.[233] Another study by Dr. Schoenthaler, the Alabama Diet-Behavior study, monitored 488 incarcerated delinquents for twenty-two months. Again there was a decrease in antisocial behavior ranging from 17 percent to 53 percent (with an average of 45 percent), just from reduction of sugar in the diet.[234] The relationship between sugar in the diet and behavior in children is clear to me. Most of us have seen this and even experienced it personally with family and friends. Yet even though it seems to be common knowledge and even clinically evident, many people still debate whether sugar is a problem. Maybe if we look more closely at those who don't believe in the direct and causal relationship, we might find that they have financial ties to the sugar industry, the pharmaceutical industry, or prison systems. Personally I think they all have drunk the Kool-Aid!

Sugar and Childhood Obesity

Don't want to be a fat man.
—JETHRO TULL

Just one soda every day increases the risk of obesity in children by 60 percent. That was the result of a study entitled, "Relation between Consumption of Sugar-Sweetened Drinks and Childhood Obesity," published in *The Lancet* in 2001.[235] Sugar from sweetened beverages adds a massive amount of sugar to the diets of our children, delivering about 9 teaspoons daily for girls and 14 teaspoons daily for boys.[236] When one considers that about 65 percent of adolescent girls and 74 percent of adolescent boys consume sugar-sweetened drinks every day, is it surprising that America is facing a childhood obesity epidemic?

In addition, a more recent study demonstrated a startling key fact about the number of calories in twenty-ounce bottles of soda, sports drinks, and fruit juices: they are virtually identical. Each twenty-ounce bottle contained 250 calories, had 16 teaspoons of sugar; in each case it would take either fifty minutes of running or five miles of walking to work off those additional calories.[237] How many children (or adults) walk five miles a day or run for nearly an hour? And we haven't even accounted for all the fast food, junk food, and candies most children consume in excess!

Our children's overall lack of physical activity and increasing computer/tablet/smartphone use are only making them more obese—on top of their consumption of sugary drinks. Unfortunately their excess weight not only increases the incidence of heart disease, diabetes, and elevated blood pressure—yes, even in young people—but also puts them at a disadvantage economically. A recent study showed that obese young males will earn 18 percent less over their lifetime than those of a normal weight. According to the researchers who carried out this study, this is roughly the same lifetime-earnings penalty as missing about three years of college education.[238]

Again, the worst part of this health crisis is that it is entirely preventable through inexpensive and simple means: offering healthier food options, reducing sugar, and requiring physical activity as part of a regular school day.

Sugar and Dental Cavities

A mouthful of rotting cavities
—BECK

I am not a dentist, but there is no dispute that sugar is bad for our teeth. The more sugary foods and drinks consumed, the higher the risk of cavities. Soda consumption nearly doubles the risk of dental cavities in children and increases the likelihood of cavities in adults.[239] The acid in soda and other sugar-sweetened beverages causes erosion of tooth enamel, often after just one sip. And the sugar in these beverages provides fuel for bacteria that cause tooth decay and have a negative impact on digestion, which starts in the mouth.

Sugar, the Immune System, and Inflammation

Burning down the house
—TALKING HEADS

Several studies confirm a strong link among high consumption of sugar, the suppression of the body's immune system, and an increased incidence of inflammatory conditions. As mentioned in "Sugar and Aging," high amounts of sugar in the diet increase advanced glycation end products (AGEs), resulting in damaged proteins. As the body tries to break these AGEs apart, immune cells secrete inflammatory messengers called cytokines. These inflammatory signals trigger a variety of mechanisms that contribute to worsening inflammation-based health problems—or "itis" conditions.

Several studies have directly correlated the consumption of sugar to the suppression of the immune system. In one study in particular, researchers assessed ten healthy people's fasting blood-glucose levels and their phagocytic index of neutrophils (a measure of an immune cell's ability to engulf and destroy invaders such as cancer). These subjects consumed 24 teaspoons of carbohydrates from glucose, sucrose, and orange juice. This amount of sugar—regardless of the source—resulted in a significantly decreased capacity of neutrophils to engulf bacteria, effectively paralyzing these soldier cells.[240]

What does this mean? It means that drinking three cans of soda, a Big Gulp, two bottles of apple juice, or two bottles of sweetened iced tea or eating three small yogurts daily feeds you enough sugar to weaken your immune system. A weakened immune system means that your body is less able to fight off invaders and repair itself, leading you to have a higher risk of chronic diseases, infectious diseases, and cancers. As an aside, complex carbohydrates from starches, surprisingly, did not have this same immune-dampening effect.[241]

More recently, a Japanese study reported that sugar causes the increase of a particular protein that inhibits macrophage activity, which appears to disrupt and weaken the immune system.[242] Bacterial invasion and infectious disease can result from elevated blood sugar, even going as far as to cause sepsis.[243] In those who have candida infections, excess sugar in the diet exacerbates the candida overgrowth; thus, ridding oneself of candida involves not just antimicrobial treatment and probiotics but avoidance of sugar.

The Unsweet History of Sugar

Stolen from Africa, brought to America
—BOB MARLEY

In the book *Sugars and Sweeteners*, authors Kretchmer and Hollenbeck estimate that in the four centuries prior to the abolishment of slavery, the transport of slaves involved twenty-two million people. Of these, twelve million were taken to the Americas. The rest died during transport or shortly after arrival. The authors state, and other historians back this up, "Sugar was responsible for 70% of the traffic of slavery."[244] This history of the sugar industry and slavery is often overlooked or not commonly known, yet it is critical to understand how this sweet crop was not so sweet to begin with.

Disparities in Sugar-Sweetened-Beverage Consumption

I think it's time to tell the truth.
—DAVID LEE ROTH

Latinos and blacks are more likely than whites to consume sugar-sweetened beverages on a daily basis.[245] This unfortunate inequality is directly influenced by a lack of grocery stores, a high prevalence of convenience stores, and the low cost of sugar-sweetened beverages compared to healthier beverages in many predominantly Latino and black communities,[246] along with a long history of marketing that targets these communities.[247] According to an FTC report titled *A Review of Food Marketing to Children and Adolescents in 2009*, the beverage industry spent $395 million—more than $1 million per day—on marketing campaigns directed at youth.[248] This is the second highest marketing budget for any consumable product.[249]

In addition to the sugary soda drinks, the US fast-food industry spends "nearly a quarter of their marketing budgets targeting youth aged 2 to 17 years," according to Arizona State University nutrition professor Punam Ohri-Vachaspati, who authored a recent study that showed, "In 2009, fast food restaurants spent more than $700 million to market their products to children and adolescents; nearly half of the amount went toward premiums such as kids' meal toys."[250] The study also determined that a majority of black communities, rural areas, and middle-income communities are disproportionately exposed to this fast-food marketing. Fast-food chains in predominantly black neighborhoods were about 67 percent more likely to use child-directed marketing—like indoor displays of kids' meal toys—than those in white areas. Each day, almost a third of children aged two to eleven years and more than 40 percent of twelve- to nineteen-year-olds consume food and drinks from fast-food restaurants. Therefore, minorities—especially children—are aggressively targeted by fast-food and beverage companies to consume unhealthy drinks and foods, which lead to obesity, diabetes, and other completely preventable health problems.[251]

Keeping Healthy Blood-Glucose Levels

Get the balance right.
—DEPECHE MODE

We should all be concerned about insulin resistance, metabolic syndrome X, and diabetes—different names for a health condition in which your blood glucose is elevated above normal levels. One must understand that blood glucose is one of the most important things to keep within the normal range, and the most current scientific data indicates that keeping it in the lower part of the normal range is better.

Most doctors screen their patients by ordering a fasting glucose test (which comes as part of their complete metabolic panel—CMP). Unfortunately, fasting glucose levels are not the best way to detect whether you have a blood-glucose problem or not. Although this test can show if your levels are very high, most people can have a normal fasting glucose and still have blood-sugar problems. Let me give you a simple analogy for this phenomenon using the stock market.

If you look at a particular stock price at this very moment, that is equivalent to a fasting blood-glucose level. It is just a snapshot in time. But stocks are always fluctuating up and down. When you take only a snapshot of a stock, you get the price of the stock at the exact time you checked it, but it could either trend up or down at any point thereafter.

A fasting glucose level is very similar—it tells only your blood-sugar level at that specific time. Your blood sugar is as volatile as the stock market, so it is best to get a test called HBA1c, or hemoglobin A1c, to get a better idea of your blood-sugar levels overall. This test gives an overall measurement of what your daily level has been averaging over the past three months. If you were to look at a three-month history of the stock that you were interested in, you would see an overall trend—taking into account more data—that would allow you to calculate whether or not your stock has gone up or down or has been stable. The HBA1c works by testing the blood-glucose levels that are attached to the hemoglobin molecule on our red blood cells. Since our red blood cells have a three-month life cycle, this tests your average daily blood glucose over that period of time.

Traditionally, medical doctors would only order an HBA1c test when a patient was diabetic. They did this to see if patients were recording their home blood-glucose levels correctly and taking their medications as directed. Patients often reported feeling guilty if they came in with their blood-glucose logbook and had elevated numbers, so they sometimes reduced their logged numbers to look like they were doing better. However, the HBA1c gives doctors a three-month average to compare against the logbook, allowing us to have more accurate pictures of patients' "real" numbers. In addition, a test called GlycoMark looks for spikes in blood-glucose levels even with normal blood-sugar levels. If the test shows high spike levels, then an investigation into the foods a patient consumes may provide an explanation for why such spikes occur. For example, someone may eat a highly refined sweet snack that causes a large spike in blood sugar, but the body may, for the time being, still have the ability to correct for it.

Integrative-medicine MDs, and most good primary-care doctors, are now ordering HBA1c tests for all their patients, as we want to detect blood-sugar problems earlier instead of waiting until patients have serious complications. That's because blood-glucose problems are not a single problem but only the first domino to fall in a series of problems that can result from this one imbalance.

Terms like "insulin resistance" and "metabolic syndrome" have been used to describe what is occurring prior to and up to the development of full-blown diabetes, which is when elevated blood glucose starts a cascade of other health problems. For example, with elevated blood glucose, one can develop high blood pressure, an increase in lipids (cholesterol), an increase in weight, and a host of other problems that are far better avoided.

The problem with conventional medicine is that we tend to treat elevated blood-glucose symptoms and the secondary problems of blood-sugar issues separately—by medical specialty. That means if someone has heart disease and elevated cholesterol levels, and that person also has elevated blood sugar, his or her cardiologists may only focus on the heart disease. The cardiologist may give statins and blood-pressure medication but will not help manage the patient's blood sugar; in his or her mind, that is an internal-medicine, family-medicine, or endocrinology problem. Without a holistic and integrative approach, a patient's care becomes disconnected, with each doctor treating separate symptoms instead of the cause of the blood-sugar problems. Let's explore this disconnection more closely.

If someone has elevated blood sugar or diabetes, they are at a fourfold increased risk of developing heart disease. Why? Because when blood glucose is elevated, insulin (the well-known hormone secreted from the pancreas that helps bring glucose into the body to be utilized as fuel) resistance develops over time because of the continued consumption of highly refined carbohydrates and processed foods (e.g., white bread, white flour tortillas, doughnuts, and pastries), highly sweetened snacks (e.g., candy bars) and sugary drinks (e.g., soft drinks), and other triggers that cause inflammation of the pancreatic cells. This inflammation in turn causes an imbalance whereby the body cannot absorb glucose into its cells, muscles, and organs, and the glucose instead remains in the bloodstream. This excess fuel—or energy—that the body cannot use is then converted to fats (both excess weight and elevated lipids/cholesterol).

Additionally, once blood sugar is elevated, there is an increase in the metabolic pathway to convert more omega-6s **(see fig. 10)**, triggering more inflammation—not only systemically but also in the endothelial (internal) lining of the arteries—leading to more cholesterol and plaque formation. This plaque formation is the body's attempt to calm the inflammation initially, but when there is chronic inflammation, the repair becomes a hindrance. This pathway of inflammation and the complications from it become a vicious cycle.

When eating the standard American diet (SAD), people obtain most of their calories from highly processed and refined foods. This in turn creates spikes in their blood-glucose levels, and over time their insulin loses the ability to bring it down.

All food has a glucose number, called its glycemic index, which tells how much your blood glucose will rise once you consume that food. White bread is the standard measurement to which other foods are compared, as it has one of the fastest glycemic indices and is the most consumed item in the SAD. White bread and similar highly refined grain foods have been "predigested;" the manufacturing process removes the whole-grain and fiber content—in addition to other core nutrients. This makes the processed grain product easier to chew, cut, slice, and pull apart, and it also increases the rate of absorption and conversion to glucose. As a result, blood glucose spikes immediately after consuming these refined foods. While that doesn't sound very appetizing, these types of foods are popular because a glucose spike gives a quick, satisfied feeling of having instant energy. But soon thereafter, energy levels crash, and you feel hungry again. And so you eat again. This rapid cycle is part of what makes these foods so "addictive."

Most people don't know it, but packaged foods are manufactured to create the fastest glucose spike and the steepest crash, timed physiologically to be almost the same, in everyone who eats them. When I graduated from medical school, I knew two students who, instead of going to a residency program, went to work for snack-food companies. After food scientists figured out the ideal artificial flavors and scents to entice us, the young doctors would conduct tests using various combinations of fats, sugars, and salts to create the quickest glycemic spike, sustain it for a certain period of time, and then end the spike with a huge crash in blood sugar. By testing blood samples of paid volunteers in private food-science laboratories, they could figure out what composition of ingredients would best create this artificial and repeatable physiological response.

You might be wondering, why would they do this? What would be the purpose? If it weren't so detrimental to human health, the work of these doctors (and the work of countless others like them) would be the pinnacle of human biological science.

These food companies conduct these tests and create their foods so precisely so that once the average teenager at school or adult in the workplace eats a snack, his or her physiology is basically *on a timed cycle to spike and crash exactly as food companies want it to*. Most of these packaged products have been calculated to create that specific rollercoaster of soaring highs followed by a massive crash—timed to happen right before the next class or workplace break. The food companies are not kidding when they tell you that they "bet you can't eat just one." They are telling you up front that if you eat one of their food products you won't be able to stop.

Many people blame the obese by labeling them as lacking willpower. But that is not always true. Most people will say that they literally can't stop eating once they start. They are experiencing a physiological response that nearly every major food company has studied, tested, and packaged to ensure continued consumption of its products. Consumers are Pavlov's dogs, and food companies are the ones ringing the bell.

It doesn't matter who you are, the strength of your willpower, how educated you are, or how rich you are. This controlled glycemic-spike-and-crash response works the same way on everyone. If I eat any of these foods—even though I know better and have a physician's understanding of the health risks—I will still have difficulty stopping myself. Because chemistry is involved, not just will power. Once your blood sugar spikes so suddenly, your insulin level must spike even more severely just to catch up. Then, once this surge of insulin attaches to the glucose and brings it into your body's cells, it drives your blood-sugar levels down not just to normal but to slightly below normal, creating the condition known as hypoglycemia—the crash. After your calculated time of feeling really good really quickly, the crash begins. Now you feel even hungrier than when you first started eating, so at your next break, you will again be at the vending machine to get another quick pick-me-up from the same snack food. This engineered physiological cycle is what makes snack-food companies some of the most profitable companies in the world.

Avoid this rollercoaster ride by not allowing yourself to get on it to begin with. That is the willpower you need. Try to learn not to put these foods into your grocery cart when you go shopping. Do what you can to replace these quick-fix foods with something that you really like that is genuinely satisfying—generally foods that don't come in a box.

Sugar and Cancer

Give me fuel, give me fire, give me that which I desire.
—METALLICA

Dr. Otto Warburg, a Nobel Laureate in medicine, discovered in the 1930s that cancer cells have a different energy metabolism compared to healthy cells. He discovered that increased cancer-cell production was related to a low-pH and low-oxygen cellular (respiration and fermentation) environment. This in turn shifts metabolic processes within cancer cells to increase glycolysis (the conversion of glucose into energy) at a higher rate than normal cells, which in turn increases lactic-acid production, creating the ideal acidic environment for the vicious cycle of cancer-cell growth. Warburg demonstrated the direct relationship between sugar intake and the risk of cancer-cell growth.[252] Since cancer cells cannot master the more complex synthesis of glucose from larger molecules, they require a direct supply of glucose. This makes the buildup of lactic acid and an acidic pH in the body, caused cancer cell's direct consumption of glucose, a diagnostic factor for cancer.[253]

Over the past decade, more and more research is investigating the role of glucose in the body as it relates to the growth of cancer. This relationship now is so widely understood that at the most recent cancer conferences I attended, discussion shifted to potentially classifying cancer as a metabolic disease. Researchers now understand that cancer exhibits certain metabolic behaviors, with its direct relationship to glucose and inflammation, that keep its cells alive, well fed, and growing.

One of the most interesting characteristics of all cancer cells (which makes cancer a metabolic disease regardless of what type it is and where it is located) is the fact that cancer cells have about ten times or more insulin receptors on them than healthy cells. This means that cancer cells uptake ten times or more blood glucose than regular, healthy cells, and one must not overlook or underestimate the relationship between them.[254]

With this understanding, over the past thirty years many integrative and holistic oncology centers around the world have been advocating low- to no-sugar diets in cancer patients, because glucose (sugar) indisputably feeds cancer-cell growth. If you know someone with cancer, encourage him or her to immediately stop any and all extradietary sugar (the only sugar he or she should consume should be that found in natural sources like fruits). Frighteningly, many chemotherapy centers provide dairy beverage products and bowls of candy to "keep up the energy" of the patients going through treatment, when in reality they are feeding their patients' cancer.

A novel approach to treating cancer that is fast becoming the most promising new cancer therapy is the introduction of metabolic inhibitors that block these glucose pathways in cancer cells, shutting them off and stimulating cell death (apoptosis). One such therapy is the invention of a novel compound called 3-BP, or 3-bromo-pyruvate. Although seemingly a simple molecule, it took over fifteen years of research to learn how to stabilize the molecule to get successful and safe results. It is a lactic-acid analog that can "trick" the cancer cells and enter like a Trojan horse through their lactic-acid transporters. Then it can destroy the cells' energy production, causing cancer-cell death internally. This therapy is more specific to the cancer cell versus normal cells (due to the difference in metabolic functioning). A renowned scientist, researcher, and patent owner (as well as good friend of mine) named Dr. Young Ko has conducted animal studies with amazing outcomes, including a few case studies that have been published in scientific literature.[255] To learn more about 3-BP, I highly encourage all my cancer patients to read the book called *Tripping Over the Truth: The Metabolic Theory of Cancer* by Travis Christofferson. He nicely details the history of cancer treatment discoveries from past to present and highlights novel therapies on the horizon. I also recommend that health-care providers read this book, as it covers many historical facts that are not usually taught to us during medical training. (However, please disregard the last few chapters on the ketogenic diet, as I am in disagreement with the use of this diet for cancer patients. The most recent scientific data has shown only seen short term benefits by switching energy metabolism due to decreasing highly refined carbohydrates and sugars, but not long term benefits without eating high amounts of antioxidants, phytonutrients and fiber – which is limited in ketogenic diets. Placing patients in a continued state of ketosis is not normal, nor is compliance easy to maintain for long periods of time. Consuming plant oils, phytonutrients and antioxidants from a plant based diet seems more natural and cheaper than taking ketogenic supplements). Only certain certified cancer clinics (outside the U.S. currently) and other countries are now able to provide 3-BP safely and correctly. Additionally, clinical trials are underway to make this new compound available for use worldwide as an effective cancer therapy without the toxic side effects of conventional chemotherapy and radiation. To keep up with the latest information about 3-BP scientific studies, clinical trials, and medical centers certified in providing 3-BP treatment, visit the official site approved by Dr. Ko, **www.3bpKo.com**.

I am also proud that these certified cancer clinics using 3BP and clinical trials are including Bosmeric-SR and other Sanjevani products (e.g., the Sanjevani Intensive Support Pack) and dietary recommendations as part of the overall cancer support protocol for their anti-inflammatory and anticancer benefits. **(See Side Notes—Sanjevani Intensive Support Pack for**

details.) This falls in line with what integrative-medicine doctors have been saying for decades: that a comprehensive and supportive treatment protocol will provide an optimum outcome and is preferable to a monotherapy or "magic bullet" approach to all health treatments.

All of this is to reiterate the point that keeping blood sugar in the normal range is important for lowering your risk of developing cancer and other chronic diseases. People who have insulin resistance, metabolic syndrome (syndrome X), or diabetes have a higher risk of developing cancer because, if they have cancer cells in their body, their elevated blood glucose creates a beneficial environment for those cancer cells to grow. For those who don't have cancer, that's even more of a reason to keep your average blood glucose levels in the optimum range—between 70 mg/dl and 114 mg/dl. This will help reduce one more risk factor—in this case a factor with influence over many potential future problems. Those who have had cancer and want to prevent recurrence should keep their average blood glucose levels between 70 mg/dl and 100 mg/dl to minimize any chance of cancer cells regrowing. This is where eating a plant-based diet and avoiding highly refined sugars, oils, and carbohydrates are key in preventing and reversing most health conditions—even cancer.

What about Natural Sugars?

Like it's only natural
—ROB THOMAS

There is a new way of thinking when it comes to the relationship of sugar to cancer-cell growth. The *form* of sugar that is ingested may make all the difference with regard to cancer growth.

According to some holistic cancer doctors, who study this in detail with their cancer patients—it's not the category of sugar, but the *form* of sugar that is important. Here's what he means.

When we eat whole plant foods like fruits, their sugar molecules are in what is called the "L-form" (meaning they rotate leftward) which is the natural form. When we take supplements like amino acids, the L-form is best absorbed by the body and, therefore, is more effective (e.g., this leftward rotation of the molecule is what the *L-* refers to in L-lysine and L-arginine). However, most highly refined sugars are converted through conventional food processing and end up in the "R-form" (right rotation). In addition, the sugar molecule from fruits is a disaccharide, which contains both fructose and glucose, but with highly refined sugary foods you get only the glucose molecules. Fructose undergoes metabolic utilization slightly differently than glucose; whereas glucose directly feeds cells (in this case cancer cells), those cells are less affected by fructose (especially in cancer-cell metabolism). Thus, these holistic cancer doctors find with their patients—as did practitioners historically who prescribed juicing, like the famous Dr. Gerson (Gerson Therapy)—that patients who consumed natural sugars from fruits (in moderate amounts) showed improved outcomes and did not worsen their condition. Mother Nature provides us safe, natural foods; therefore, it is most likely that cancer patients (as well as everyone else) can consume natural sugars from fruits in moderation without exacerbating their health conditions. It's only when sugar comes in the form of processed juices (which add more glucose) and refined carbohydrates that it provides a detrimental outcome, since our body may metabolically use this refined sugar in a negative way. This is an area that needs further research, but it will most likely be validated; as experience shows again and again, "nature nurtures," whereas "man-made, processed, and refined" usually harms.

Many patients ask me why most doctors and oncologists do not seem to understand the relationship between blood sugar and cancer growth. My guess is that they are simply practicing what they learned from those before them and are not looking at cancer as something that comes from within someone; instead, they look at it as a foreign invader (and are trained to wage "a war on cancer"). Thus they focus on recommending surgery or giving chemotherapy and radiation to "blast it or kill it" at all costs. But trying to kill cancer with toxic therapies without including the body's own immune system in the process is somewhat willfully ignorant of basic physiology. In addition to conventional treatments, we should use all measures possible that incorporate the body's own natural defenses and strengthen them along the way. This approach only improves the success of treatment and the survival of the individual, regardless of what type of treatment the person elects to pursue.

Many doctors (even oncologists) think that the idea that cancer is a metabolic disease or is strongly related to blood glucose is a strange concept. Yet these doctors actually demonstrate this principle every day in practice. When a cancer patient gets a PET scan to see if the cancer has metastasized (spread from one site to another, like colon cancer spreading to the bone or lungs), the PET scan itself uses the same mechanism as the metabolic effect of glucose on cancer cells! During a PET scan a radioactive tracer is attached to a glucose analog that is injected into the body. As this tracer travels throughout the body via the bloodstream, if there are cancer cells (or an infection), then those cells grab onto the tracer, since it has a higher receptivity to the glucose molecule. The radioactive tracer concentrates into the area with cells that grab onto it and causes the area to light up on the scan. In other words, the only places in the body that take up the radioactive marker are those that are more *metabolically active*. This demonstrates very simply that cancer is a metabolic disease. The PET scan has been used for over thirty years; it is ordered hundreds of times daily across the United States, yet we tend to forget how this test actually works and what it tells us about cancer-cell metabolism. We just deliver toxic treatments to the affected areas and never investigate the nature of why and how that cancer exists.

Many of my cancer patients have asked their oncologists and doctors the same question: "Does sugar affect my cancer?" Most of these patients report being told that "sugar plays no role in cancer growth" or cancer metabolism. I then instruct my patients to ask their doctors, "If sugar does not play a role in cancer, how does a PET scan work?" If their doctor can't figure out this connection, as described above, they might be interested in looking for another doctor who does.

Cancer doctors around the world (and now a few in the United States) have understood this concept very well for years, and they have innovated groundbreaking approaches to put this metabolic understanding into practice. When cancer patients receive conventional chemotherapy, although they may receive different types of chemicals for different types of cancer, those chemicals basically affect every cell in the body, similar to the way antibiotics work. Thus, if we are treating breast or colon cancers, chemotherapy affects not only those sites but also every part of the patient's body from the toes to the top of the head. In consequence, although chemotherapy kills the cancer cells, it kills many, many healthy cells as well. This is why many patients who undergo chemotherapy die: not from their cancer but from the cancer treatment. It's a truth about cancer treatment that isn't talked about too widely—that it's a battle of endurance. A majority of cancer patients die from the toxicity of the chemotherapy and the damage to healthy cells in the body during the treatment. Not to mention the fact that conventional cancer treatments of chemotherapy and radiation therapy increase inflammatory markers such as NF-kB and other inflammatory factors that also increase the recurrence of cancers.[256]

Chemotherapy also eradicates the natural probiotics in the GI tract, and it is an order of magnitude more effective than antibiotics in doing so. This is why it is imperative for cancer patients to take large doses of probiotics (I recommend *Sanjevani Complete Probiotic Powder Formula*) to help heal their guts, improve their immune-system functioning, help keep them from worsening leaky gut, and reduce the severity of their weight loss/cachexia.

Over the past few years, research has shown that although chemotherapy can kill cancer cells, it also causes severe damage in the body and triggers other mechanisms for cancer growth elsewhere (by lowering immune-system functioning, stimulating protein synthesis of new cancer cells, and stimulating a few other mechanisms, such as the increase or release of CXCL1 and CXCL2, WNT16B, c-FLIP, Bcl-xl, IAP-I and IAP-2, XIAP, and Survivin. The turning on or increasing of these factors may explain why those who receive chemotherapy have higher cancer-recurrence rates and also higher chemotherapy-resistance rates.[257]

New cancer therapies on the horizon, such as 3-BP, focus on using the metabolic pathways that cancer cells utilize and targeting those functions directly, essentially turning them off, thereby shutting off the cancer cells' ability to grow, without harming healthy cells in the body. As baby boomers continue to age, I feel hopeful that this big segment of the population will demand more innovations in cancer treatments.

Artificial Sweeteners—Are They Effective and Safe?

> *All that's artificial*
> —ERASURE

Artificial sweeteners have been marketed for years as safe or healthier alternatives to sugar. Research does not support either of these facts.

Let's look at the example of diet soda. A common misperception is that diet soda helps people lose weight by reducing the calories in sodas to nothing or virtually nothing. Studies—including a study at Johns Hopkins Bloomberg School of Public Health[258]—have shown repeatedly that diet-soda drinkers increase their risk for a number of health issues. They think they are making a smart choice when they are actually not. The Johns Hopkins study discovered two important factors that contribute to the negative impact that diet soda has on overall health:

1. Diet-soda drinkers generally don't make any other changes to their diet.
2. Obese or overweight people are more than twice as likely to drink diet soda as adults at a healthy weight.

Therefore, changing from regular to diet soda has very little effect on a person's dietary choices overall. The sad aspect of this behavior is that overweight or obese people want to lose weight and think that diet soda will help them; in actuality, it may cause them to gain weight (which in turn makes them purchase more diet sodas—helpful only to the soda manufacturers). In fact, many studies now show that to be the case.[259]

If diet soda has zero or few calories, how does one gain weight or have trouble losing weight when drinking it? The zero calories are not the problem; the problem with artificial sweeteners is that they are not glucose, a molecule that your body recognizes as the main source of fuel. Even though artificial sweeteners taste sweet to our tongues, in our stomachs it's a different story. Artificial sweeteners do not trigger the receptors for identifying glucose in the stomach, so the stomach tells the brain to eat more food.

So, diet soda won't help you *lose* weight. Is it at least safe to drink? Not necessarily.

Most artificial sweeteners, like the pink packet (saccharin), the blue packet (aspartame), and the yellow packet (sucralose), have animal studies as well as human data that catalog a variety of side effects. Some are minor and some can be major, such as migraine headaches, visual disturbances, increased seizure risk, increased muscle pains—even increased risk of developing certain types of cancer. As a doctor, I recommend that you avoid these products as much as possible. The documented side effects are just not worth it when there are alternatives.

Stevia, for example, has been shown over many decades of use worldwide to be without health risks. Stevia is a non-nutritive natural sweetener derived from a leaf that has about three hundred times the sweetness of sugar but does not increase blood-glucose levels. In fact, some data indicates that stevia might have some other health benefits as an anti-inflammatory, antihypertensive, antihyperglycemic, antitumor, antidiarrheal, and diuretic, and it may even have immunomodulatory effects. Although stevia is not bad for you, I would not recommend it for medical conditions, but I would also not be concerned about the intake of it.

The only problem with stevia, as with all sweeteners as described above, is that it can lead you to consume more calories, since your stomach does not receive the glucose signal when you consume stevia; therefore, you might still eat more food with a stevia-sweetened beverage—but without any harmful side effects. Therefore, if you choose to sweeten your beverage, you can use stevia, but sparingly, so it won't lead you down the path of consuming more food that you don't need or crave to have only sweet flavors.

The Question of Salt

Searchin' for my lost shaker of salt
—JIMMY BUFFETT

In addition to recommending that my patients lower their consumption of refined and artificial sugars, I also encourage them to be cautious of the high amounts of added salt in packaged and restaurant-prepared foods.

Everyone knows that excess salt consumption contributes to elevated blood pressure, swelling, and fluid retention, as well as other negative health outcomes. But how much salt are we actually consuming? The recommended daily intake of salt *should not exceed 2,300 mg*. Those with high blood pressure, African Americans, or those over the age of fifty-one should be consuming an even lower amount—around 1,500 mg per day.

Here are a few examples of the amount of sodium in classic frozen meals, which we all have heard of or consumed:

Jimmy Dean Breakfast Bowl—Pancakes and Sausage Links with Syrup:
1,000 mg of sodium, 710 calories, and 34 g of fat

DiGiorno Small Size, Supreme Traditional Crust:
1,330 mg of sodium, 770 calories, and 32 g of fat

Boston Market Buffalo-Style Chicken Strips with Macaroni and Cheese: 1,500 mg of sodium, 680 calories, and 31 g of fat

Banquet "Extra Helping" Salisbury Steak Dinner:
2,363 mg of sodium, 646 calories, and 40.5 g of fat

Hungry Man (Swanson) Classic Fried Chicken:
2,869 mg of sodium, 960 calories, and 45 g of fat

You can see that most of these common, classic frozen meals have at least half or more of our total recommended daily amount of salt (not to mention almost half or more of our daily calories and fat). Although this sounds frightening to some, these meals actually contain less salt than you get when you go out to eat—which many people think is healthier. Below is a current list of the "top 10 saltiest meals" at common chain restaurants:[260]

10. Chili's Boneless Buffalo Chicken Salad:
3,730 mg of sodium

9. Cheesecake Factory Sunrise Fiesta Burrito:
4,600 mg of sodium

8. Chili's Chicken Crispers—Honey Chipotle Style:
4,910 mg sodium

7. Applebee's Sizzling Skillet Shrimp Fajita:
5,140 mg of sodium

6. TGI Friday's Jack Daniel's Ribs and Shrimp (without sides):
5,140 mg (add 980 mg of sodium if with fries)

5. Chili's Texas Cheese Fries:
5,310 mg of sodium

4. On the Border Firecracker Stuffed Jalapeños with Original Queso:
5,760 mg sodium

3. PF Chang's Dan Dan Noodles:
6,190 mg of sodium

2. Applebee's Appetizer Sampler:
6,260 mg of sodium

1. PF Chang's Hot and Sour Soup Bowl:
7,980 mg of sodium (or more than *three days' worth of sodium*—the sodium equivalent of forty-four bags of Doritos Cool Ranch tortilla chips!)

If these are the amounts of unhealthy ingredients in classic frozen meals and popular dishes at chain restaurants, what do you think we are eating when we go to all-you-can-eat buffets?

This is why we are so unhealthy in America: too much sugar, fat, and salt, along with large amounts of animal proteins and GMO foods. If you have diabetes or are overweight, a typical American diet might be the reason.

If your doctor has told you that you have essential hypertension, you now should understand there is nothing essential about it. There is always a trigger to being unhealthy; we just have to explore and investigate what is causing our problems. As I hope you're realizing as you read this book, the food we eat daily is most of what causes our health problems.

Is All Salt the Same?

> *The salt of the earth*
> —THE ROLLING STONES

The short answer is no. Unfortunately, many scientists and doctors believe that salt is salt, but the type of salt, its source, and the way it is processed do make a difference.

Most salt that you see in a saltshaker is not good for you and may cause you harm. We have all used the common brand of table salt that has the girl with the umbrella on it. Although used for decades as a common food ingredient, this type of salt is processed with other chemicals and really should be used for deicing your driveway—not for adding to your food.

Regular table salt is 97.5 percent sodium chloride and 2.5 percent chemicals like moisture absorbents, as well as iodine. It's dried at over 1,200°F, and this excessive heat alters the natural chemical structure of the salt. This makes a big difference in how it affects the body.

When consumed in large amounts—as seen with classic frozen and popular restaurant meals—this typical table salt causes increases in blood pressure, swelling and water retention, joint pains, and kidney and gallbladder stones. When you look at those table-salt crystals under a microscope, their shape is irregular. This is the result of chemical cleaning, which in turn causes the body to use more energy to break up the sodium and chloride molecules. This in turn causes the body to use more intracellular water to neutralize and get rid of this excess salt—up to twenty-three times more water per single gram of sodium chloride.[261]

Many countries commonly use mined salts, such as Himalayan salts and even sea salts, for their "table salt." Sea salts are wonderful; however, they can also be problematic. Ocean waters are often contaminated with chemicals, mercury, PCBs, and other toxins. The purity of the water used for sea salt is often not regulated or filtered. On top of that, 89% of all the sea-salt producers now refine their salt.[262] This can make a difference, especially when it comes to the cheap "sea salt" used in fast-food, restaurant, and packaged-food industries.

I prefer to use Himalayan salts, or pink salts that are mined from the Himalayan Mountains. These sources are about 250 million years old and contain no artificial chemicals. When you look at the Himalayan salt crystals under a microscope, you will see wonderful crystalline shapes that are completely unlike regular table salt. These crystals provide better assimilation and absorption, along with optimum cellular utilization. In addition to organic natural sodium, Himalayan salt also contains around ninety different trace minerals. These trace minerals are important for cellular functions, and thus using this type of salt, rather than regular table salt, offers some health benefits.

The benefits of natural Himalayan crystal salt include:[263]

- Regulating the water content throughout your body
- Promoting healthy pH balance in your cells, particularly your brain cells
- Promoting blood-sugar health and helping to reduce the signs of aging
- Assisting in the generation of hydroelectric energy in cells in your body
- Enhancing absorption of food through your intestinal tract
- Supporting respiratory health
- Promoting sinus health
- Preventing muscle cramps
- Promoting bone strength
- Regulating your sleep
- Supporting your libido
- Promoting vascular health

In conjunction with water, this type of salt is actually essential for the regulation of your blood pressure—especially when taken in a preparation called *sole*, which is a special concentrated mixture of Himalayan salt water that, used daily, can lower high blood pressure.[264] For this effect, however, please closely follow the sole protocol, as it is very specific. Just using crushed Himalayan salt will not do the trick—only the concentrated solution as described. **(See Side Notes: Sole Protocol.)** In my practice, I have many patients who have successfully lowered their blood pressure with this simple addition to their diet—as strange as it may seem to use salt to lower blood pressure!

I would recommend switching your regular table salt to Himalayan salt (pink salt). Over time, you should notice a striking difference in how you feel—and it also tastes great. A little goes a long way, so you don't have to use as much as regular table salt, and you can either use it granulated or crush it in a grinder. Like eliminating soda, making the change to pink salt is a simple switch with noticeable health benefits.

CHAPTER 11

STEP 9: Stress Reduction through Meditation and Yoga

I'm in meditation high above.
—QUEENSRYCHE

I do yoga and Pilates.
—MADONNA

n addition to eating an organic, non-GMO, plant-based diet; avoiding food sensitivities; taking Bosmeric-SR; avoiding processed sugars and salt; and keeping blood-glucose levels normal, another important factor in staying healthy is reducing stress—ideally through meditation and yoga.

Most MDs and health professionals recommend daily exercise routines that include a combination of cardiovascular exercise (like walking on treadmills or jogging) and strength training (like weight lifting). But I take a slightly different point of view.

General exercise helps keep the body in motion, but it is not always the best or most effective way to maintain your health. Exercise is a state of physiology, not a state of health. Just because someone exercises, that does not automatically mean he or she is healthy. Exercise does improve certain physiological parameters, but it does not negate all the unhealthy lifestyle behaviors and dietary factors that we may choose.

How many of us know people who go to the gym and exercise daily and still have to take blood-pressure, cholesterol, antianxiety, and antidepressant medications? How many of us know people who go to the gym and exercise daily who still have had stents placed inside their arteries and suffered heart attacks? If everyone is exercising all the time, why are we not all healthy? Why do we still have to take medications?

Now, don't get me wrong; I am not trying to tell people to stop exercising! I'm asking them to change the way they look at improving their overall health, the types of exercise they are doing, and the overall goal they are trying to achieve. Many people think that going to the gym and working out will somehow cancel out the cheeseburger, fries, cookies, candies, alcohol, and tobacco they consume. This is a false belief. Although exercise does improve certain physiological aspects, such as our physical strength and speed or our heart-rate capacity, it does not directly lower cholesterol, reduce inflammation, or even lower stress in most people. As with conventional medicine, the typical exercise "standard of care" does not help us as much as we once believed it did.

The problem with conventional exercise is that it puts the person in a greater *sympathetic* state rather than a *parasympathetic* state. With our current hectic and stressed lifestyles, we need to be in more of a parasympathetic state. I will explain what these states mean.

Commonly known as the "fight-or-flight response," the sympathetic state readies you to either engage with someone or something (fight) or retreat or run away (flight). The parasympathetic state is our state of relaxation. These two biological states, inherent to all of us, have many physiological effects. Here are some examples of what happens to your body during both states.

Sympathetic vs. Parasympathetic Response

I'm so excited.
—Kiss

Take a deep breath and relax.
—Enigma

Physical manifestations of the sympathetic state include the following:

1. Increased heart rate
2. Increased respiratory rate
3. Increased blood pressure
4. Increased adrenal hormones (epinephrine, norepinephrine, cortisol)
5. Movement of blood from the abdomen to the extremities
6. Increased thickening of platelets (acutely)
7. Vasoconstriction (squeezing of the arteries)

Physical manifestations of the parasympathetic state include the following:

1. Decreased heart rate
2. Decreased respiratory rate
3. Decreased blood pressure
4. Decreased adrenal hormones
5. Movement of blood from the extremities to the abdomen
6. Normalization of platelet function
7. Vasodilation (relaxation of the arteries)

Let's first take a look at the sympathetic state, otherwise known as our fight-or-flight response. This is an inherent, primitive biological response. When confronted with a situation, you will either engage (fight) or retreat (flight). For example, if you were to encounter a threat—if someone with a gun approached you in a dark alleyway—you would either try to defend yourself (fight) or run away (flight). When actively engaging in the fight-or-flight response, your body increases your heart rate, breathing, and blood pressure. It releases hormones like epinephrine and norepinephrine to make you move quickly. While in this response state, your body also anticipates potential physical damage; it tries to decrease possible swelling by releasing cortisol (your own steroid that acts like prednisone). Your platelets get sticky (acutely) to help increase clotting in case you bleed during the fight. Blood also travels away from the abdomen to go to the arms and legs to deliver a boost if you have to strike or run.

The sympathetic response allows us to survive, as it helps us manage potentially dangerous situations. But the problem with most Americans (and most of the industrialized world) is that our entire lives comprise a sympathetic state. We live in what I call *sympathetic overdrive.*

We all go to work and have a stressful or busy day; we drink coffee to stay alert, stimulating the release of stress hormones (like adrenaline); we experience stress from our commute to and from work; and then when we get home we watch the news, which makes people even *more* stressed. We check our mail or e-mail and find mortgage payments along with credit-card and insurance bills waiting to be paid. The more health-inclined among us go out for a run or go to the gym. But, remember, although this can improve overall physiological responses in our bodies, ordinary exercise is not necessarily healthy; it *is a state of physiology, not a state of health*. The general misperception is that everyone can have a stressful day or unhealthy diet and then "work it off" via exercise. This is not necessarily true. Exercising when in a sympathetic state does provide the benefit of increasing cardiovascular function, strength, and metabolism, but achieving these results is not directly related to actually *being* healthier. Let's explore this further by looking at the typical day again.

Most people wake up stressed out from not having a good night's sleep; they drink their morning cup(s) of coffee or energy drink(s), go to a stressful job, eat unhealthy highly processed and sugary foods to keep them going, and then come home or go work out at the gym. The problem with this scenario is that most people lead themselves from one sympathetic state to another without balancing themselves out by entering a parasympathetic (relaxation) state for at least a portion of the day.

Here is a classic example of this problem. In 2008, I had four male patients who all exercised in the morning before going to work. They went to the gym early and ran on treadmills while watching the financial news. None of them drank or smoked, and all had very good BMI or ideal body weight. These men were not diabetic, nor did they have high blood pressure. But they ate a standard American diet and did not participate in any parasympathetic activities.

With regards to their cardiovascular health, one had elevated cholesterol but did not believe in treating it with prescriptions or natural therapies and wasn't worried about it; another had elevated cholesterol that he controlled with a statin medication (i.e., Lipitor) given by his cardiologist; the third had elevated cholesterol but had had a side effect from the statin medication, so he was using omega-3 products that brought his levels into the normal range; and the final man had normal cholesterol levels to begin with. He had no increased cholesterol and thus was not on medication or taking omega-3s. All these men were of a similar age and had similar jobs—they were all pension and financial managers. They all had been in the field for over twenty-five years and had managed their clients' finances and retirement funds. When the stock market and economy started to tank in 2008, especially at the peak of the crash, all four men, after exercising at the gym and watching the financial markets fall, started to have chest pains; all of them went to the ER and were diagnosed with heart attacks.

Now, you might think that some of the men were already at risk—especially the one with elevated cholesterol who was not taking anything to control it. But the other two men whose cholesterol levels were controlled by medication or natural therapies—and even the man who had normal levels to begin with—all had heart attacks. How do we explain this?

This is a clear example of the *excess sympathetic state* that we are putting ourselves in through the typical stresses of our modern lives. When these men went to the gym in the early morning after drinking their coffee, they were all running on their treadmills while watching the financial markets crash. As the markets continued to fall, each of them had an increase in his sympathetic activity ("fight") response during an activity (running on the treadmill) that is already highly sympathetic ("flight"). Their heart rates were already at a high level from exercise, and their bodies' responses to the stressful news created an even greater sympathetic response that made their blood platelets stickier. The fact that all of these men had inflammation in their arterial walls (due to the standard American diet) only heightened their sympathetic states. The result: heart attacks.

Although exercise and activity are good for our physiological health, we must not think of them as ways to balance inflammation or stress, but as occasional strong initiators. Remember, exercise is a state of physiology, not a state of health. We need to improve both our inflammation and our physical stamina simultaneously. Addressing only one does not necessarily correct the other. Exercise and diet are only part of the picture—the part that gets all the press. Most of us are missing our fundamental human need for relaxation and true rest.

Activities like yoga and meditation are ideal for initiating a relaxed, parasympathetic state. To start, let me briefly introduce you to the many benefits that yoga can bring to your life.

Many people think that yoga is just stretching, or an easy exercise. In truth, yoga is the yolk, or union, of a practice that includes breathing (pranayama) and postures (asana) that lead one to a state of meditation. Yoga is an intense exercise, as it combines physical, mental, and spiritual aspects into one practice. The medical and health benefits have been clinically shown.

The Benefits of Yoga[265]

Doing yoga in the evenings
—TIM MCGRAW

There are myriad reasons to take up a yoga practice. There are nearly as many different types of yoga as there are benefits to your well-being.

Mental-health benefits

- Reduce stress and prevent stress-related illnesses
- Reduce anxiety and increase GABA
- Reduce depression (up to 45 percent)
- Improve insomnia
- Improve concentration
- Improve mood
- Improve memory
- Reduce PTSD symptoms

Physical-health benefits

- Reduce back pain (up to 42 percent)
- Reduce arthritis pain
- Reduce fibromyalgia pain
- Reduce inflammatory markers (NF-kB)
- Reduce weight
- Reduce blood sugar
- Reduce blood pressure
- Increase flexibility

- Increase strength
- Reduce asthma attacks
- Reduce allergy symptoms
- Increase lung function
- Improve digestion and elimination
- Reduce irritable bowel symptoms
- Improve pregnancy outcomes
- Improve immune-system function
- Improve sexual function and libido
- Increase longevity

Spiritual-health benefits

- Increase quality of life
- Increase well-being
- Increase higher levels of consciousness
- Increase inner peace and focus

Personal financial benefits[266]

- According to studies on patients practicing yoga, decreased use of antinausea, antianxiety, sleep, and pain medications saves, on average, $469 per patient per hospitalization (three days).
- In a small oncology unit of twenty-four beds, improvements credited to yoga accounted for a total savings to the hospital of $443,781 annually, which in turn yields a personal savings to the public by decreasing the health-care costs that hospitals pass on through their patients.

So, as you can see, there are many reasons to do yoga—even if you also partake in conventional exercise. But if you do yoga correctly, you won't need conventional gym exercises. Yoga costs nothing to do at home, or you can take a yoga class instead of joining a gym, which will generally save you hundreds of dollars a year.

Yoga is an exceptional exercise in that you can gain all the benefits of conventional exercise—like increased strength and improved cardiovascular health—and also improve flexibility, balance, focus, and concentration.

Focus and concentration are extremely important, especially as we get older. I usually recommend yoga a few times a week, in addition to walking, for an effective exercise regimen. If done correctly, this is all you need to do to truly improve your health and well-being parameters.

Most people have trouble with yoga because they believe you have to be fit or know something about yoga to go to a class. This is definitely not the case. You do need to find classes that have a certified yoga instructor who can help guide you at whichever level or with whatever limitations you may have; all yoga postures and techniques can be modified to the individual. Good yoga instructors teach students of all shapes, sizes, and abilities because they understand that the benefit of yoga comes from the practice—not just the outcome.

At Sanjevani, Maureen Sutton teaches our patients yoga—all of whom have various health limitations or conditions—and they all benefit greatly from the practice. With an experienced yoga instructor, you should feel comfortable coming to a yoga class regardless of any physical limitations, temporary or otherwise.

There are, however, some forms of yoga that I generally suggest that people avoid. These include hot yoga or chain yoga studios that have levels that you must pay to achieve and are pressured into. These are not real yoga practices but franchises (I call them "McYogas") and trendy fusion practices (e.g., yoga blended with martial arts, dance, etc.) marketed through gimmicks. They mislead those who want to pursue yoga as a complete practice joining body and mind. Just as I have been advocating eating real food, you should also practice authentic yoga in order to gain the benefits and reach the full potential of the practice.

Most likely I will get "heat" for saying this, but you should avoid hot yoga because it gives a false sense of flexibility due to the heat. Hot yoga is the form of yoga that results in the most injuries due to tendon microtears and overstretching that are less likely when practicing yoga at room temperature. But there's a reason why it is popular. Most Americans believe that if they sweat, they are working out; they have a "no pain, no gain" attitude. This is not a yoga concept but an American marketing concept (leveraged by a very successful Indian). If yoga is taught and practiced correctly, it is much safer than going to a gym and lifting weights or using machines. Nothing is safer than working with your own body against gravity. Hot yoga, unfortunately, bucks this trend.

The routine practice of yoga can also be used along with conventional exercise; those who do both will notice improvements in their conventional exercises. Conventional strength training (using machines) predominantly increases strength but not flexibility or balance—and we need all three for optimum fitness. The rests between postures during yoga place the body in the parasympathetic state instead of keeping it in the sympathetic state, as conventional training does. But yoga alone can build muscle, tone, strength, flexibility, and balance. When you practice yoga routinely, you will feel refreshed, light, and relaxed afterward—not exhausted, tired, or even more stressed. Yoga doesn't bring only the body into a parasympathetic state; it does the same to the mind, helping calm and focus our thoughts. This relaxed state of body and mind easily prepares one for meditation.

Meditation naturally follows in the footsteps of the routine practice of yoga. Like yoga, meditation is something that many people in the West have misunderstood.

Meditation comes in many forms and techniques: from simple mindfulness to specific practices that help focus the mind and expand the consciousness. All vary in technique or approach, but the benefits are similar and many.

A common misconception about meditation is that it is a religious practice. Religion has nothing to do with meditation (although many Eastern and Western religions incorporate meditation). Instead meditation is something that everyone—regardless of gender, race, or religion (or lack of religion)—can practice. There are many ways to meditate, and Maureen Sutton, elder and medicine woman for Sanjevani, will teach you a variety of meditation techniques in the next book in our Sanjevani Integrative Medicine Health and Lifestyle Series. But let's take a look at just a few of the benefits of maintaining a meditation practice.

The Benefits of Meditation[267]

If I go there real late, let my mind meditate
on everything to be done
If I search deep inside, let my conscience be my guide
Then the answers are sure to come
Don't have to worry none.
—NORAH JONES

Meditation has been clinically proven to deliver the following benefits:

- Positively impacts the expression of genes and protein markers of inflammation, including a number of genes regulated by the inflammatory transcription factor NF-kB, C-reactive protein (CRP), and IL-6
- Lowers stress and fatigue associated with painful rheumatoid joint disease and other chronic-pain conditions
- Lowers stress hormones such as cortisol
- Relieves depression
- Improves memory and multitasking abilities
- Relieves anxiety
- Reduces blood pressure and blood-sugar levels
- Increases gray matter (the size and complexity of brain tissue) in areas of learning, memory, and emotion regulation
- Increases telomere length (the parts of our genes involved with longevity)
- Reduces medical costs (up to 11 percent in one year and 28 percent in five years)
- Decreases mortality (23 percent), decreases death due to cardiovascular problems (30 percent), and confers a *significant* decrease in cancer mortality (49 percent)

In addition to the amazing benefits listed above, a recent study from Harvard University and the University of Sienna found that the effects of meditation move beyond the cultivation of self-awareness, improvement of concentration, and protection of the heart and immune system—meditation can actually alter the physiology of the human brain.[268]

Consistent meditation practice can also help alleviate symptoms of anxiety and depression in people who need it most.[269] The Italian scientists selected twenty-four subjects who had never meditated before and guided them through an eight-week meditation course. Subjects completed a two-and-a-half-hour session each week. During this session they learned various elements and styles of meditation. In addition, subjects meditated daily on their own for forty-five minutes. MRIs and psychological evaluations were performed before and after the meditation program. The data concluded that the subjects experienced a thickening in the part of the brain responsible for perception and emotions. These positive changes to the brain strengthen our natural defenses against anxiety and depression.[270]

The question is, why aren't you meditating? It doesn't matter which type of meditation you choose (there are, of course, many kinds and many instructors); it's the actual practice that is important. Some people use mantras, which are "sacred" sounds or chants that help the person get into the meditative state faster; some use guided imagery; and some simply count backward and focus only on the process of counting. There really is no wrong way to meditate.

I have many patients who tell me that they find it too difficult to meditate or find that their mind has trouble focusing. If this sounds like you, a natural supplement called *Sanjevani L-Theanine* can help bring you into the meditative state quickly. It contains the patented form of L-theanine at a 200 mg dose. This natural amino acid comes from the green-tea leaf; it is *not* EGCG (the antioxidant component of green tea), nor is it the caffeine component. This amino acid brings the brain into the theta-wave state, which is the state in which you are the most relaxed and aware. It is not a sedative, but it keeps the mind focused and turns down the background noise of our environment. Athletes call this state of mind the "zone." Meditators call it the "meditative state."

When your brain is in the theta-wave state, you are less stressed, more relaxed, and more focused. I recommend *Sanjevani L-theanine* to many of my patients who have anxiety and stress or who need to improve their focus. It helps those who have wandering minds in conjunction with trouble sleeping, and I also recommend it for patients who have trouble quieting the mind when they try to meditate. Sanjevani L-Theanine is like meditation in a pill. Once people have help experiencing this calm, focused state, it encourages them to learn how to meditate so they can experience it by themselves—without any pills, and whenever they want.

There are ways to take true relaxation to the next level, and one of those involves using what is called a "float tank" for a meditative experience like no other.

Sanjevani REST Pod

So I can rest my head
—GREEN DAY

I recommend every single person try something called floatation therapy. At Sanjevani, we have our REST (Restricted Environmental Stimulus Therapy) Pod, which is the next generation of float tanks, and it provides amazing deep relaxation and pain relief to hundreds of my patients.

The tank looks like something high-tech from the Apple Store; its bright white and rounded design provides an inviting and safe environment. The tank is spacious; it is filled with 1,200 pounds of pharmaceutical-grade magnesium salts, similar to the Epsom salts used in a bath but hundreds of times more concentrated. The tank also contains ten inches of structured water kept at the same temperature as the skin of your body. With the large amount of salt in the water, your body becomes buoyant and you actually float, similar to the way people float on the Dead Sea.

This ultrahigh concentration of magnesium and filtered, structured water absorbs through your skin and raises your intracellular-magnesium levels. Raised intracellular-magnesium levels lower pain by relaxing muscles and joints. The zero-gravity-like environment of the REST Pod enhances this effect, which also lowers blood pressure, calms the mind, and places the brain in the theta-wave state within mere minutes. One hour in the float pod provides the healing and rest equivalent of five to six hours of deep sleep.[271]

Floatation therapy has been around since the 1960s, but the newer tanks have been modernized and improved for comfort, cleanliness (the Sanjevani REST Pod has a high-tech filtration system designed by the Ministry of Defense in the United Kingdom that cleans the pod between each use), and therapeutic outcomes (via heated water and soundproof materials, with sound- and light-therapy options available). Many doctors will soon highly recommend the noninvasive and nonpharmacological use of floatation therapy for helping people with many health conditions. While they're not yet as popular in the United States, certain centers with these floatation pods in England and Europe serve over one hundred thousand people annually.

An article titled "Integrative Pain Management for Optimal Patient Care" in the American Academy of Pain Management journal *The Pain Practitioner* detailed the therapeutic and health benefits of using the REST Pod float tank to help treat the following conditions: [272]

- Anxiety and depression
- Sports and back injuries

- Chronic pain
- Sore muscles
- Arthritis
- Insomnia
- Attention deficit hyperactive disorder
- Asperger's and autism-spectrum disorders
- Mental fatigue and overall stress

The Sanjevani REST Pod float tank offers immense pain relief and immediate relaxation. This instant deep-relaxation state allows the body to recover from stress and to enter deeper REM sleep following the session. It stimulates blood flow through all the bodily tissues, causes the body to release natural endorphins, and moves the brain into alpha- and theta-wave states associated with relaxation, meditation, and healing responses. Benefits carry over from one session to the next with progressive improvement. The majority of our patients (70 percent) report achieving full pain relief during a float session, and most report that the positive effects from their session last for three days and up to one week later.

People who use the float tank include those who have chronic pain or insomnia, CEOs, and weekend warriors.

Here are a few testimonials:

At times I would nod off in the middle of conversations with friends either standing or sitting. It was embarrassing and I became frustrated and resorted to taking two, maybe three different medications just to knock myself out. I would often go running miles in the middle of the morning just to try to exhaust myself, but that led to me suffering injuries that took forever to heal because my body had no down time for restoration and tissue repair. I felt hopeless. I became obsessed with trying to find a sleep solution so I began blogging and reading blogs, only to find hundreds of other sleep-deprived people going through the same thing. Nothing worked and it became a vicious cycle. I would pace the floor and stop and stare at my bed each night like it was something I should throw out. I'm a forty-six-year-old male, who suffered from chronic insomnia for years. Since visiting Sanjevani and trying the REST Pod, my sleep has drastically improved. I'm no longer taking harmful pharmaceutical medication that led to my abuse and addiction. I've cleansed my liver and started taking nothing but natural sleep supplements, which were purchased at Sanjevani. I practice good sleep habits that have also helped increase the number of hours of sleep that I am currently getting. Prior to visiting Sanjevani, I logged ten to twelve hours of sleep per week and now I sleep six to seven hours per night! Sanjevani helped me return to natural REM sleep and abandon my use and sometimes abuse of pharmaceutical sleep medication. I thought I would never be able to achieve natural REM sleep. Thank you, Sanjevani.

—Robert W. | Albuquerque

I'm almost six months post-op for surgical repair of a badly broken ankle—three plates, thirteen pins. Floating in the REST Pod was the first time since the accident that I have been completely pain-free. In fact, it was a strange sensation to have my foot and ankle feel normal, because I had become so accustomed to low-grade pain that I forgot what it was like to not have any. The whole experience was relaxing and blissful, and I felt like all the stress just drained away. I was impressed by the large size of the sleek, high-tech pod. This is not a claustrophobia-inducing tank; it's more like a giant egg with lots of room inside. I was reassured by the meticulous filtration and indeed the filter system kicked on at the end of my float. A great experience, I highly recommend it.

—Susan T.| Albuquerque

I broke my leg in seven places. The constant pain made me feel depressed and unable to sit up for any length of time. After only one float in the pod, I felt complete relief from pain! So I floated again and was able to completely relax. I no longer feel consumed by pain, my mood has lifted, and I feel ready to get back to my life.

—Nickie D. | California

I also use the Sanjevani REST Pod every two weeks or so, especially when I have trouble sleeping due to traveling across the country giving lectures and consulting. I was always a light sleeper, but ever since the end of my medical training, I have been even more sensitive to sleep disruptions. For many years I was always on alert from being on call every three days. About three years ago, while I was attending an integrative-medicine conference in another city, I found out that there was a float center nearby. Maureen recommended years ago that we have a floatation tank at Sanjevani, but I had never tried one. Then one evening after the conference, I left the cocktails-and-snacks event and went for a float instead.

I was impressed from my very first session. For the next three days, I slept so hard that I told Maureen, "the last time I slept this good was prior to going to medical school." I knew from that moment on that this would be a great treatment for my patients and for members of our community. We have had amazing results with something so simple yet so effective for every person who uses it.

For those with pain and chronic inflammatory conditions or even insomnia, the Sanjevani REST Pod is a great place to bring them back into the parasympathetic state naturally, without any side effects or worries about prescription-medication interactions. If you are in the Albuquerque area, I invite you to try a float session; if you are not, I recommend you find a REST Pod similar to ours in your area. For more details or to book a float session, please visit **www.floatabq.com**.

To enhance the benefits of the float session, I recommend using **Sanjevani Magnesium Chelate** (an easily absorbed form of magnesium that does not cause the usual loose bowel movements seen with other forms, such as magnesium oxide). If one takes two capsules (150 mg each) or our powder daily, especially after floating, it can help maintain the levels and lasting effects of the magnesium absorbed through the skin in the REST Pod. For those who want to help improve memory function or who have low blood flow to the brain, I recommend trying our **Sanjevani Magnesium L-Threonate Forte**, which uses a patented form of magnesium (from MIT) that has been shown to cross the blood-brain barrier and increase synaptic density of neurons in the brain. This comes as a powder and should be started slowly, at half a scoop daily at bedtime for two weeks, and then it can be increased to one scoop. Between the two forms of magnesium, one can improve upon the wonderful benefits of floatation and help keep the body in that balanced and calm state for longer periods of time.

BIO-WELL and BIOCOR

I feel your energy.
—BEYONCÉ KNOWLES

We all have stress, some more than others. We all have energy, some more than others. We are all balanced, some more than others. We all have these attributes, but how do we measure whether our stress, energy levels, and body are balanced? A simple educational tool at Sanjevani can provide that answer for you. It is called a Bio-Well.

An international team led by Dr. Konstantin Korotkov has developed Bio-Well.

Dr. Korotkov is a professor of physics at Saint Petersburg Federal Research University of Informational Technologies, Mechanics, and Optics in Saint Petersburg, Russia. He is a leading scientist internationally renowned for his pioneering research on the human energy field. Professor Korotkov developed the Gas Discharge Visualization (GDV) technique, based on the Kirlian effect, in 1995. The Bio-Well brings this powerful technology to market in a more accessible way than ever before. GDV technique is the computer registration and analysis of electrophotonic emissions resulting from the placement of different objects, including biological (specifically the human fingers), in the high-intensity electromagnetic field on the device lens. Its unique software translates and transmits the information back in graphical representations to show energy, stress, and vitality evaluations. It then maps the images to different organs and systems of the body and shows the function as being high, normal, or low. In addition, it taps into Chinese energy meridians and the Indian chakra energy system.

This technology has been verified by eighteen years of clinical experience and clinical studies by hundreds of medical doctors with many thousands of patients in Russia and all over the world. The scanning process is quick, easy, and nonintrusive. It provides real-time feedback on which factors—positive and negative—affect a person's energy state.

In the United States, Bio-Well is not considered a medical instrument but an educational tool providing biofeedback. It gives you an impression of your energy field and allows you to see its day-to-day transformation and the influence of different situations upon your condition. I use this on patients to demonstrate how balanced—or more importantly, how imbalanced—they are on an energetic level. This correlates very well to their current health state, even when all routine blood tests and imaging seem normal. You might have had a similar experience. You feel tired, exhausted, and out of balance, yet all your blood work (e.g., thyroid, blood sugar, and blood pressure) and imaging are normal. You might even exercise regularly and have a healthy diet yet still feel unwell. Or, more commonly, your conventional blood tests are abnormal in correlation with your symptoms, but even with the standard medical recommendations, you still feel unwell. This is where the Bio-Well can help. It can provide subtle educational information—guidance that is unique to you—that is vital to improving your sense of well-being and overall health. After learning which areas are imbalanced, which need be to lowered or strengthened, professionals can then provide a personal lifestyle plan.

Many alternative and holistic health-care providers use muscle testing to help shape their clinical decisions. The problem with this method is that using one's own energy can be very subjective; the labels (words and images) written on a bottle of supplements being tested can influence the tester; and the materials being tested can easily influence the outcome due to its subjectivity. Thus the test is not as sensitive or specific as people believe it to be. With the Bio-Well one can actually demonstrate, through reproducible scientific calculations and measurements, whether certain products (or therapies) actually affect your energy field for better or for worse. One can then help guide patients, through a variety of traditional energy systems (Chinese and Indian), to an understanding of what they need to do to create that balance.

Yoga, meditation, floatation therapy, exercise, guided imagery, eating better, and taking the right type of natural supplements can help improve your biofeedback test results, and practitioners can continue to perform evaluations to help you keep optimizing your energy fields.

Although I recommend the lifestyle changes above, there is another way to provide even more specific benefits, and it is called the BIOCOR. It is an accessory to the Bio-Well for balancing the human energy field utilizing information taken from the Bio-Well. It translates the information that has been analyzed by the Bio-Well into music with specific healing frequencies used to balance your energy systems through positive biofeedback. Balance and harmony of your energy systems are created simply by listening to your music through special headphones provided during the therapy.

I highly recommend that you try to get an evaluation yourself and see how well you are doing with your balance, energy, and stress levels. If your levels are great, continue on with your current routine. If they are not, then we (or your health-care provider) can help with healthy lifestyle changes **(see Side Notes: Bio-Well and BIOCOR)**.

CHAPTER 12

STEP 10: Love, Happiness, Social Relationships, Faith, and Spiritual Practices

> *All you need is love.*
> —JOHN LENNON

And love is all you need. This holds true for every being on this planet. Yet so many people are not taught to love or to be compassionate or, perhaps most critically, how to receive love.

We are bombarded with hollow values. Reality shows and professional sports market competition—only one can win. We all have been sold the idea that "greed is good." This Wall Street mantra has given only false hope, leading us into a place where we are not as well off as we used to be, both financially and spiritually.

It may seem strange for a physician to talk about love as an integral part of your health, but at the very least I recommend that you take a moment to explore the values and virtues for which you work daily. Whom do you love? Who loves you? How are you serving your neighbors? Do you allow people to give to you? Do you ask for help? Would those people closest to you still love you if you had no money or if you were in poor health?

It's easy to get caught up in the *extrinsic* values we think are important: status, wealth, and image. Our society correlates those things with security and stability and, therefore, sees them as valuable. And to some extent, having wealth and status can be beneficial. Yet when we look a little deeper (and the research bears this out), people who focus on extrinsic values are almost always the unhappiest with their lives. They overwhelmingly report that they are living life without love.

Social media drives the illusion home, as people position themselves to look as if they are extraordinarily happy all the time. And think of all the movie stars and pop stars, with all their wealth and fame, who still end up in rehab or who lose their star status because of drugs, alcohol, suicide, or bad behaviors. We obsess about these people because we see their inner destruction mirrored in our own lives.

We all need to take the time to really explore our *intrinsic* values: community, service, and connection to our true selves. These priceless values provide more happiness, and more happiness in turn improves our overall health. Any doctor should be able to tell you that feeling unhappy—which depresses the body and mind—is counterproductive to a patient's well-being. Living a more fulfilled life and feeling happier may be as simple as shifting priorities. Here are a few recommendations for improving your feelings of happiness and, therefore, your health as well.

Start things off with positive, uplifting, and affirming media. I recommend kick-starting your inner exploration by watching a film called *Happy: The Movie.* It asks people the world over, "What makes you happy?" with surprising and truly delightful results. That intrinsic values are held in the highest regard the world over—far above money or status—may be the most surprising revelation from the film. In fact, one small country instituted a new indicator of progress instead of GDP (gross domestic product); they did this after discovering that, as GDP rose, happiness decreased overall. They called this new metric GNH (gross national happiness), and its measurement of the country's progress takes into account societal values and services that make everyone, regardless of income or ability, truly happy. It's pretty incredible.

Volunteer to help the less fortunate. A simple and fulfilling way to create more happiness in your life is to gain perspective—not to negate your experiences or feelings but to provide new sources of strength. I recommend starting by participating in more community events through volunteer work or providing a necessary service to those in need. When you share your experiences and wisdom with others, before you know it you will feel happier in ways you never imagined. Learning to love others—even those you may not like or with whom you may disagree—is critical to feeling more connected in the world in an age when we can customize the types of people we interact with. This is, of course, easier said than done, but try to practice this approach—even if it's only for a day.

Let go of resentment and anger. When it comes to illness, it is critically important that you not hold on to anger or resentment. Holding on to anger or resentment, however justifiable, only drains your immune system and may actually worsen or accelerate your disease, whatever that may be. Find constructive ways to release your anger and resentment, such as journaling, meditation, physical release (through yelling or crying in a secure, secluded area, but note that I do not recommend sympathetic exercise or activities like martial arts for this purpose, as they may lead to a higher likelihood of injury), or find a supportive therapist or group that allows you to vent constructively.

Live in the present. Instead of merely getting through your day, learn to *live it.* Try to be aware of your surroundings and your environment in the moment. Avoid living in the metaphorical bubble of social media without being social in "real life." Humans are meant to socialize and to live in groups—not alone. See if you can communicate directly (when you can) instead of e-mailing or texting.

Create your own community. Although many of us feel that we have community through social media, nothing can replace being part of a real community. Direct contact with others provides love, support and improves your confidence. This "extended family" of people with whom we share the same beliefs and interests is very important for our mental and physical health. If you don't feel like you have community, go to your local religious, spiritual, educational or community center and see what type of activities, services, and meetings they offer. If you don't find one you like, create your own community, as I am sure there will be many people just like you who are seeking the same but waiting for someone else to do it.

I get asked almost every day, "How do people stay happy and healthy and achieve their dreams?" Outside of hard work, patience, and good family and friends, I do my best to follow the ten steps outlined in this book. In addition, I perform an "intention board" exercise yearly to focus on bringing goodness to those around me and to myself.

An intention board, sometimes called a "treasure board" or a "vision board," is a way to help you visualize your goals and intentions. It only requires a large poster board, some glue (usually a glue stick, hopefully nontoxic), a dozen or more magazines that you like to read—such as travel, health, cooking, hobby, social, or news magazines—and a couple of hours of your time. Use the magazines to find words, phrases, and pictures that interest you or resonate with you on any level. Cut or tear out these words and pictures and set them aside, and within an hour or two, you will have dozens of words and pictures. Once you feel like you have enough, glue them to the poster board in any order or fashion you choose. Some people make a collage with added decorations, while others simply place their pictures and words on the board in random order.

There is no right or wrong way, and you don't have to be artistic. The purpose is to keep your goals and intentions top of mind by making them visible physically—not only in your mind. When you've finished, place the poster board somewhere that you will see every day—in your bathroom near your mirror, for example. Wherever you put it, make sure you look at it for at least two minutes. Start at the top and briefly scan the images and words to get to the bottom, and do it every morning and evening.

This practice of looking at your intention board helps seed the positive words and images into your consciousness. The law of attraction spurs action, and the items and actions you put on your intention board should start to occur within the year. It is perhaps important to note here that this is more than simply *wishing* to have a better life, or to attain your goals, or to feel happier. This exercise is a *practice of mindfulness* that causes conscious and unconscious focus and attention on that which you want most. This helps you create your reality through your thoughts, words, and choices—like practicing a new song on the piano every day. At first it feels like work, but eventually the song becomes second nature and you start to consciously and unconsciously make the perfect choices to play the right notes every time.

Every year at Sanjevani, we create intention boards with our patients, and the practice has become very popular. In our (albeit anecdotal) experience, about 70 percent to 80 percent of the items on an intention board come to fruition if people practice viewing it daily for two minutes in the morning and two minutes in the evening.

But what about the other 20 percent to 30 percent of items on an intention board? If you create an intention board yearly, you will start to see that those other items occur, but in different years; consciousness and time are infinite, although we may have only put these ideas on a "calendar" in the moment.

I know this all might sound strange, but it has only had positive, helpful results. I have had some of my most successful (and even most conservative) patients create an intention board, and they tell me they attribute their success and happiness to this activity. Placebo or not, I am happy to suggest something that may help a patient emotionally and spiritually. Wishing for things to happen is a passive activity; visualizing through an intention board is cementing the intention into our minds and getting it out into the world, whether we realize it or not. Perhaps intention boards could be called "springboards" for their ability to help people visualize and actualize a happier, more fulfilling life. It's a meaningful way to take action, and I encourage even the biggest skeptics to try it at least once.

In addition to love, happiness, developing social relationships and community, one must also try to strengthen their faith or spiritual practices. Your faith or spiritual practice is an important part of health and healing. Remember optimum health is the balance of all parts—body, mind and spirit. Whatever you believe in, I encourage you to utilize that belief system or practice as part of your overall daily regimen. At ONAC of Sanjevani, I can formally address and encourage my patient's belief system and spiritual practice as part of my overall recommendations. Most people forget that many hospital centers have names such as Presbyterian, Methodist, St. Agnes, St. Christus, St. Joseph's, Jewish, and so on. Many people think those names are just titles on buildings and forget that these institutions grew from a religious or spiritual foundation. However over time those belief systems were separated from medicine. Unfortunately, in most conventional medical institutions, doctors are taught to keep this aspect separate from medicine. For example, in most hospital centers we call upon the religious or spiritual representatives for the patients only once all therapies have failed and the patient is about to pass away. I disagree with this approach. I believe that when a patient is admitted, as part of the initial team of providers for the patient, their religious or spiritual representative should also be included at the beginning to help encourage, support, and guide the patient to their own healing. This should be part of the initial treatment plan, not an afterthought when nothing is left to offer the patient.

Even if you do not have a religious or spiritual practice, I advise you to cultivate your own inner strength and core beliefs. Learning to love one another, your community, and yourself will help improve and develop your awareness and consciousness. Filling yourself with love and giving unconditional love to others will lead you to better health and lifestyle choices.

CHAPTER 13

Summary: Moving Forward and Taking Action

I will choose a path that's clear; I will choose freewill.
—RUSH

At Sanjevani Integrative Medicine Health and Lifestyle Center, we have helped thousands of patients and people in our community, one at a time, with one-on-one education and support, in starting plant-based diets and natural therapies. Most importantly, we strive to be a model of the values that we hold so true.

Most people did not just wake up with their diseases or problems. Thus at Sanjevani we emphasize the daily practice and conscious effort to be mindful of what we put into our bodies and minds. This practice, along with how we interact with others and our environment, results in tangible and practical health care. There are no quick fixes in life, although most people are seeking them; instead, there are real and permanent solutions that are easy to attain with a willingness to practice and the desire to start feeling better. For some people this occurs immediately, and for others it takes some time and patience.

Patients that follow the Ten Steps to Optimum Health and Longevity experience amazing results, such as reversal of their chronic diseases (even cancers), elimination of their prescription drugs, improved cognition, improved libido, deeper sleep, increased energy, and overall improvement of their happiness. The conventional medical system would describe these incredible outcomes as miracles. We call them daily occurrences that everyone can achieve with a little practice, some persistence, and the attempt to follow your true path in life.

I hope that now that you are finished with this book, your path toward meaningful lifestyle changes and control of your health will become a priority. Remember, at the end of the day all you have is your health. No matter how rich or poor you are; what political party you align yourself with; or what race, religion, or gender you are—what defines you is how happy you are and what quality of life you enjoy. All of this is based on how healthy you are and how healthy you can become.

Let's review briefly the **Ten Steps to Optimum Health & Longevity**:

1. Eat an organic, non-GMO, plant-based anti-inflammatory diet.
2. Test what triggers inflammatory responses in your body.
3. Detoxify: clear the toxins.
4. Avoid smoking.
5. Avoid NSAIDs—the unknown danger.
6. Decrease inflammation through the use of supplements like Bosmeric-SR.
7. Increase immune-system functioning.
8. Maintain healthy glucose levels and decrease sugar in the diet.
9. Reduce stress through meditation and yoga.
10. Embrace love, happiness, social relationships, faith, and spiritual practices

So now that you are educated on the Ten Steps, the only question I have is, when do you plan to start implementing them? If you utilize these steps, your health conditions can improve, resolve, and even reverse. You can turn your health around right now or whenever you decide to feel happier, healthier, and more fulfilled. I hope that this book will change not only your life but also the lives of your family and friends. I encourage you to share this information and become an example of wellness and an advocate for change.

It has to start somewhere
It has to start sometime
What better place than here?
What better time than now?
—RAGE AGAINST THE MACHINE

Best of health,
Sunil Pai, MD

Side Notes

Functional Medicine

As defined by the Institute of Functional Medicine, functional medicine addresses the underlying causes of disease using a systems-oriented approach and engaging both patient and practitioner in a therapeutic partnership. It is an evolution in the practice of medicine that better addresses the health-care needs of the twenty-first century. By shifting the traditional disease-centered focus of medical practice to a more patient-centered approach, functional medicine addresses the whole person, not just an isolated set of symptoms. Functional-medicine practitioners spend time with their patients, listening to their histories and looking at the interactions among genetic, environmental, and lifestyle factors that can influence long-term health and complex, chronic disease. In this way, functional medicine supports the unique expression of health and vitality for each individual.[273]

Acid Blockers

Over the past twenty years or so, those who practice holistic or integrative medicine have come to understand (from a basic understanding of the role of stomach acid) that the long-term effects of using acid blockers cause both macronutrient and micronutrient deficiencies.

Dozens of published clinical studies have demonstrated long-term problems with acid blockers (proton-pump inhibitors, or PPIs).[274] These include decreased calcium absorption and a nearly tripled risk of hip fracture. The latter risk was discovered through correlation when ordering routine bone-density screenings for postmenopausal women and elderly men. In addition to increased incidence of hip fractures, older men and women taking acid blockers also were twice as likely to develop pneumonia, three times more likely to get a potentially deadly infection from C. *difficile*, and more likely to develop anemia and gain significant amounts of weight. In addition, the studies have also found that acid blockers decrease vitamin B12, iron, and magnesium.

Although my fellow integrative physicians felt vindicated to see evidence that our theory was correct—that low stomach acid decreases the body's ability to break down the nutrients in our foods, leading to malnourishment and related disorders—it was still an egregious oversight by the majority of doctors. They assumed that a lack of calcium absorption was due to the acid blockers, which led to the deficiency. But most failed to realize that it was not calcium alone that was decreasing bone density but all its cofactors—like vitamin K1, K2, boron, silicon, magnesium, vitamin D, and other nutrients—involved in bone metabolism.

In integrative medicine, we use an understanding of basic nutrition and deduce that the blockage of one nutrient does not happen in isolation (healthy bones are the result of a variety of nutrients—not calcium alone); blockage always affects multiple nutrients.

On top of that, other side effects—such as headache, diarrhea, abdominal pain, nausea, or a rash—occur in 1 percent to 5 percent of patients taking prescription Prilosec. The Prilosec OTC package insert doesn't mention these side effects; only the prescription form does, despite the fact that Prilosec OTC is the same twenty-milligram dose as the standard prescription. The Prilosec OTC package insert also *omits several subtle yet significant side effects*, including joint, muscle, and leg pains. These side effects are infrequent but can be troublesome—especially if they are mistaken for arthritis or fibromyalgia and then treated with additional drugs. Proton-pump inhibitors are the third-largest class of drugs sold in the United States, with over one hundred million prescriptions written per year (which, obviously, does *not* include millions of OTC purchases) correlating to about 20 million people[275]. That means there are at least about *one million people* suffering significant side effects from acid blockers, on top of the malabsorption of nutrients and increased risk of hip fracture and infections. When you include OTC sales, that number could easily triple.

The biggest problem with the proton-pump inhibitors is that they produce a rebound effect after you stop taking them. When you block your acid pumps with medication, your body still wants to produce acid to help break down the foods you eat. Every time you smell or think about food, your stomach anticipates eating soon thereafter and starts producing acid to prepare for digestion. Acid blockers shut the proton pumps in such a way that, once you stop taking the medication, the valves open wide and create an overproduction of acid—the rebound effect. This creates *more* heartburn, *more* reflux, and *more* GI symptoms. This rebound is so pronounced that it makes people think they need to keep taking medication, since without it they have worse symptoms. The problem with this rebound effect is that it creates positive reinforcement of a negative behavior; people think acid blockers are solving their problem when they are only masking the symptoms.

Proton-pump inhibitors are very powerful, and they can have a rebound effect after as little as one week after stopping the medication. This is why you might want to think twice when you're offered a "one-week free trial" of a prescription acid-blocker medication. After the free week, you may be visiting your doctor to ask for refills of your prescription because your heartburn and GI symptoms got worse when you stopped taking it! And don't forget to read the fine print: drugs like Prilosec are intended to be used for *no more* than fourteen days (that's fourteen pills)...but they are sold in packages of twenty-eight and forty-two pills!

Another interesting aspect about the use of acid blockers is the reason they used to be prescription-only. Each drug has a patent that lasts eleven years before becoming a generic. This means that when the patent expires, a $238-per-month Prilosec prescription goes down to $28 per month and becomes an OTC medication. Why does the price go down so dramatically? Why, when it was once so important to have a prescription from a doctor, is it suddenly available at convenience stores? What purpose did the prescription serve in the first place?

In my opinion, once a drug loses its patent protections and thus the ability to charge a high price, the pharmaceutical company switches its focus and spends most of its marketing dollars not on "patients" but on "customers." The doctor's role for the first part of a drug's history is mainly to assist in the branding of the product to patients. It's not about ensuring safety (this is assessed before a drug goes to market) or making sure it is recommended, with medical guidance, only to those who need it; it's about maximizing the profits from the patented and nonpatented "lifecycle" of a drug. Remember, once the drug goes generic, it no longer requires medical guidance. This happens overnight. So for eleven years the drug must be carefully prescribed and controlled, and then people can simply purchase it OTC, as much as they want, without medical supervision. Funny how that works.

Sanjevani Acid-Blocker Support

Before weaning off any acid-blocker medication (e.g., Zantac, Pepcid, Prilosec, Prevacid, or Nexium), consider testing for food and gluten sensitivities (both IgE and IgG4) and eating an organic, non-GMO, plant-based diet. In addition to appropriate diet and lifestyle changes, I would recommend (for one to two months) the following to reduce rebound side effects and to heal the stomach:

1. **Sanjevani Zinc Carnosine 75 + Glutamine:** One tablet twice daily between meals. This special form of patented zinc will help heal gastritis and lower acid irritation without keeping stomach acid from digesting food. The glutamine will provide multiple benefits to the internal mucosal lining of the entire GI tract. Take this for one month after stopping the acid blockers.
2. **DGL Plus Ginger:** Deglycerized licorice plus ginger in chewable wafers. Chew one to two wafers prior to meals.
3. **Guna Reflux or Stomach**: Twenty drops twice daily in water or your drink of choice. The biotherapeutics in this product help stomach functioning and decrease reflux without blocking acid production and causing rebound effects. This supportive treatment should be used while taking acid blockers and for one month after stopping them.
4. **Heartburn Free (Enzymatic Therapy)**: Take as directed on the bottle. Benefits may last up to six months to control symptoms. Do not use if you are experiencing severe gastritis or stomach ulcers, or if you have an allergy to citrus or orange.
5. Eat more **alkaline foods** and drink **alkaline water**.

Dr. Pai's Recommended Laboratory Testing

When one has GI problems like stomach pain or indigestion, I recommend obtaining an *H. pylori* AB test to rule out a bacterial infection or ulcer. This can be done by blood if it's the first time testing), but if you have had a previous infection and recurrent symptoms, then you need a breath test or stool test.

If you have symptoms of GERD, heartburn, gas, bloating, diarrhea, or constipation (i.e., IBS), then I would suggest the following tests:

A. **Dr. Pai's IgE & IgG4 Food Panel.** This will show both the immediate (within one hour) and delayed (from a few hours up to four days later) food inflammatory sensitivities. This panel covers 50+ of the most common foods in the Standard American Diet ranging from almond through wheat including both animal and plant proteins.

B. **Dr. Pai's Celiac Panel, which includes gluten/gliadin screenings (reticulin antibodies/tissue transaminase/gluten IgA, gliadin).** This test will show whether there is inflammation from eating gluten/gliadin, which are the compounds found most abundantly in wheat products. It also tests for the severe condition of celiac disease (which affects about one out of every hundred people). If this test result is positive, then you can get inflammatory reactions that last from one week up to three months after ingestion of the offending foods. With these results, if positive, you need to strictly avoid gluten/gliadin.

C. **CDSA (Comprehensive Digestive Stool Analysis) 2.0 or GI Effects.** This stool test will show how much of the general good probiotics you have in your GI tract. It will also tell whether there is any bad bacterial overgrowth and whether these overgrowths constitute infections (pathogens). In addition, the GI Effects test will look for candida and parasites. If any unwanted microbes are present, they will be tested for sensitivities and resistance to common antibiotics and natural therapies so that doctors can use only the most effective therapeutic agents. It will also show if there are any problems with inflammation; digestion of fats, proteins, and carbohydrates; and so on.

D. **Candida Panel:** If one does not get the stool test above or just wants Dr. Pai's Food and/or Inhalant-Allergy Panel, then a blood test can check for candida IgA, IgM, and IgG. That test helps tell us whether the patient has current, past, or chronic overgrowth or infection. If it is positive, then I would recommend using my Natural Antimicrobial Support if you prefer natural therapies over prescriptions. If, however, you choose a prescription, I would advise using Nystatin orally, which predominantly stays in the GI tract, and not fluconazole (i.e., Diflucan), which spreads systemically.

E. **NutrEval nutrition evaluation.** If you have had surgery that involved the removal of any part of the GI tract, then this test will help show the levels of your vitamins (A thru Zinc), minerals, digestive enzymes, CoQ10, alpha-lipoic acid, glutathione, amino acids, omega 3-6-9s, and even toxic elements (i.e., heavy metals). If you have any deficiencies, this test will then provide the ideal supplement dosage for you and list the types of foods those nutrients are found in, allowing you to eat more to get these nutrients directly from your diet—not just from handfuls of pills.

When one has inhalant or seasonal allergies—which usually involve sensitivities to grasses, weeds, trees, molds, dust mites, cockroaches, cats and dogs, and so on—or has asthma or any lung disease that is treated with antihistamines (e.g., Benadryl, Zyrtec, or Claritin), steroids (nasal sprays, such as Flonase or Nasonex, or oral steroids, such as prednisone), or montelukast (i.e., Singular), I would recommend not only tests A and B above, but also **Dr. Pai's Inhalant Panel**, to test for inhalants. This panel contains thirty-four inhalants, including grasses, weeds, trees, molds, dust mites, and animals, that cross-react with two hundred other species. It can be modified to include local environmental allergens specific to your area.

Manufacturing of Probiotics

Not all probiotics are the same. Since they are dietary supplements, most (approximately 90 percent) are *only guaranteed potency at the time of manufacture, not at the time you take them.*

This corresponds to most products having only 10 percent to 30 percent (confirmed by independent testing) of the potency that is advertised on the label by the time you take the product. If a probiotic is not acid-stable (few advertise themselves as such), then most of the probiotics will be destroyed by stomach acid and, thus, will not reach the small and large intestine, where they are mainly needed.

A good rule of thumb when it comes to probiotics is to be wary of proprietary blends. When not stating on the label specifically how much of each species of probiotic is in the product—instead listing only the total amount of the "proprietary blend"—manufacturers tend to put the largest amount of the probiotic first and the smallest last. That enables a manufacturer to include 95 percent of the first probiotic ingredient (sometimes a less expensive and, usually, a less effective strain) and smaller percentages of the remaining probiotics. They do this to keep production costs very low without the consumer knowing exactly how much of each probiotic strain is in the product. Although most probiotics on the market are not harmful, because they are not formally regulated, most of them are not clinically effective.

The ideal label for probiotics includes each amount of every species and the total amount in CFU (colony-forming units) **(see fig. 39)**.

Supplement Facts

Serving Size 1/4 Teaspoon (1g) • Servings Per Container 60

Amount Per Serving

Probiotic Blend (100+ billion CFUs) in a base of inulin (derived from chicory root) and proprietary polysaccharide complex		1 g*
Lactobacillus rhamnosus	24.0+ billion CFUs*	
Bifidobacterium bifidum	20.0+ billion CFUs*	
Lactobacillus acidophilus	12.0+ billion CFUs*	
Lactobacillus casei	10.0+ billion CFUs*	
Lactobacillus plantarum	8.0+ billion CFUs*	
Lactobacillus salivarius	8.0+ billion CFUs*	
Bifidobacterium longum	4.0+ billion CFUs*	
Streptococcus thermophilus	4.0+ billion CFUs*	
Lactobacillus bulgaricus	4.0+ billion CFUs*	
Lactobacillus paracasei	2.0+ billion CFUs*	
Bifidobacterium lactis	2.0+ billion CFUs*	
Bifidobacterium breve	2.0+ billion CFUs*	

*Daily Value not established.

Other ingredients: None.

Figure 39: Ideal Label for Probiotics: Includes each amount of every species and total amount in CFU (colony-forming units)

The typical label for probiotics **(see fig. 40)** does not list each amount of every species and provides total amount in milligrams instead of CFU. Therefore, amounts of each species can vary within the product and the total amount of CFU (potency) cannot be easily compared.

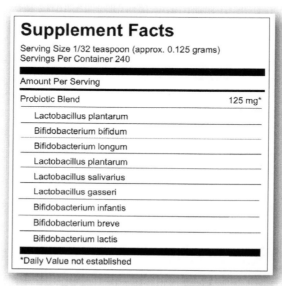

Figure 40: Typical label for probiotics

Most probiotics also contain dairy ingredients. This can be a problem for those with dairy allergies, especially those with IgE immediate reactions. Although companies can claim "dairy-free" on the label, in reality the FDA allows the definition of "dairy-free" to contain up to 5% dairy ingredients. There have been cases of children exhibiting worsening symptoms—even anaphylactic reactions—when using probiotics following treatment with antibiotics, even when the parents, knowing their child was allergic to dairy, chose a product labeled dairy-free. Even a small amount of dairy can, for certain individuals, be enough to cause problems.

At Sanjevani, our probiotics are manufactured using the most stringent standards. As a physician who practices integrative medicine, I recommend probiotics for people for their overall health, but I understand that when I do so, I have to ensure that my patients are getting the full benefits (and no harm) from these important supplements.

That's why I personally made sure that *our probiotics are guaranteed for potency and purity at the time that you take them* (not only at time of manufacture) *and hold their potency up to one year after the expiration date* when kept at room temperature. We have our probiotics *manufactured with acid-stable technology that prevents the probiotics from being destroyed by stomach acid*, allowing them to release into the small and large intestine. In addition, our probiotics are 99.99 *percent dairy-free*, defined as having less than two parts per million of dairy protein, rendering them safe for those with dairy allergies. It was important to me that we provide a probiotic with twelve clinically validated probiotic species and offer potencies from twenty-five billion **(Sanjevani Complete Probiotic Formula)** to one hundred billion CFUs per serving **(Sanjevani Complete Probiotic Powder Formula)**. Even though our probiotics are stable at room temperature, all probiotics are best if kept refrigerated. Be skeptical of probiotics that state that they don't need refrigeration, are in the form of pearls, or are freeze-dried. These are likely all wastes of your money. It all comes down to quality in manufacturing that adheres to the strictest standards. Unfortunately, most probiotics miss the mark.

Furthermore, one should avoid taking formulated probiotic yogurts. Although some may have specialized probiotic strains, most manufacturers pasteurize and heavily process the yogurt, which has a tendency to decrease the viability of the probiotics. Although some companies may add them afterward, they add very little, as they do not have to list the amount. Thus, they too are not as clinically effective as they want you to believe. According to their clinical studies, one must consume this yogurt three times daily, costing an average of forty to sixty dollars a month.[276] In addition, these types of yogurts contain all the usual colors, artificial sweeteners or corn syrups, casein protein (procarcinogenic promoter), whey protein, hormones (endocrine disruptors), and antibiotics that are not good for you anyway. In addition, they also contain 80–110 calories and 4–12 g of dairy protein per serving. Thus having the recommended three servings a day will add 240–330 calories and 12–36 g of dairy protein to your diet.[277] In my opinion, that's not good for those trying to lose weight or lower their risk from dairy consumption. It is cheaper to stick to taking an effective probiotic supplement, like **Sanjevani Complete Probiotic Formula**, than to take in additional dairy protein (non-organic with hormones), calories, fat, sugars (non-GMO), and all the other chemicals and preservatives in processed foods like "enhanced" yogurts.

You may have noticed the explosion of probiotic products on the markets—especially from companies that make OTC pharmaceutical products or generic supplements. This is because these companies already have slotting allowances or shelf space, available in pharmacies and health-food stores, due to them having a large share of products already in these stores. This prohibits many smaller competing companies and products from entering the marketplace, since they cannot pay these stores for the shelving space. Some larger companies actually threaten stores, stating that they will pull all their products if the stores carry a competitor's product (especially if that product may be better).

When considering purchasing a probiotic product from a big pharmaceutical or food company, ask yourself simple questions like:

"Why is a company that sold me antacids, stool softeners, and acid blockers for the last twenty years only now selling me probiotics?"

"Shouldn't companies that claim to be specializing in GI health have been providing these products over the last twenty years?"

"If this big pharmaceutical company is now telling me that probiotics are good for my GI health, why have they been selling me symptomatic treatments all this time?"

"If they really care about my GI health, why are they selling me only one or two strains of probiotics in small potencies, and why are these not acid-stable?"

This issue pertains not only to generic pharmacy or grocery-store probiotics but also to OTC probiotics that claim to be "recommended by GI doctors."

Why are these big companies selling such inferior probiotics at all? Companies that dominate the marketplace already have millions of marketing dollars and influence what stores sell. They are not interested in resolving your health issues. If they were, you would not buy their other products for symptomatic treatments. Hence, it is in their best interest (or their shareholders' best interest) to sell a substandard probiotic that does not give you complete clinical benefits; it means you will take their other GI products to help regulate your condition.

Remember that almost all generic probiotics on the market will never cause harm, but they also won't have much true clinical benefit for you. For the most potent, pure, and effective probiotics, I recommend **Sanjevani Probiotic Formula Powder** or **Sanjevani Probiotic Formula (capsules)**. Sanjevani Probiotic Powder can be taken ¼ teaspoon daily (up to three times a day for those with active colitis, diarrhea illness, or undergoing chemotherapy or radiation therapy) sprinkled on food. It is four times more potent than our capsules thus provides more cost savings for those who need maximum support. Sanjevani Probiotic Formula capsules can be taken one to two daily for maintenance and those who prefer capsules for convenience. Both can be taken with or without food.

Natural Antimicrobial Support*

For those who have allergies or sensitivities to antibiotics such as penicillin, sulfa, or Floxin drugs, here is what we use at Sanjevani to provide antimicrobial-supportive therapy:

A. **Argentyn 23.** This is a hydrosol of silver that is better absorbed and more effective than regular colloidal silver products. It is very effective for infections like bronchitis. It can be used orally or topically (it comes in a gel also), or it can be nebulized for lung infections. The dose taken orally is very specific, so follow the directions on the bottle or from your health-care provider. You should only take this product for the same duration as an antibiotic course; do not take it daily as a preventive product.

B. **Oreganol P73 Super Strength.** This is a very strong antimicrobial herb.* We offer it in a five-day pack (similar to a Z-Pak) for minor upper-respiratory infections, *H. pylori*, and candida infections.* Patients take one softgel twice daily with food.

C. **Sanjevani Urinary Tract Support Formula.** Great to use for minor urinary-tract infections at the start of symptoms. Patients take one capsule twice daily with food for seven to ten days.

Even though the above are natural antimicrobials, like antibiotics, they also negatively affect probiotics in our GI tracts. Therefore, I recommend taking

Sanjevani probiotics **(see Side Notes on Probiotics)** at a different time during the day—usually around two hours before or after—when taking any of the above products. In addition, I strongly recommend taking some of the immune-support products **(see Side Note: Sanjevani Immune-Support Protocols)** to strenghten your body's own defense and repair mechanisms for optimum results. As with all products above, please consult with your healthcare provider prior to use for individual guidance and evaluation.

Sanjevani Immune Support Protocols
Some of my favorite immune-system boosters follow:

A. **Sanjevani Vitamin D3 (capsules or liquid).** Vitamin D3 is a simple yet effective vitamin that keeps your immune system functioning optimally. It comes in 5,000 IU capsules or liquid 1,000 IU per drop. I recommend 1 capsule or 5 drops daily with your largest meal to increase absorption since it is a fat-soluble vitamin (better absorbed with healthy fat like organic coconut oil, olive oil, avocado, nut butters, and organic ghee). Remember the goal for your Vitamin D3 levels should be between 50–100 ng/ml on your blood test.

B. **Sanjevani Beta-Glucan 300** is an all-natural formula that uses Beta 1,3 glucans, scientifically proven to support, balance, and boost the immune system. Beta glucans are a naturally occurring long-chain polysaccharide purified from the cell walls of baker's yeast. Our beta glucan is intensely purified through a patented process to create Beta-1, 3D Glucan. This form of beta glucan is *biologically active* and easily absorbed through the Peyer's Patches in the small intestine. From here it is taken into the body to bind to a specific site on the immune cells called the CR3 receptor (sometimes called Mac1 or CD11/C18). CR3 stands for complement receptor number three; these receptors are found on a variety of different immune cells, which are the soldier cells of our immune system (white blood cells), also known more specifically as macrophages, neutrophils, eosinophils, monocytes, natural killer (NK) cells, and others. By binding to these specific receptor sites, it activates these immune cells. Through this activation it places those soldier cells on "high alert" to look out for foreign substances (i.e., viruses, bacteria, cancer cells) that they see as non-self. This process is referred to as immune modulation, not stimulation. Therefore beta glucans fine-tune these solider cells to improve their actions to help trap, consume, and destroy foreign substances that do not belong in the body. Beta Glucan modulates or activates but doesn't over stimulate, which is key to the safety of the compound. Research shows that our Beta-1, 3D Glucan is a highly effective immune modulator.[278]

Sanjevani Beta Glucan 300 provides the best quality, potency, and purity of beta glucans commercially available. It is produced with a minimum of 83 percent Beta-1,3D Glucan content, with no harmful contaminants. In comparative studies with competitor products in the beta glucans market, our source outperformed all others. It has been tested side-by-side with all the best-known, most widely available immune supplements and modulators and has been shown to outperform all of them.[279] This included better phagocytosis of neutrophils, stimulation of Interleukin-2, stimulation of antibody response, increased superoxide production, and increase in IFN-γ (interferon gamma). The purity, biological activity, and the potency of Sanjevani Beta Glucan 300 surpasses all others. I recommend 2 capsules daily on an empty stomach for thirty minutes for general health maintenance. For those with cancer or chronic health conditions, one capsule for every fifty pounds of weight.

C. **Sanjevani Immune Formula.** This natural formula has a combination of AC-11 and larch arabinogalactan that not only enhances immune responsiveness but also promotes the body's natural capacity to repair DNA. AC-11 is a patented water-soluble extract of *Uncaria tomentosa* that has numerous and varied beneficial effects on immune cells. Its ability to repair damaged DNA helps to counteract cell damage caused by oxidative stress that results from environmental influences and aging. Arabinogalactan polysaccharides derived from the larch tree stimulate certain beneficial immune cells (macrophages and natural killer cells) and cytokines (part of the body's natural defense system), resulting in a potent immunomodulating effect. This supplement can be taken twice daily with food when one is sick, dealing with a chronic condition that causes one to be prone to infections, or having trouble recovering from chronic

illness. You can also use it for prevention; for example, take one tablet before going into an area where you are at risk for exposure to
illness (such as going to a concert, taking a cross-country flight, or
going to the mall during the holiday season).

D. **Sanjevani Complete Probiotic Formula (pills or powder).**
Sanjevani probiotics have guaranteed potency and purity at the
time that you take them—not just at the time of manufacture—and
hold their potency for up to one year after the expiration date (when
kept at room temperature). We manufacture our probiotics with
acid-stable technology that prevents stomach acid from destroying
the probiotics, enabling their release into the small and large intestines. You can take our probiotic with or without food, making it a
convenient option for those on the go. In addition, our probiotic is
99.99 percent dairy-free, containing less than two parts per million of
diary protein, making it safe for those with dairy allergies.

We provide twelve clinically validated beneficial bacteria species
and offer potencies ranging from 25 billion CFUs per capsule to 100
billion CFUs per serving of powder. Even though our probiotics are
stable at room temperature, all are best if kept refrigerated. For general health, I recommend taking one capsule once or twice daily—
depending on your bowel function (or dysfunction). For those with
IBS, colitis, or heavy use of antibiotics, or for those who are dealing
with chemotherapy or radiation therapy for cancer, I recommend
1/4 teaspoon of the powder once or twice daily—or more if needed.

D. **Sanjevani Vegetarian Strengthen.** This non-GMO and plant-based
protein shake contains the full amount of amino acids for an easy-to-
digest protein. It is predominantly made from a combination of pea
and rice protein that provides an amino-acid score of 100 percent and
digestibility score of 98 percent.[280] This vegetarian protein is naturally
obtained by simple water extraction, which keeps all the nutritional
qualities intact and provides a particularly high content of lysine, argi-
nine, and branched-chain amino acids, which are essential nutrients
that help protein synthesis (keeping and increasing muscle mass).

This fructose-free shake also includes ingredients that promote
overall gastrointestinal health and support the body's natural ability to detoxify and respond to inflammation and chronic disease.

A serving contains 21 g of protein in addition to natural immune-supportive ingredients. It is a highly concentrated source of immunoglobulins (40 percent IgG), bioactive proteins and growth factors called ImmunoBoost (which are derived from whey peptides but filtered so that less than 1 percent of the dairy proteins remain—thus providing a vegetarian formula). It possesses three times more immunoglobulin G (IgG) and total immunoglobulins than colostrum and has twice as much cysteine—an important amino acid for maintaining glutathione levels. Compared to colostrum alone, ImmunoBoost delivers fifteen times the level of transferrin and lactoferrin. In addition, it contains OncoDefense, a patented form of glucoraphanin derived from broccoli-seed extract, which has been shown to have beneficial effects on antioxidant activity, detoxification, cellular metabolism, and cell-life regulation.[281] It also contains larch arabinogalactan, an immune strengthener and prebiotic.

      Note: For cancers patients, substitute **Sanjevani Immunoglobunin IgG powder** instead to avoid any additional glutamine in diet.

E.   **Sanjevani HistaPlus Formula.** Quercetin is potent antioxidant flavonoid that is found in plant pigments in many fruits and vegetables. Quercetin acts like an antihistamine and an anti-inflammatory, and may help protect against allergies, heart disease, hypertension, and cancer.[282] Quercetin can also help stabilize the cells that release histamine in the body and thereby have an anti-inflammatory effect. Quercetin can provide real benefits for allergy sufferers. Sanjevani HistPlus Formula delivers the right dose of an optimum form of quercetin along with adding beta glucan. This combination offers synergistic effects that may be especially supportive of healthy immunologic responses during exposure to allergens or irritants. Combined use of both agents may assist in modulating inflammation, maintaining serum IgE levels in the normal range, and stabilizing mast cells and basophils. Both ingredients help balance the ratio of T helper 1 (Th1) to T helper 2 (Th2) lymphocyte responses to a variety of pathogens. Animal studies have shown them to support immune surveillance and response to neoplasms.

F.   **Megaway or Cannabiseology Shake.** See **Plant-Based Health Shakes** section.

G. **CBD (Cannabidiols):** CBD is the active and main constituent of industrial hemp oil. Unlike cannabis that is used for recreational or medical purposes, CBD derived from industrial hemp oil has only trace amounts of THC (usually less than 0.3 percent) and thus one does not get "high" from taking it since the psychogenic component THC is barely detectable. CBD from industrial hemp oil is legal in all fifty states and can be obtained without a medical cannabis card. CBD has many health benefits including anti-inflammatory, antiseizure, anticancer, and immune-balancing properties.[283] I have been successfully using CBD in my practice for years and lecture on the subject at integrative cancer conferences, where I teach other doctors how to effectively offer CBD to their patients. It comes in sublingual drops and a concentrated paste. We carry a variety of brands for which the industrial hemp is grown in Europe, and each batch is third-party tested for purity, potency, and contaminants. Some are organic with no preservatives or flavors, some with MCT oil and stevia. Our CBD products also have different CBD percentages ranging from 15 percent to 25 percent and certain types provide CBDa, which contains natural terpines, which provide additional anti-inflammatory pain-relieving benefits. Please see **www.cbdproducts.org** or contact our office for details at **www.sanjevani.net.**

Books and Movies

For a different take on health and happiness that is in line with the topics covered in this book, I highly recommend the below list of books and movies.

Books:

1. Greger, Michael, *How Not to Die,* (New York, Flatiron Books, 2015).
2. T. Colin Campbell, PhD, and Thomas M. Campbell II, MD, *The China Study,* (Dallas, BenBella Books, 2006)
3. Travis Christofferson, *Tripping Over the Truth: The Return of the Metabolic Theory of Cancer Illuminates a New and Hopeful Path to a Cure,* (Rapid City, CreateSpace Independent Publishing Platform, 2014).
4. Bruce Lipton, *The Biology of Belief: Unleashing the Power of Consciousness, Matter, & Miracles,* (New York, Hay House, 2008).

5. Michael Pollan, *The Omnivore's Dilemma*, (New York, Penguin Books, 2007).

6. Michael Pollan, *Cooked: A Natural History of Transformation*, (New York, Penguin Books, 2014)

7. Michael Pollan, *Food Rules: An Eater's Manual*, (New York, Penguin Books, 2009).

8. Martin L. Rossman, *Fighting Cancer from Within: How to Use the Power of Your Mind for Healing*, (New York, Holt Paperbacks, 2003).

9. Bharat B. Aggarwal, PhD, and Debora Yost, *Healing Spices: How to Use 50 Everyday and Exotic Spices to Boost Health and Beat Disease*, (New York, Sterling, 2011)

10. Dean Ornish, MD, *Reversing Heart Disease—*

11. Caldwell Esselstyn, Jr. MD, *Prevent and Reverse Heart Disease: The Revolutionary, Scientifically Proven, Nutrition-Based Cure*, (New York, Avery, 2008)

Movies:

1. *The Quest for the Cures…Continues* and *The Global Quest Continues* www.TheTruthAboutCancer.com—Series from Ty Bollinger

2. *Genetic Roulette: The Gamble of Our Lives*, The Institute of Responsible Technology (Jeffery Smith), www.geneticroulette.com

3. *Fast Food Nation: The Dark Side of the All-American Meal*

4. *Forks Over Knives*

5. *Food, Inc.*

6. *Fat, Sick, & Nearly Dead*

7. *Statin Nation*

8. *Thrive*

9. *King Corn*

10. *Earthlings*

11. *Pink Ribbons, Inc.*

12. *Bought*

13. *Happy, The Movie*

14. *FeedTheWorld.info* (movie about Glyphosate/Roundup and its effects)

15. *Plant Pure Nation*

Growing an Inexpensive Garden and Growing Boosters

Everyone who can should grow a garden. It is surprisingly easy, even if you haven't done so before, and starting off small is the way to go. But once you start getting accustomed to growing some of your food, you will appreciate nature in a different light. You will also benefit from the direct nutrition, and, in a way that changes people's minds about vegetables, you will taste the difference.

Planter barrels used for planting trees are perfect for starter gardens. Commercial landscaping stores and nurseries offer them very inexpensively. They run under fifteen dollars and are made of plastic with holes for drainage. Best of all, they will last for decades. The next step is to get natural organic soil called Fertilome, which is nutrient rich with humic acids and organic seeds. Choose plants appropriate for the mixture of sunlight and shade you have available. To help grow your garden, you can use an amazing product called **Fruitland Plant Stimulator**, which is organic based. It contains high amounts of humic acids that give all the trace minerals that will make your plants grow. You need no toxic chemicals. You will see improved growth when using this natural and safe product.

You can even use hay bales (for around seven dollars), dig deep holes about six inches by six inches across, put soil and seeds inside the holes, and water. This method will only last one season before you have to dispose of the hay bale, but it can give you a season of learning about growing plants. I prefer the planter barrels, since they are sturdier and less messy. If nothing else, you can get a small planter box and just start growing herbs. Eventually you will have fresh herbs and some (small) vegetables that you can use daily in your meals. Having your own garden puts nature's pharmacy at your door.

Safer Alternatives for Weed and Bug Control

A safe alternative for getting rid of weeds in your garden or lawn is a product called **Essential Vinegar**. This works incredibly well—without resorting to toxic chemicals. You may have to apply it more frequently than commercial weed-control products, but as a trade-off, you won't have to worry about health problems from using it or just being around it.

For your home or workplace, consider using a product called **Essentria IC3 Insecticide Concentrate**. A little goes a long way, so be sure to follow the directions. You will have to get a spray bottle and dilute it with water, but it works well against spiders and insects, including ants. It uses natural oils like rosemary, geraniol, and peppermint—and it smells like root beer! It's safe for pets, so we use it at our clinic, and I use it at home.

If you have a small place or area of concern and do not want to use a spray at all, you can take aspartame (NutraSweet), mix with a small amount of sugar, and sprinkle it around where ants enter the building. The ants will eat the aspartame along with the sugar and die! If you research the historical discovery of aspartame, it was initially being studied as an insecticide. When the head of the lab asked the research scientist to "test it," he misunderstood and thought he was told to "taste it." Voilà! An artificial sweetener was born. But it's a far better (and safer) insecticide!

Microbe Blast (available at sanjevanistore.com) is a safe and effective product that is great for use on plants to eliminate fungus and molds. It is an all-natural plant-based product that uses a proprietary blend of pollinated plant esters and is processed using a highly advanced proprietary method. This produces a high pH, and through its unique properties, the product acts as a catalyst to assist the body in degrading unhealthy proteins and the chemical bonds that hold them together. It is a superconcentrated product, so follow the instructions on the insert; it has to be diluted to certain concentrations for different applications. I use it not only for the plants in my garden but (at a different dilution) for oral care for brushing teeth.

Omega-3 Recommendations

In over fifteen years of recommending omega-3 oils to thousands of patients, I have finally found a company that meets all my standards. The company is called Ascenta. After learning about the company and how they use only sustainable practices through strict governmental-agency regulations, follow the Council for Responsible Nutrition's guidelines, offer only high-potency products using natural triglyceride forms, and have plant-based softgels and liquid options, I was truly impressed.

Their Pure Check–branded potency and purity testing of each bottle of their oil (they provide third-party testing results online via a number on the bottle) has set the standard for real transparency. No other company has gone through that many quality checks, and no other company stands by their testing for potency and purity. They also run an environmentally friendly company that uses "green credits" for energy and donates to environmental causes.

Ascenta offers the first high-potency, clinically dosed, plant-based omega-3. As a vegan, this really captured my attention. When I met with the founder and heard his story—he restored his health by using fish oil—and learned about his drive to raise the bar for industry standards and improve the quality of omega-3s for everyone, I was stunned by how similar his passion was to my own when I developed Bosmeric-SR. I couldn't believe that I found another company that was small and personal, had a social and environmental consciousness, and was not afraid to enter a market dominated by large corporate entities that, in my opinion, are more about quantity than quality.

I myself use and recommend **NutraVege**, the plant-based omega-3. It has been a great addition to my practice and for my patients moving toward a plant-based diet.

The company offers liquids in addition to softgels, and their liquids taste crisp, clean, and light, with natural flavors of citrus, mango, and green apple. You have to taste it to believe it; the one for children even tastes like bubble gum—and all without artificial flavors, colors, or preservatives.

Liquid omegas aren't for everyone, so for those who prefer softgels, I recommend the following:

NutraSea +D: Two softgels contain 750 mg EPA, 500 mg DHA, and 1,000 IU of Vitamin D3

For those who prefer liquids and want more servings per bottle, I recommend the following:

NutraVege: One to two teaspoons daily. Two teaspoons contains 550 mg SDA (precursor to EPA), 400 mg DHA, and 1,000 mg of GLA. Citrus flavored.

NutraSea + D liquid: One teaspoon (5 ml) contains 750 mg EPA, 500 mg DHA, and 1,000 IU of Vitamin D3. Citrus flavored.

NutraSea: One teaspoon (5 ml) contains 750 mg EPA and 500 mg DHA. Mango flavored. I recommend this for those who want to change up the flavors so they don't get bored.

For those with high triglycerides, other lipid abnormalities, or severe inflammatory conditions:

> **NutraSea HP liquid:** One teaspoon (5 ml) contains 1,500 mg EPA and 500 mg DHA. Citrus flavored. This product also comes in softgels, but you would have to take four softgels daily, so I recommend the liquid. It is easier to take the increased amount, and you get ten more servings per bottle for the same price.

For those who have higher DHA needs for cognitive and behavioral conditions:

> **NutraDHA liquid:** One teaspoon (5 ml) contains 800 mg EPA and 500 mg DHA. Citrus flavored.

For children:

> **NutraKids liquid:** One teaspoon (5 ml) contains 320 mg EPA, 200 mg DHA, 50 mg GLA, and 500 IU Vitamin D3. Bubble-gum flavor (natural).

For pets:

> **Canine Omega-3 (dogs):** One teaspoon of meat-flavored oil daily provides 740 mg EPA and 460 mg DHA.
> **Feline Omega-3 (cats):** One teaspoon of fish-flavored oil daily provides 185 mg EPA and 115 mg DHA.
> **Equine Omega-3 (horse):** One teaspoon of apple-flavored oil daily provides 4,200 mg EPA and 2,600 mg DHA.

If you want to get the highest potency and safety of a plant-based omega-3 product (and the product I take daily), I recommend the NutraVege. To order any of the omega-3 products, please visit www.sanjevanistore.com.

Water Filtration

For general devices for your home and office, visit **www.sanjevani.net** and look up **Water Filtration Systems**. We have linked to a company that has a variety of options that can accommodate every filtration need and situation—whether you have city, rural, or well water—and suggest different types of removal processes for different contaminants. For most homes I would recommend a Total Solution Water Purification System (I use the Iron Total Solution Purification due to the high iron content of the water in my area). For those who cannot afford a full system, they also have small units for your home, shower, and sinks. This company also has additional reverse-osmosis-water-filter donations for people on reduced incomes with medical conditions and provides applications for those who may qualify.

After filtering your water, I highly recommend "structuring" it for maximum health and environmental benefits, especially for those with chronic health conditions **(see Side Notes: Structured Water)**.

Structured Water

"Organized" or "energy-enhanced" water—or, as it has more recently become known and understood, "structured water"—refers to water in its natural state that has not been subjected to the damaging effects of the modern phenomena of pipes and toxic chemicals. The best water-structuring device that I have researched (and use) is called Crystal Blue. Its structuring unit's unique design accomplishes one of nature's greatest miracles of regeneration and renewal by mimicking the natural spiraling motions and hydrologic cycles of water. This creates a measureable increase in water's ability to hydrate plant and animal tissues, penetrate soils, and conserve water. This technology employs an innovative application and advanced understanding of the vortex phenomenon. It uses the dynamic characteristic of the water itself to create a natural action that works at the molecular and quantum level. These specially designed units alter the molecular structure of the water, activating and retaining the healthful benefits of minerals and energetic characteristics. By enhancing the water, it allows "clusters" of water to form in perfect geometric shapes with the unique ability to receive, store, and convey information and bioelectric energy. When this structured water is consumed, it penetrates throughout the entire body, revitalizing and regenerating each and every cell. This action therefore causes people, plants, and animals to grow healthier and better. When you drink it, you will feel more refreshed, and the water will taste better. When placed in the house, the water will feel naturally soft, especially in showers, baths, hot tubs, and pools, all without the need for harsh chemicals and salts.

Research and university studies conducted with commercial structured-water devices over a decade have demonstrated significant favorable advantages in agricultural use, from increased yield of produce and healthy plant growth to decreased water consumption. A recent report from a leading agriculture university in India stated that after a two-year-cycle study, the Crystal Blue structured-water devices increased yield by 40 percent!

Crystal Blue Water Structuring Units are a quantum leap forward in the science of structured water over anything I have seen before. They are manufactured using only the finest grade surgical stainless steel, pure copper, and precision ground glass and quartz including a proprietary blend of broad-spectrum organic components, rare earth elements, and semi-precious mineral components. Placing this perfect combination under ten thousand pounds per square inch of pressure causes it to generate vastly greater amounts of pure electromagnetic energy and life-enhancing resonant frequencies.

I have been using Crystal Blue for the past few years at our office and home, and I have experienced amazing results. It seems very simple and easy to use and install, but it really works. If you are interested in learning more about structured water and using the best units that are available, please visit Crystal Blue Enterprises at **www.crystalblueent.com**. We are a distributor for Crystal Blue Enterprises products, so if you would like to order personal, home, or agricultural units, or if you have any other questions, please contact us at **www.sanjevani.net**.

Humic and Fulvic Acids

The following information has been provided by my colleague Dr. Dan Nuzum, who specializes in manufacturing and formulating humic- and fulvic-acid products, which we use at Sanjevani. "Our fulvics are a water-extraction process from multiple humics, all very good sources of bioactive carbon compounds.

A yellow to yellow-brown humic substance that is soluble in water under all pH conditions. We have in our arsenal quite a few of these fulvics and bioactive carbon compounds. All of the four primary organic macromolecules—nucleic acids, proteins, carbohydrates, and lipids (important ones, such as triglycerides, phospholipids, cholesterol, and steroids)—contain carbon, hydrogen, and oxygen. We have built these around bioactive carbon compounds with active carbon-rich polydisperse polyanions. Our lab list comprises liquids and powders that we use in our products and provide as raw material for many other companies. We have both powdered fulvic-acid and humic-acid extracts that are 100 percent pure fulvic acid and humic acid. These have massive surface area, carbon, hydrogen, and oxygen and are excellent delivery systems for our products. Our liquid products are certified at a 3.8 percent fulvic on the classical laboratory analysis, which is extremely high in the field.

"The most powerful feature of our products at Anwei labs is the bioactive carbon compounds and the stabilized molecular oxygen that is concentrated in our products.

"These active carbon compounds are a proprietary complex with highly stable molecular oxygen. We do not use hydrogen peroxide or ozone, which are unstable forms of oxygen. In our (fulvic) bioactive-carbon-compound hybrids, such as The Chelator and The Oxygenator, the active carbons are highly concentrated, and the molecular oxygen is driven up. Yet, the oxygen is still very stable and will not gas off. We have one product that has 1,100 ppm molecular oxygen in a stabilized state that is readily available to the body on contact. By nature it consists of 100 percent organically complexed, nano-sized, negatively charged ionic molecules that can easily penetrate human tissues and cells. For this reason, these highly bioactive carbon compounds on the cellular level provide innumerable biochemical and metabolic detoxification functions. In addition to carrying essential carbon, hydrogen, and oxygen to the cell, it has been shown that fulvic acid may be an excellent natural chelator of toxins and can reduce them to a harmless state. Fulvic acid is effective at neutralizing and detoxifying a wide range of toxic materials, heavy metals, and other pollutants. It is essential to wash away the waste and toxins that cells produce. Oxygen cleans and detoxifies the blood and tissues; it burns off cellular waste. It is essential in combating invading microorganisms. Oxygen soothes inflammation and pain. The presence of oxygen helps tissues heal. It also helps us deal with stress better, calming the nerves. Without enough molecular oxygen, tissues accumulate toxins from metabolic waste. There could also be a chronic low-grade infection by viruses, bacteria, candida yeast, and/or larger parasites. Any of these give off toxins as well.

"The fulvic and humic acid bioactive carbon compounds that we produce are carbon, hydrogen, and oxygen (CHO) molecules that carry such an enormous amount of energy that they enhance virtually everything they are bonded to. Our bodies are 96 percent carbon, hydrogen, and oxygen and little less than 4 percent minerals. Mineral assimilation without chelation is only about 10 percent effective. Don't let your nutrients that do not get assimilated in your body get flushed down the toilet. A good fulvic complex increases retention, absorption, and utilization of all the nutrients in food, vitamins, and supplements. Due to the higher concentration of active carbons, fulvic can extend the time that the carbon, hydrogen, and oxygen remain active in the body. A balanced electrochemistry is a requirement in the human body. Using a good source of active carbon, hydrogen, and molecular oxygen will give an effective food source for the beneficial aerobic bacteria. The body will fundamentally have the means to repair itself. When fulvic with active carbon, hydrogen, and high molecular oxygen encounter free radicals with unpaired positive or negative electrons, it supplies an equal and opposite charge to neutralize the free radical. We believe that our technology with fulvics, humics, and bioactive carbon compounds are untouchable in quality and design."

I recommend using **Equalizer Concentrate** 3–5 sprays 2–3 times daily in beverage of choice (available at sanjevanistore.com). I take it daily in my morning smoothie to give me an energy boost as well as enhance the absorption of my other supplements and foods. **Note**: Do *not* take humic and fulvic acids with prescription medications such as chemotherapy, SSRIs, anxiety meds, thyroid meds, blood-pressure and glucose medications, or other pharmaceuticals that have a very precise dosage or therapeutic window of efficacy, as they may be absorbed better than expected and cause side effects from being too strong. However, if taken about two hours way from the above you may obtain the benefits without concern of negative drug interactions.

Cosmetics and Body-Care Products

Why do our body- and skin-care products contain so many chemicals? Most people understand that the FDA regulates our foods and drugs (though some would question to what extent). There are regulations in place, and we are grateful to have them in many instances, but they definitely can be improved and enforced. Dietary supplements, for example, are not regulated like drugs, but the FDA has provided GMPs (Good Manufacturing Practices) and guide-lines that reputable manufacturers should follow. But the FDA does not pre-screen to determine whether or not a supplement should be on the market.

Most Americans think that their cosmetic products—including cosmet-ics and everything we put on our body to clean or make ourselves smell better—are regulated by the FDA...but they are *not regulated*. In fact, one of the biggest lobbying groups (behind oil and gas, pharmaceuticals, and insurance) is the cosmetics industry. Most of us believe that when we pur-chase a skin-care product, someone has reviewed it to ensure that it con-tains no dangerous ingredients; this is a completely false belief. There are few to no regulations for the production and manufacturing of the ingredients in body-care products.

How can this be? Isn't there an FDA for that? *No.*

With all the various large government regulatory agencies, isn't there one to oversee the products that we put on our babies, children, grandpar-ents, and ourselves? *No.*

In fact, the cosmetics industry has been lobbying against regulation—and has largely succeeded. What does this mean, then? *Buyers beware!* Yes, beware of the hundreds of chemicals that are in our body-care products and cause inflammation, irritation, immune dysfunction, and even cancer.

Wait—how are these chemicals in our products? It's easy—let me explain. When large companies produce chemicals, they also produce waste chemicals in the process. The question of what to do with these waste prod-ucts—many of which are classified as hazardous and cannot be disposed of directly, but only by expensive waste-management options—led industry lobbying groups to devise an effective and cost-efficient way to dispose of these toxic ingredients.

Lobbyists for these chemical corporations got Congress to provide tax credits to other companies who purchase these waste products and use them as "inert fillers." For example sometimes in order for a company to produce one pound of product, they may also produce ten pounds of waste materials that they have to dispose of. This is, again, a very costly process due to the hazardous nature of the waste chemicals. Instead, another company will take these toxic ingredients off the original company's hands for a tax credit and use them as inert ingredients (fillers) in their body-care products. They add these products to dozens of different brands of shampoos, conditioners, soaps, and cosmetics.

When you look at the products in your bathroom, do you ever wonder why there are so many ingredients in your shampoo? Why are the ingredient names almost impossible to say, and why does it seem as if you need a PhD in chemistry to understand what they are? Trust me—they are not there to make your shampoo lather better, make your hair shinier, or help clear away dirt and oil. They are just fillers classified as inert ingredients. As long as they are not classified as active ingredients (which must be reviewed for health claims and regulated for use), the inert ingredients do not have any purpose but to fill the bottle. Chemical companies produce so much of this stuff that we have no other place to put it but in more personal-care products. This is not a conspiracy; it's how business runs in the cosmetic and body-care industry in the United States today.

According to the CDC and EWG, the average person in the United States has *over 700 nonhuman chemicals in his or her blood*; newborn babies' cord blood has over 287 chemicals, of which 180 can cause cancer in humans or animals. Of the 700 chemicals in an average person's blood, 217 are toxic to the brain and nervous system, and 208 cause birth defects or abnormal development in animal tests. All from putting cosmetics on the body! While it may seem improbable that we absorb enough chemicals to have any effect, consider the use of lipstick; the average woman consumes (not intentionally but through mucosal absorption and reapplication) about *three to seven pounds* of lipstick by the time she reaches retirement age. Over time, our cumulative body burden harms the body's repair mechanisms, decreases immune function, and increases inflammation and cellular dysfunction.

We allow more than *hundreds of known carcinogens* in our body-care products in the United States, but many countries have banned and outlawed the use of the same chemicals in their products. Other countries have removed known carcinogens from products, but they remain in similar products sold here in the United States. Therefore, a lipstick here can contain dozens of dangerous chemicals, but when sold overseas in other countries—like Australia, Japan, and some EU countries—it is actually free of these hazardous ingredients. It all depends on which countries will allow the use of those hazardous chemicals. So far the United States is leading this race.

The largest companies that sponsor health-focused events (such as a marathon, walk-a-thon, or race) often sell products in conflict with that event. If, for example, their products (whether cosmetics, food, or pharmaceuticals) were investigated for their correlation to the cause promoted by the sponsored event, one might find a closer relationship than the company might like to admit. But this is not a new tactic; it's simply another way corporations like to distract the consumer. If we associate their product with helping a health-related cause, we will never realize that the product itself might be contributing to the health issue that requires a "cure." Remember, you might sponsor a race for the "cure," but the race never ends and there is never a real finish line in sight. Be careful of what you are being led to believe or run and walk for.

Case in point: before you purchase a product that has a pink ribbon on it, check out the documentary *Pink Ribbons, Inc.* or read the book *Pink Ribbons, Inc.: Breast Cancer and the Politics of Philanthropy*. The obfuscation of health dangers by corporations is well established in our economy.

Of course, many books, investigational reports, and documentaries have uncovered the same incestuous relationship between corporations and "health awareness" activities as marketing tools. Although I commend the public for participating in such events, as they are only trying to help others, I feel I have a duty to point out that they are being misled. I want only for each person to play a direct role in improving the system—not just attending a race that may be promoting corporate agendas instead of actually helping the cause.

Sinus Polyps and Surgery

If you are getting a nasal polypectomy from an ENT surgeon, make sure your doctor only removes the polyp directly and does not "Roto-Rooter" the entire sinus cavity, as this will decrease the ciliary (tiny hairs in the mucous lining) function in the sinus cavity. This ciliary functioning is crucial to helping move out the mucous that carries the pollens, dust, and anything else that we breathe into our digestive tract.

As with all types of surgery, the surgeon/doctor can bill more for a needlessly comprehensive procedure. Therefore, whether fully indicated or not, doctors commonly "take it all out." This is done for two perceived benefits:

1. To avoid any additional issues with the area (this thinking encourages nonessential surgery in an effort to decrease the likelihood of reoccurrence of the dysfunction or problem)
2. To be able to bill insurance companies and, therefore, charge the patient more for the procedure

The ciliary function is very important to keeping our respiratory tract healthy. We move about one and a half liters of mucous daily, and these tiny hairs (which, similar to those in our lungs, are easily damaged from smoking) play an important part in the cleaning of our airways. Surgery always damages cilia. Although surgery removes polyps and clears the sinus (confirmed on a CT scan or MRI), it often causes drainage problems thanks to functional damage to those hair cells. Most people after sinus surgery feel immediate relief but over time can end up having increased symptoms—with no conventional surgical options remaining. At this point, they are put on antihistamines and steroid nasal sprays for the rest of their life. An important yet simple way of helping clear the sinus cavity from allergies and irritation can be found in chapter 4. Hopefully, if you follow this protocol, use Bosmeric-SR, change your diet to eliminate causes of inflammation, and test for and treat your allergies, you will be able to avoid sinus surgery—as most of my patients are able to do. For those who already have had surgery, this protocol will help resolve any reoccurrences of sinus polyps and symptoms.

Exelon Patch

The Exelon Patch (and other Alzheimer's drugs such as Aricept) is aggressively marketed and prescribed for treatment of mild to moderate Alzheimer's disease (at a cost of approximately three hundred dollars per month). While on the surface this treatment seems promising, the way it is marketed disturbs me greatly.

When I see its commercials on TV, they show caregivers of aging parents holding a patch (with writing that says, "We're Fighters."). These commercials state that the patch "may improve overall function and cognition" and that "your loved one can get a 30-day free trial." Yet they immediately also state, "It does not change how the disease progresses," and "Hospitalization and rarely death have occurred from wearing more than one patch at a time." Then it lists the common side effects, which include nausea, vomiting, agitation, application-site reaction, diarrhea, urinary-tract infections, anorexia, dizziness, insomnia, weight loss, tremor, depression, anxiety, hallucinations, stomach pain, fatigue, muscle weakness, headache, drowsiness, vertigo, and allergic-contact dermatitis. (You can read the full list of side effects on ExelonPatch.com.) The commercial then states the likelihood of these side effects may increase when dosage increases or if one weighs less than 110 pounds. One of the problems with the Exelon patch, in my opinion, is that these side effects occur in a targeted population that cannot appropriately communicate if they obtain those side effects.

The slogan at the end of the commercial states, "Your care. Together with ours," and the title on the website reads, "A celebration of love between real caregivers and their loved ones."

To me, this campaign is a direct play on caregivers' emotions. Yet, if the drug companies really cared, wouldn't they endeavor to give you a drug that would not have so many side effects? How many of our parents and grandparents already have stomach problems (most elderly patients are on acid blockers like Prilosec), heart problems (most are taking statins, blood-pressure medications, blood thinners, etc.), difficulty breathing (many are taking medications for COPD and asthma), or bladder problems (many are on medications for urinary problems)? Thus, most elderly people are already at risk for a potential side effect.

But here is the secret to putting a medication with such wide-ranging side effects on the market: if your parents or grandparents experience these side effects, they will have difficulty telling you because of their Alzheimer's condition. How convenient that is for the drug company! The drug causes many common side effects that decrease the quality of life, but the people taking it can't make sense of why they are feeling so poorly.

Here is the other secret: once a patient experiences these side effects, conventional medicine will simply prescribe another medication to counteract those symptoms. The more medications, the more side effects for the patient. Patients then experience so many common side effects that their doctors can't figure out what is causing their symptoms, and this leads to the all-too-common downward spiral of health and quality of life. Yet, drug companies play on our fear of "not caring for our loved ones" unless we give them medications, so they offer a thirty-day free trial. But once people start something like the Exelon Patch, doctors usually never stop giving it, and thus they take this medication until they pass away—all under the guise of helping Alzheimer's sufferers.

Since the introduction of these types of medications, not once have I heard from family members that these medications made a big difference in their loved one's quality of life. But they do tell me that they feel pressure to state that they *do* see a difference, as they do not want to feel that they are not doing enough for their family member. I find it shameful that caregivers are put into this position, feeling helpless and desperate to depend on drugs that don't change the outcome of this terrible disease.

Absolute Risk Versus Relative Risk with Statins and Other Medications

When research is conducted and the data is presented, you should under-stand a few key words to make sure that you comprehend the real benefits of taking the medications. You need to know the difference between absolute and relative risk. Relative risk is how much risk is reduced over five years, which is the time period used in clinical studies. A 50 percent risk reduction would mean one out of two people would not have acquired the disease or problem if they took this treatment. However, this relative risk reduction is often misused (unintentionally and intentionally) to steer doctors and patients toward giving and receiving treatments. The more important factor to clarify is the absolute risk, which is the number of people one must treat in order to get the stated risk reduction. Let me give you two examples that have similar risk reductions of about 50 percent. Statins (e.g., Lipitor) and hormone blockers (e.g., Tamoxifen) both advertise to doctors and patients that they offer a 50 percent risk reduction in heart disease or reoccurrence of estrogen-positive receptor breast cancer. Now at first that sounds quite impressive. That means one out two people who take these drugs may prevent the disease from occurring. So most people take these drugs thinking that they will be part of the 50 percent that benefits. But here is the tricky part of clinical studies data—the absolute risk. Again, this is the number of people one must treat to get the 50 percent reduction in one out of two people. So if you look at the absolute risk for statins, one must treat four hundred people for five years in order to get the 50 percent risk reduction between just two people! Therefore, that means with the statins 399 people in over five years will not get that benefit.

Using the example of Tamoxifen, an estrogen blocker commonly used for preventing breast-cancer reoccurrence, among one thousand women, nineteen would be expected to develop breast cancer over the next five years. Therefore, if all those women took Tamoxifen, only nine of those women would avoid breast cancer. However, Tamoxifen is expected to cause twenty-one additional cases of endometrial cancer, thirty-one cases of cataracts, twenty-one cases of blood clots, and twelve cases of sexual problems. More than five hundred of the thousand women would naturally develop menopausal symptoms such as hot flashes, vaginal dryness, dry skin, and changes in vaginal discharge or irregular menstrual cycles.[284]

Be careful with how you are being sold and guided with pharmaceuticals said to treat chronic diseases and cancer when those drugs have serious side effects. Always make sure you ask about absolute risk, and then you can make a better-informed decision about whether you feel lucky enough to be among the few who actually benefit.

Preemptive Protocols for Food Allergies

Avoidance of the foods you're allergic or sensitive to is the best form of protection from food allergies (especially with severe IgE immediate reactions). However, social and environmental situations can make it difficult to avoid every food you are sensitive to all the time. Therefore, in addition to using Allergy-Drops Therapy or SAAT, I recommend the following to help preempt the inflammatory response and lower the flare once the food is ingested:

(Note: You should take these before eating the foods that you may have sensitivities to in order to help start the process of protection and support before foods can trigger inflammation.)

1. **Bosmeric-SR:** Two caplets at the beginning of the meal.
2. **Sanjevani Complete Digestive Enzyme Formula:** Contains a full spectrum of enzymes at clinical potencies, including a patented enzyme that helps break down gluten/gliadin proteins (helpful for those with wheat sensitivities/allergies). Two caplets prior to ingestion of the meal/foods.
3. **Sanjevani Complete Probiotic Formula (capsules or powder):** One to two capsules or less than 1/4 teaspoon at the beginning of the meal.
4. **Sanjevani HistaPlus Formula:** One capsule prior to meals for those who get runny nose or congestion when exposed to certain foods.

Plant-based Health Shakes

We successfully use the following different plant-based health shakes at Sanjevani.

1. **Sanjevani Vegan Sustain:** Our standard plant-based health shake made from non-GMO pea and rice blend with Aminogen, a plant enzyme that enhances protein digestibility and absorption, and Artinia chitin-glucan, a novel fiber that supports antioxidant systems in the body. It also contains high-potency vitamins and activated forms of B vitamins and Albion TRAACS chelated minerals. You can add organic veggies and fruit to taste and organic alternative milk (soy, almond, or coconut) if you want more protein, and you may water it if you want low calories. Contains 17 g of protein and 6 g of fiber per serving.
2. **Sanjevani Vegetarian Strengthen:** A plant-based health shake similar to the one above but with additional ingredients, including ImmunoBoost (immunoglobulins derived from less than 1 percent dairy—thus vegetarian instead of vegan) for supporting immune function, OncoDefense (patented form of SGS broccoli-seed extract) for supporting detoxification and liver function, MCT (medium chain triglycerides), and fiber complex. This shake is reserved for those with chronic or severe health conditions, such

as colitis flare or cancer, and those recovering from surgery. Contains 21 g of protein and 8 g of fiber per serving.

Note: Cancer patients substitute **Sanjevani Immunoglobulin IgG powder** to avoid any additional glutamine in diet.

3. **MegaWay Shake**: Our organic, raw, vegan, power-meal plant-based health shake, which contains seed proteins including hemp, golden flax, black chia, pumpkin, and sunflower seeds. Also has turmeric, goji berries, raw cocoa, alfalfa leaf, wheat grass, ashwagandha, red maca, cinnamon, and luo han guo. Contains 24 g of protein and 17 g of fiber. We recommend adding coconut milk or alternative milk beverage with some fruit. This can be used as a meal replacement if needed.

4. **Cannabiseology Shake**: The same as the above organic vegan raw shake but with added CBD (cannabidiols) at eight or 15 mg per serving. The CBD is verified by third-party laboratories and contains less than 0.3 percent THC. Thus it provides *no* psychotropic (high) effect but only the health benefits from the industrial hemp oil. This is legal and available in all fifty states.

Detoxification Support Protocols

The best form of complete detoxification is called *panchakarma*. At Sanjevani, we offer an integrative-medicine approach to panchakarma; we add additional therapies that, based upon clinical outcomes, have adjunct or supportive properties that improve upon this traditional Ayurvedic detoxification program. For those interested in a personalized panchakarma program, please contact our office. We also include Ayurvedic foods made specifically for your health condition and your dosha. For those unable to have panchakarma at Sanjevani, we have designed general detoxification protocols that everyone can use.

We first incorporate a variety of plant-based Ayurvedic food made specifically to each person's health condition (and dosha). One may start these foods prior to and after the program. We also may add a small amount of plant-based health shakes, in addition to specific supplements, as part of your unique Ayurvedic detoxification protocol—all of which are based upon your overall state of health (see below). These individualized Ayurvedic detoxification protocols integrate Ayurvedic medicines along with plant-based nutrition that includes protein, fiber, phytonutrients, vitamins, and minerals, in addition to adaptogens and antioxidants. These formulas help balance out the main bodily systems: digestive, circulatory, respiratory, urinary, endocrine, nervous, structural, immune, and emotional/mental.

Panchakarma seeks to augment the body's natural detoxification response with specific nutrients, minerals, and amino acids, in addition to comprehensive homeopathic formulas that use nosodes, sarcodes, metabolic and immune factors, and gemmotherapy—all of which support detoxification and drainage pathways, thus improving health and rejuvenation mechanisms.

Here are the enhanced panchakarma protocols I recommend (if one does not have access to Ayurvedic cooking):

General Health Maintenance:

1. **Sanjevani Vegan Sustain:** See **Plant-based health shakes,** *or*
2. **MegaWay Shake (vanilla mocha bean or triple creamy cacao):** See **Plant-based health shakes.** One scoop daily with organic soy, almond, or coconut milk and some organic fruits and veggies.
3. **Organic Spirulina:** Half teaspoon daily in shake above.
4. **Organic Clean Chlorella:** Half teaspoon daily in shake above.
5. **Sanjevani Liver Formula Forte:** One capsule daily at night. If elevated liver enzymes, may increase to one capsule three times daily with food.
6. **Equalizer Concentrate:** Liquid Fulvic Acid. Three to six sprays in shake above.

Weight Loss or Insulin Resistance/Diabetes:

1. **MegaWay Shake (vanilla mocha bean or triple creamy cacao):** See **Plant-based health shakes.** One scoop daily with organic soy, almond, or coconut milk and some organic fruits and veggies.
2. **Organic Spirulina:** Half teaspoon daily in shake above.
3. **Organic Clean Chlorella:** Half teaspoon daily in shake above.
4. **Sanjevani Berberine:** One capsule three times daily with food.
5. **Sanjevani Liver Formula Forte:** One capsule daily at night. If elevated liver enzymes, may increase to one capsule three times daily with food.
6. **Equalizer Concentrate:** Liquid Fulvic Acid. Three to six sprays in shake above.

Chronic Inflammatory Diseases, Cancers, or Injury:

1. **Sanjevani Vegetarian Strengthen:** Two scoops in organic soy, almond, or coconut milk with organic fruits and veggies. This contains ImmunoBoost from immunoglobulins (contains less than 1 percent dairy and thus is vegetarian, not vegan) and SGS (patented broccoli-seed extract), Aminogen (a proprietary plant enzyme blend to ensure breakdown and absorption of amino acids), and prebiotics, along with 21 g protein (pea and rice based) and 6 g of fiber. **Note:** Cancers patients substitute **Sanjevani Immunoglobulin IgG powder** to avoid additional glutamine in diet.

2. **MegaWay Shake:** See **Plant-based health shakes** or, for autoimmune diseases, cancer, or severe illness, use:

3. **Cannabiseology Shake:** See **Plant-based health shakes**.

4. **Organic Spirulina:** Half teaspoon daily in shake above.

5. **Organic Clean Chlorella:** Half teaspoon daily in shake above.

6. **Sanjevani Liver Formula Forte:** One capsule daily at night. If elevated liver enzymes, chemotherapy, chronic use of antibiotics or antifungals, exposure to environmental toxins, heavy use of alcohol, or liver disease, may increase to one capsule three times daily with food.

7. **Equalizer Concentrate:** Liquid fulvic acid. Three to six sprays in shake above. **NOTE:** Do *not* take fulvic-acid or humic-acid products with chemotherapy or with medications that lower blood pressure or with psychiatric medications, as they will make the effects stronger. You may take this product one and a half hours after medications.

As always, be sure to consult with your physician before starting any new dietary supplements or detoxification protocols.

Therapies to Help with Anxiety, Depression, and Insomnia
In addition to neuro-acupuncture (provided by Dr. Pai—**see Side Note: Neuro-Acupuncture**), the following devices are used successfully at Sanjevani to help with anxiety, depression, and insomnia:

1. **Sanjevani REST Pod (floatation therapy)**—see **chapter 11.** For details, visit **www.abqfloat.com.**

2. **Alpha-Stim:** This is an FDA-approved device for anxiety, insomnia, and depression. It uses microfrequencies in a patented waveform that amplifies some neurological-system activities and deactivates others in a fine-tuning process called neuro-modulation, which then places the brainwaves in the alpha-wave pattern in as little as twenty minutes. Alpha waves produce feelings of calmness, relaxation, and increased mental focus. The neurological mechanisms that occur during the alpha state appear to decrease stress effects, reduce agitation, stabilize mood, and regulate both sensations and perceptions of particular types of pain. Alpha-Stim can produce beneficial effects after a single treatment. Evidence for this abounds in fMRI, LORETA, and EEG mechanistic studies and clinical double-blind, randomly controlled medical, psychological, and dentistry studies.[285] For more details, visit **www.sanjevani.net** and look up Alpha-Stim.

3. **NT-3000 for treatment by auriculotherapy.** This is a specific microfrequency device used in Auriculotherapy (applied to ear acupuncture points) that works successfully on different phases of diseases from acute to chronic. It is painless and is delivered by Dr. Pai directly in addition to neuro-acupuncture protocols. For more details, visit **www.sanjevani.net** and look up NT-3000.

In addition to the devices and treatments listed above, you can also use the following Sanjevani natural therapies. Please ensure you speak to your health-care provider if you are taking any prescribed medications for such conditions so that he or she can monitor you symptoms.

1. **Sanjevani L-Theanine:** Recommended for anxiety, stress, and insomnia. The patented form of L-theanine at 200 mg helps place the brain in the theta-wave state, which is the "meditative state," better known in athletes as the "zone," when they are performing at high competitive levels. This amino acid is derived from green tea (without caffeine or the EGCG) and lasts about twenty-four hours. Take one capsule twice daily up to two capsules twice daily with food. This helps lower stress and improve focus and concentration. It is not a stimulant and

helps one also obtain better sleep if the mind wanders at night. It has no rebound or addiction and thus can be used daily or during times that require focus, attention, and calmness.

2. **Sanjevani 5-HTP SR:** Recommended for depression or severe insomnia. 5-HTP is an amino acid that is the precursor to serotonin production. For that reason, it provokes the body to produce more serotonin, uplifting the mood when a person's serotonin levels are low. One hundred milligrams per capsule is provided in a sustained-release form to maintain optimum balance. May be used along with SSRIs (with medical guidance) to help lower the side effects when weaning off prescription drugs. One capsule twice daily with food.

3. **Sanjevani GABA Plus:** Gamma aminobutyric acid is an amino acid that helps lower anxiety and OCD symptoms by its inhibitory function on neural overactivity. Our GABA Plus adds inositol, glycine, and taurine to support brain function and maintain optimum balance. One capsule twice daily between meals on empty stomach.

4. **Sanjevani Melatonin SR:** Higher dose (5 mg) in a sustained-release form of melatonin, our natural sleep hormone. The sustained-release form is especially helpful for those who frequently awaken at night; it keeps them asleep the entire night. One capsule one hour prior to bedtime. Plan at least seven hours of sleep. Because of its sustained-release action, not to be taken as a rescue remedy in the middle of the night.

5. **Sanjevani REST Pod: see section on Sanjevani REST Pod for details.**

Curcumin C3 Complex* In Bosmeric-SR

Bosmeric-SR contains the patented Curcumin C3 Complex, which has the highest number of human clinical studies and is used in more universities, research centers, and hospitals than any other brand. It also is GRAS approved, is supported by safety-dosage limit studies, and has been used for over twenty years by millions of people worldwide. Some companies that claim higher bioavailability are actually measuring the metabolites of curcuminoids, such as glucuronides, not curcuminoids themselves. Studies have recently shown these metabolites *not* to have anti-inflammatory effects. Thus, such providers are delivering only a lower percentage of curcuminoids.

	Bosmeric-SR®	BCM-95® Curcumin	Longvida
Curcuminoids	250mg	400mg	250mg
Bioavailability claim (higher absorption than regular form of curcumin	20 times	6.75 times	65 times
Dosage Equivalent to Curcumin	5000mg	2700mg	3250mg
Enhanced Absorption System	Bioavailability enhancer: BioPerine™	Micronization and Turmeric Oil	Solid lipid particles
GRAS Status	Curcumin C3 Complex™ and BioPerine™ are GRAS affirmed	N/A	Only self affirmed
Mechanism	Inhibition of Glucoroniation in GI tract. Thermogenesis by BioPerine™	Unproven phenomenom of extra intestinal absorption	Lipid based formulation
Peer reviewed research articles	Over 30	2	3 clinical studies
Maximum safe dosage limit	Curcumin C3 Complex™ 12 grams per person daily	No chronic toleration study available	No chronic toleration study available on human services
Allergens	None	Turmeric Oil	Soy lecithin
Sustained Release	8 Hours Sustained Release	N/A	N/A

Figure 32: Comparison Curcumin C3 Complex in Bosmeric-SR* vs. others

	Bosmeric-SR®	NovaSOL® Curcumin	Turmeric Extract
Curcuminoids	250mg	6% (30mg Curcumin in 500mg formulation)	?
Bioavailability claim (higher absorption than regular form of curcumin	20 times	185 times	N/A
Dosage Equivalent to Curcumin	5000mg	5.5g	N/A
Enhanced Absorption System	Bioavailability enhancer: BioPerine™	Curcumin micronisate and micelle using Triacetin Panodan, Silicon dioxide, Tween 80	N/A
GRAS Status	Curcumin C3 Complex™ and BioPerine™ are GRAS affirmed	N/A	?
Mechanism	Inhibition of Glucoroniation in GI tract. Thermogenesis by BioPerine™	No specific mechanism cited	N/A
Peer reviewed research articles	Over 30	2 (one human, one animal study)	?
Maximum safe dosage limit	Curcumin C3 Complex™ 12 grams per person daily	No chronic long term study available to assess safety	?
Allergens	None	?	?
Sustained Release	8 Hours Sustained Release	N/A	N/A

Figure 33: Comparison Curcumin C3 Complex in Bosmeric-SR* vs. others

The following comparison data on BCM-95, Meriva, Longvida and Novasol was provided by Sabinsa Corporation (the patent holder of Curcumin C3 Complex) at time of writing.

BCM-95

1. BCM-95 claims to provide highly bioavailable curcuminoids using turmeric *oil*, whose history of use and safety are still questionable.
2. BCM-95 does not have GRAS status and cannot be added in food as a legal food additive. Curcumin C3 Complex, on the other hand, has FDA GRAS status.
3. BCM-95 uses turmeric oil without defining its composition, but that composition could affect both the stability and safety of products that contain BCM-95.
4. Independent studies have shown that, when used along with curcuminoids, turmeric oil tends to reduce the protective benefits of curcuminoids in the arthritic model, thus reducing the efficacy of this composition in comparison to curcuminoids when used alone.[286]
5. Bioavailability claims are based on a small and insignificant number of subjects, thus raising question on the results themselves.
6. In the absence of any proven mechanism of action by which turmeric oil enhances bioavailability, the unproven phenomenon of "extraintestinal absorption" has been held responsible for bioavailability, but this is highly debatable.
7. Unlike most arthritis studies, which are double blind, the only efficacy-based study done on rheumatoid arthritis subjects with BCM-95 was single blind, only making it more vulnerable to biased results.
8. Compared with results from curcuminoids studies done in the past, results from the arthritis clinical study on BCM-95 did not show any significant difference in end point results, in length of treatment required or duration of improvement, or higher compliance or safety outcomes.
9. Claims of enhanced bioavailability in BCM-95 have not been experimentally verified by independent researchers, nor have claims of improvements in efficacy of curcuminoids.

10. The number of independent studies supporting the clinical efficacy of the BCM-95 combination is nil. Turmeric oil and its main component ar-Turmerone have been long recognized and used as insect repellant.

Meriva

1. Meriva is a phospholipid complex of curcuminoids (20 percent); hence Meriva contains only 20 percent of the desired curcuminoids.
2. Phospholipid complex formation is a technique used by pharmaceutical scientists to improve solubility and absorption.[287] In 1999, a scientific paper was published by Central and Food Technological Labs in India showing the influence of phospholipid formulation of curcuminoids.[288] Also another publication in 2006 clearly demonstrated the absorption of curcuminoids with phosphatidylcholine.[289] So, we do not believe this is a novel or patentable concept.
3. The published paper on Meriva did not show or comment on the useful phase I metabolites of curcumin.[290] An example of a phase I metabolite is tetrahydrocurcuminoids, found to be similar in action to curcuminoids.
4. The phospholipid complex on oral administration increased phase II metabolites, that is, predominantly phase II metabolite of a minor curcuminoid, demethoxycurcumin (DMC 15–17 percent component of 95 percent curcuminoids). These phase II metabolites have never been studied, and their pharmacological effects and toxicity profile on continuous usage is unknown.
5. A recent study[291] has shown the glucuronides of curcuminoids, that is the phase II metabolites, lack biological activity similar to their parent molecule. The study's authors pointed out very clearly the inability of glucuronides to cause "mitotic catastrophe," a key parameter to destroy tumor cells:
   - Showing twenty-nine times more of an inactive metabolite (or a metabolite of unknown pharmacologic activity) and making a claim for bioavailability is not relevant.
6. Curcuminoids are good and safe material. But increasing the bioavailability of any substance indiscriminately could be counterproductive. An intravenous injection of curcumin along with phospholipid

complexes (liposomes) that will theoretically give the maximum bio-availability has resulted in hemolysis (destruction of red blood cells) in dogs. See http://www.signpathpharma.com/styled-4/. Curcumin C3 Complex has been shown to be safe up to 12 g per day orally.

7. The statement that Meriva increases bioavailability of curcumin is technically wrong. Meriva, if at all, increases the bioavailability only of curcuminoid metabolites (the glucuronide and sulfated metabolites of curcuminoids, with unproven beneficial activity), not curcuminoids per se. The paper on Meriva,[292] acknowledges that, stating, "Free curcumin could not be detected in any of the plasma samples in accordance with previous studies."

8. GRAS (Generally Recognized As Safe) Affirmation: Meriva is self affirmed-GRAS certified. However, Curcumin C3 Complex from Sabinsa is the only curcumin to have GRAS status approved by the FDA, which further validates its safety.

9. US Status: Meriva is a new entrant with minimal supportive research and clinical data. Curcumin C3 Complex is considered an Old Dietary Ingredient, as it was sold and marketed prior to October 1994. Curcumin C3 Complex has a rich legacy of research and clinical documentation spanning nearly two decades. Meriva also seems to vitiate the ratio of absorption of curcuminoids in a distorted way and the long-term effects of such phenomenon are yet to be evaluated.

Longvida

Reasons to choose Curcumin C3 Complex over SLCP (Solid Lipid Curcumin Particles) Longvida:

A. SLCP contains only 20–30 percent of curcuminoids. Actual composition of inert material used not disclosed.

B. Very limited studies showing clinical efficacy have been done and published on the SLCP composition.

C. Safe dosage of 42 g per day for human consumption of SLCP is based on an incorrect extrapolation of NOAEL dosage in rats.

D. Using the FDA guideline in calculating human-equivalent dosage from animal study, it was found that daily dosage in humans for Longvida is only 6.1 g per day, which contains only 20–30 percent of curcuminoids (1.2–1.8 g).

E. Bioavailability of SLCP is based on a three-subject study (in each arm).

F. Human study did not conclusively prove the sustained availability of curcuminoids in the gut. Not all the arms of the study using Longvida showed sustained availability (note: $t_{1/2}$ given in table 4).[293]

G. Though free curcuminoids were claimed to be present in the plasma,[294] sample preparation exposed the plasma to high temperature of 70°C, which can easily hydrolyze the glucuronides, giving a faulty observation of free curcuminoids.

H. No clinical study has been done on the SLCP to show the efficacy of the product in comparison to the regular grade of curcuminoids, hence any bioavailability claims to enhance efficiency of the product are unproven.

NovaSol

Following are important points regarding a study on the micronized powder and liquid micelle-curcumin product NovaSol.

1. The study[295] uses the beta glucuronidase to break down the curcumin conjugates in the blood, thus defeating the whole purpose of studying the bioavailability of unaltered pharmacologically active curcuminoids. The study probably measures mostly inactive glucuronides.

2. Micronized and micelle-based curcumin formulations do not inhibit the biotransformation of curcuminoids, which is the limiting factor for improving bioavailability; instead these formulations just load the body with more inactive glucuronide metabolites of curcuminoids.

3. Delivery system of powdered curcumin is not ideal for comparison, especially with curcumin not soluble in the water.

4. The micelle composition contains 7 percent curcuminoids. To reach the normally recognized dosage of 500 mg of curcuminoids, patients will need to ingest 7 g every time.

5. In this 7 g, 6.3 g will be Tween, an emulsifier. According to the CFR 21 (part 172), describing the limitation of use of Tween 80—(a) as a solubilizing agent in pickles or pickle products the maximum amount of the additive cannot exceed 500 ppm (b) for vitamin-mineral preparations containing calcium caseinate, the maximum intake of polysorbate 80 shall not exceed 175 mg from recommended daily dose of preparation. For preparations without calcium caseinate, it should still not exceed 475 mg.

6. From this study no clinically effective dosage can be derived, and no clinical studies are cited to demonstrate any clinical/health benefit of such physical formulation.

Boswellin PS in Bosmeric-SR

	Bosmeric-SR®	5-Loxin®	BosPure®
Boswellic Acid (by HPLC)	20-30%	40-45%	40-45%
Total number of Boswellic Acids	4 Major Boswellic Acids	6 Boswellic Acids	3 Boswellic Acids
Acetyl-11-keto-B-Boswellic Acids (AkBBA)	10-12%	30%	10%
Major Component	AkBBA and Polysaccharide (PS)	AkBBA	10% AkBBA B-Boswellic Acids Absent
Actives from Gum	Present	Absent	Absent
Content of Polysaccharide (Polysal/PS)	20-30%	Absent	Absent
Water soluble for immediate onset	Yes	No	No
Optimum ratios of Boswelic Acids + AkBBA + PS	Yes	No	No

Figure 34: Boswellin PS in Bosmeric-SR vs. others

	Bosmeric-SR®	Boswellia Extract
Boswellic Acid (by HPLC)	20-30%	?
Total number of Boswellic Acids	4 Major Boswellic Acids	?
Acetyl-11-keto-B-Boswellic Acids (AkBBA)	10-12%	?
Major Component	AkBBA and Polysaccharide (PS)	?
Actives from Gum	Present	Absent
Content of Polysaccharide (Polysal/PS)	20-30%	Absent
Water soluble for immediate onset	Yes	No
Optimum ratios of Boswelic Acids + AkBBA + PS	Yes	No

Figure 35: Boswellin PS in Bosmeric-SR vs. others

Bosmeric-SR contains the exclusive Boswellin PS formulation. No other product available contains this new form of boswellia that contains PS—polysaccharide or Polysal. Polysal provides a synergistic benefit to the boswellic acids and AKBBA, making the product stronger than each of the individual ingredients alone. Research shows the specific ratios of each have been chosen to enhance the total benefits. With this unique patented ingredient, it also provides a fast-acting (water-soluble) absorption within twenty minutes, unlike any other boswellia extract.

Ginger Elixir Recipe

This ginger elixir is one of the special foods that I learned through the Chopra Center. For those with weak digestion who need to take enzymes to help them digest food, this ginger elixir is a great natural premeal tonic, taken in a shot glass to stimulate digestive function and appetite. It's perfect for those who are undergoing panchakarma or a detoxification program.

Ingredients:

1 three-to-four-inch piece of unpeeled fresh organic ginger root
4 to 6 organic lemons
1 cup purified water
¾ cup raw organic honey (for those who are strict vegans, organic agave nectar can be substituted)
¼ tsp. organic crushed black pepper

Cut the ginger into ½-inch pieces. Using a powerful juicer, push the ginger through the juicer and juice enough to make 1 cup. In a citrus juicer, juice the lemons to make 1 cup of juice. Combine the juices in a large bowl. With a wire whisk, mix the water, honey, and black pepper into the ginger and lemon juice. Whisk until blended. Store in a pitcher or glass jar in the refrigerator.

Recommended use: One ounce twice daily, ten minutes before meals.

Ginger in Bosmeric-SR

	Bosmeric-SR®	Ginger Extract
Standardized (Percentage of Gingerols)	20%	?
Wildcrafted Pesticide Free	Yes	?
Protected from degrading other ingredients	Yes - Through Bilayered technology	No

Figure 36: Ginger comparisons in Bosmeric-SR vs. others

Research shows that gingerols are one of the most important compounds from ginger extract. Most products are not standardized at all. For those that are, the range may be between 2 percent and 10 percent. Bosmeric-SR provides ginger extract at 20 percent, which is the highest available in a dietary supplement. Also, the other ingredients in Bosmeric-SR are protected and their potency ensured through its specialized bilayered technology. This helps protect the potencies of the other ingredients in Bosmeric-SR. Other products contain ginger in capsules, which degrade the potency of the other ingredients over time.

BioPerine in Bosmeric-SR

Only BioPerine used in Bosmeric-SR is guaranteed to be standardized to 95 percent piperine. All other generic black-pepper extracts are not. Also, each caplet of Bosmeric-SR contains the optimum clinical dose of BioPerine for enhancing absorption, 5 mg, unlike other products that use between 1 and 2 mg.

	Bosmeric-SR®	Black Pepper Extract
Standardized to 95% Piperine	Yes	No
Wildcrafted Pesticide Free	Yes	?

Figure 38: BioPerine comparisons in Bosmeric-SR vs. others

BEMER Physical Vascular Therapy Device

Physical Vascular Therapy is the new, patented waveform classification of the next generation of pulsed-electromagnetic-therapy (PEMF) devices called BEMER. Although PEMF devices are very popular in doctor's offices, pain clinics, and homes, very few are supported by published studies; the exception is BEMER, which has been used for over fifteen years in Europe. The digital device is easy to use, safe, and highly effective.

BEMER research and technology has achieved breakthrough results in affecting the smallest vessels in the body. The core of BEMER Physical Vascular Therapy is a patented multidimensional signal structure that effectively stimulates restricted or impaired arterioles, venules, and capillaries.* It supports one of the body's most important control mechanisms for prevention, healing, recovery, and regeneration processes, and it can be easily and safely used in your office or at home. BEMER can also be effectively used for:

- General enhanced blood flow,
- Enhanced nutrient supply and waste disposal,
- Enhanced cardiac function,
- Enhanced physical fitness, endurance, strength and energy level,
- Enhanced prevention
- Enhanced concentration, mental acuity, stress reduction and relaxation,
- Enhanced quality of life

The BEMER Pro Set comes with a programmable LCD computer unit with a body mat. Also included are attachments for focus areas, such as a pad for wrapping around the shoulder, knees, or feet and a spot applicator to focus on smaller areas. Additionally it comes with an LED light applicator for helping skin conditions.

Patients can purchase a BEMER directly, or a health clinic can use it in their practice. If needed, financing options are available through outside financial institutions that provide zero-interest payment plans.

For those who use BEMER at home, after using it twice daily (eight minutes per session) for about six, weeks, they can then use a sleep mode that specifically improves the immune system. No maintenance on the

BEMER is needed. The device penetrates through clothing, so you just take off your shoes and lie on the mat (or you can place it on a chair or bed). Everyone in the family can use it. It even comes with a wall mount that allows you to hang the module unit next to the bed for treatment rather than keeping it on the nightstand or office table. It also comes with a PEMF-measuring tool that will test how strongly the fields are emitting and where on the mat the energy field is most concentrated. Finally, it comes with international plugs for use in other countries and even a car charger for those who travel.

After reviewing the information, if you would like to learn more or speak to someone about whether it may be right for you as an individual or in a clinic setting, visit **www.sanjevani.net** and look up BEMER. On that web page, there are presentations about BEMER that provide more detail on the health benefits and uses, as well as options to purchase.

Neuro-acupuncture

Neuro-acupuncture is a specialized form of acupuncture that is delivered to certain parts of the scalp. The world-famous doctor of oriental medicine, considered the Father of Neuro-Acupuncture (and the third most famous acupuncturist in China), is my teacher and friend Dr. Jason (Jinsun) Hao. Neuro-Acupuncture works best for neurological disorders such as Parkinson's, stroke (with weakness and paralysis), multiple sclerosis, pain syndromes (such as peripheral neuropathy), cerebral palsy, and other health conditions. We have formed a 501-c3 nonprofit organization called Neuro-Acupuncture Institute (of which I am currently the vice president) where we provide training programs for MDs, DOMs, and acupuncturists. The results are quite amazing, and I will write about it more in detail in another book. A documentary film called *Modern Day Miracles* will soon be released to educate the public about how effective yet simple this technique is. It can improve many conditions for which conventional medicine has nothing to offer. For more information about obtaining this type of specialized acupuncture as a patient, or to enroll in a training program as a health-care provider, please look up Neuro-Acupuncture at **www.sanjevani.net**.

Peripheral Neuropathy Protocols

If you are a health-care provider, I highly recommend that you read my chapter on peripheral neuropathy in *Integrative Medicine*, fourth edition, by Rakel, published by Elsevier. I have written the specialty chapter about peripheral neuropathy in all 4 editions of this excellent medical textbook. This is a great overall basis to start with integrative medicine when you are first introducing new evidence-based therapies that you may not have experience with.

Each natural therapy such as yoga, neuro-acupuncture, physical vascular therapy (BEMER), botanicals (i.e. curcumin, cannbidiols), supplements (i.e. benfotiamine, alpha-lipoic acid, acetyl l-carnitine) is supported by clinical studies in Europe—as I describe in detail, along with other helpful therapies, in my chapter in the integrative medicine textbook. I usually start with these and obtain the best benefits. Please consult with a health-care provider for guidance or make an appointment at Sanjevani if you decide to take any of the below.

1. Bosmeric-SR: Two caplets twice daily with food.
2. Sanjevani Benfotiamine: 150 mg twice daily with food. May increase to 300 mg twice daily if needed.
3. Sanjevani Alpha Lipoic SR: 600 mg sustained-release alpha-lipoic acid daily. May increase up to three times daily with food. If diabetic, monitor blood glucose, as it will help improve glucose utilization.
4. Sanjevani Acetyl-L-Carnitine: 500 mg twice daily and titrate to 1,000 mg three times a day if needed. Note: higher doses may cause loose bowel movements.
5. BEMER Treatment: Three to four times a week for twenty minutes. For best clinical results, ten minutes twice daily at intensity level three for thirty days, along with above Sanjevani supplements.
6. Neuro-Acupuncture: Every two weeks.

Sanjevani Intensive Support Pack

Following the success I have had at Sanjevani with my integrative medicine approach, I combined a variety of our products with some new additions in a Sanjevani Intensive Support Pack for patients with cancer and chronic diseases. It contains all of our Sanjevani-formulated products including: Ashwaganda Extract, Histaplus, Co-QH, Ester-C, Green Tea Extract, Liver Formula Forte, Immune Formula, Multivitamins, Trans-Resveratrol, and Reduced L-Glutathione. This convenient pack helps improve compliance and also provides cost savings. I have formulated these products in terms of potency, purity, and amounts in collaboration with Dr. Young Ko to improve and enhance the outcome from 3BP treatments. The Sanjevani protocols for certified 3BP cancer clinics will be the Sanjevani Intensive Support Pack, Bosmeric-SR, Sanjevani Beta Glucan 300, Sanjevani Complete Probiotic Formula, and Sanjevani Proteolytic Enzyme Formula. This protocol can be used for support for other cancer therapies such as 3-BP, PNC-27, IPT, Sono-Photo Dynamic Therapy, Rigvir, Hyperthermia, immunotherapies, Gerson, stem-cell therapy, protein and peptide therapy, and so on. It can also be used for use with conventional oncological care. **Note:** Please consult with a health-care provider or integrative-medicine MD to assist you with guidance on use of the above support protocols during your cancer treatment. Sanjevani Intensive Support Pack and above products are available at **sanjevanistore.com.**

Sole Protocol

Take Himalayan salt crystal (stones), place one stone in a large glass pitcher of purified filtered water (structured water is best), and wait a few hours for it to dissolve. Continue to add one stone at a time until the stone does not dissolve. Once the stone does not dissolve, the water is saturated at the optimum concentration to balance ionic composition of the trace elements. Sole is then complete and ready to use. Take one teaspoon daily (it will taste salty). This will help those with high and low blood pressure to assist the body to maintain homeostasis. For more details, check out the book *Water & Salt. The Essence of Life: The Healing Power of Nature.*

Bio-Well and Biocor

I have been using the Bio-Well for many years with great success. Now that the technology is cloud based, it is simple and easy to use with continued improvements incorporating more data than ever before on Chinese meridian and Indian chakra energy systems. It has provided my patients and me with guidance on subtle energy changes otherwise undetectable during routine evaluations. Thus it has become an important educational tool for including the human energy field as an important part of health and healing.

The following information has been provided by: Professor, Dr. Konstantin Korotkov, National University of Informational Technologies, Mechanics, and Optics, Saint Petersburg, Russia; and Krishna Madappa, president, Institute for Science, Spirituality, and Sustainability, Taos, NM.

Revolutionary Instrument to Measure Energy Fields of Life

Human Energy Field (HEF) is the most sensitive reflection of physical, emotional, and, in some cases, spiritual conditions of a person.

We take measurements from ten fingers of both hands and using sophisticated software create an image of HEF. The physical principle is based on Gas Discharge Visualization (GDV) process, well described in many publications.[296] Interpretation is based on connection of fingers with different organs and systems of the body by traditional Chinese medicine and the Indian chakra energy system and has been verified by twenty years of clinical experience by hundreds of medical doctors with many thousands of patients.[297] GDV is certified as a medical instrument in Russia (but not in the United States—it is an educational biofeedback tool). It gives information about the human energy field and allows one to see its day-to-day transformation and the influence of different situations and stimulus to the HEF and hence to the condition of a patient.

Recently together with the Gaiam, a company based in the United States, a new instrument—Bio-Well—was developed that uses an Internet-based server for processing data and presenting results to the end user. This makes all operations much easier and user-friendly and opens up broad perspectives for the implementation of the bioelectrography approach into medicine, psychology, and life sciences. It allows direct, real-time viewing and analysis of changes in human energy fields since the data is quantified and analyzed by sophisticated software. Because the results are obtained so rapidly, it has become an "express method" not only for analysis but also for detecting abnormalities that require more detailed investigation. Most importantly, since this technology and the protocols used are standardized, Bio-Well results obtained by different investigators can be compared with reliability.

The Bio-Well device is based on the stimulation of photon and electron emissions from an object when it is placed in an electromagnetic field and subjected to brief electrical pulses. This process is called "photo-electron emission" and has been thoroughly studied with cutting-edge electronic techniques. The emitted particles accelerate in the electromagnetic field, generating electronic avalanches on the surface of the dielectric (glass) plate in a process called "sliding gas discharge." The discharge causes a glow from the excitement of molecules in the surrounding gas that is constantly measured. Voltage pulses stimulate optoelectronic emissions that are amplified in the gas discharge, and light produced by this process is recorded by a sensitive CCD (charge coupled device) camera that converts it into a colored computer image, or bio-gram. Data obtained from the fingers of both hands are converted into a human energy field image using proprietary sophisticated software.

This technology has extraordinary implications for all health-related fields, including conventional as well as complementary or alternative therapies. A comprehensive review of these varied Bio-Well applications can be found in a book coauthored with Dr. E. Yakovleva from Moscow Medical University. [298] Research with the Bio-Well device is currently being carried out at universities and research institutes worldwide in medicine, "energy medicine," athletic training, biophysics, parapsychology, and other disciplines.[299] One of the strongest applications of the Bio-Well technology is evaluation of well-being of people, which allows for use in a lot of health-related applications.

For those who have chronic health issues or many imbalances, the BIOWELL information can then be directed into the BIOCOR. The BIOCOR is biofeedback listening device that provides the combination of Music with Frequency healing based on your data from the BIOWELL. It is transformed into your own custom healing music that helps provide balance to the body as you listen to it. The BIOCOR can be purchased for listening at home on a computer or on a smartphone (or it can be used as a therapy session in an office). Your health-care provider would conduct routine evaluations from the BIOCOR to continue to evaluate and monitor your energy fields and then reprogram your personal music therapy. Then you can listen at home at your leisure (if purchased) or in the office during a therapy session.

For more information about the Bio-Well and BIOCOR, visit **www.bio-well.com**. Currently at Sanjevani, we are a distributor and help train health-care providers on how to use this tool in their practice. If you or your office is interested, please contact our office at **www.sanjevani.net**.

REFERENCES

1. Yasumichi Arai et al., "Inflammation, but Not Telomere Length, Predicts Successful Aging at Extreme Old Age: A Longitudinal Study of Semi-supercentenarians," *EBiomedicine* (July 2015), doi: 10.1016/j.ebiom.2015.07.029.

2. D Murro, "Annual U.S. Health Care Spending Hits $3.8 Trillion," *Forbes*, February 2, 2014, http://www.forbes.com/sites/danmunro/2014/02/02/annual-u-s-healthcare-spending-hits-3-8-trillion/.

3. B Burkrot, "U.S. Healthcare Usage and Spending Resumes Rise in 2013," *Reuters*, April 15, 2014, http://www.reuters.com/article/us-spending-rise-idUSBREA3E06Q20140415.

4. "Explaining High Health Care Spending in the United States: An International Comparison of Supply, Utilization, Prices, and Quality." The Commonwealth Fund, May 3, 2012, accessed December 19, 2015, http://www.commonwealthfund.org/Publications/Issue-Briefs/2012/May/High-Health-Care-Spending.aspx.

5. Centers for Medicare and Medicaid Services. National Healthcare Expenditures Data, last modified December 3, 2015, https://www.cms.gov/research-statistics-data-and-systems/statistics-trends-and-reports/nationalhealthexpenddata/nationalhealthaccountshistorical.html.

6. S Woolf and L Aron, *U.S. Health in International Perspective: Shorter Lives, Poorer Health*, National Academies of Sciences, January 2013, accessed December 19, 2015, https://iom.nationalacademies.org/~/media/Files/Report%20Files/2013/US-Health-International-Perspective/USHealth_Intl_PerspectiveRB.pdf.

7. S Bezruchka, "The Hurrier I Go the Behinder I Get: The Deteriorating International Ranking of U.S. Health Status," *Annu Rev Public Health* 33 (2012): 157–73.

8. "Bloomberg ranked countries based on the efficiency of their health-care systems. United States Ranks 46 out of 48 nations." *The Advisory Board Company. The Daily Briefing.* August 19, 2013. https://www.advisory.com/daily-briefing/2013/08/28/bloomberg-ranks-the-worlds-most-efficient-health-care-systems.

9. B Mintzes et al., "Understanding and Responding to Pharmaceutical Promotion: A Practical Guide," *World Health Organization/Health Action International Collaborative Project* (2011), http://haiweb.org/wp-content/uploads/2015/05/Pharma-Promotion-Guide-English.pdf.

10. C Rands et al., "8.2% of the Human Genome Is Constrained: Variation in Rates of Turnover across Functional Element Classes in the Human Lineage," *PLOS Genetics* (July 24, 2014).

11. P Anand et al., "Cancer Is a Preventable Disease That Requires Major Lifestyle Changes," *Pharm Res* 9 (2008): 2097–116.

12. Bruce Lipton, *The Biology of Belief: Unleashing the Power of Consciousness, Matter, & Miracles* (New York, Hay House, 2008).

13. K Alison et al., "Use of and Mortality after Bilateral Mastectomy Compared with Other Surgical Treatments for Breast Cancer in California, 1998–2011," *JAMA* 312, no. 9 (2014): 902–14.

14. Union of Concerned Scientists, "Ensuring the Harvest: Crop Insurance and Credit for a Healthy Farm and Food Future," (Cambridge, UCS Publications, 2012), accessed December 19, 2015, http://www.ucsusa.org/food_and_agriculture/solutions/expand-healthy-food-access/ensuring-the-harvest.html#.Vnhm4xorLEY.

15. Infographic:"Plant the Plate," Union of Concerned Scientists, 2012, accessed December 19, 2015, http://www.ucsusa.org/food_and_agriculture/solutions/expand-healthy-food-access/plant-the-plate.html#.Vnhl-BorLEY.

16. Union of Concerned Scientists, "Ensuring the Harvest: Crop Insurance and Credit for a Healthy Farm and Food Future," Appendix, page 29 (Cambridge, UCS Publications, 2012), accessed December 19, 2015, http://www.ucsusa.org/sites/default/files/legacy/assets/documents/food_and_agriculture/ensuring-the-harvest-full-report.pdf.

17. Union of Concerned Scientists, "Failure to Yield," *Evaluating the Performance of Genetically Engineered Crops* (Cambridge, UCS Publications, 2009), accessed December 19, 2015, http://www.ucsusa.org/sites/default/files/legacy/assets/documents/food_and_agriculture/failure-to-yield.pdf;
    Union of Concerned Scientists, "Ensuring the Harvest: Crop Insurance and Credit for a Healthy Farm and Food Future," *Evaluating the Performance of Genetically Engineered Crops* (Cambridge, UCS Publications, 2012), http://www.ucsusa.org/sites/default/files/legacy/assets/documents/food_and_agriculture/ensuring-the-harvest-full-report.pdf;
    Institute for Responsible Technology: "10 Reasons to Avoid GMOs," accessed December 19, 2015, http://www.responsibletechnology.org/10-Reasons-to-Avoid-GMOs); American Academy of Environmental Medicine, "Position Paper on GMO Foods," accessed December 19, 2015, http://www.aaemonline.org/gmopost.html.

18. Union of Concerned Scientists, "Failure to Yield," *Evaluating the Performance of Genetically Engineered Crops* (Cambridge, UCS Publications, 2009), accessed December 19, 2015, http://www.ucsusa.org/sites/default/files/legacy/assets/documents/food_and_agriculture/failure-to-yield.pdf.

19. American Academy of Environmental Medicine, "Position Paper on GMO Foods," accessed December 19, 2015, http://www.aaemonline.org/gmopost.html.

20. John Fagan, Michael Antoniou, and Claire Robinson, "GMO Myths and Truths: An evidence-based examination of the claims made for the safety and efficacy of genetically modified crops and foods," 2nd

ed., version 2.0, May 19, 2014, Earth Open Source, accessed December 19, 2015, http://earthopensource.org/earth-open-source-reports/gmo-myths-and-truths-2nd-edition/

21.   N Swanson et al., "Genetically Engineered Crops, Glyphosate and the Deterioration of Health in the United States of America," *Journal of Organic Systems* 9, no. 2 (2014),

http://www.organic-systems.org/journal/92/JOS_Volume-9_Number-2_Nov_2014-Swanson-et-al.pdf.

22.   Diego Martinez, "What Are We Eating?" *Daily Infographic*, last modified November 11, 2010, http://www.dailyinfographic.com/what-are-we-eating-infographic.

23.   Environmental Working Group, "EWG's 2015 Shopper's Guide to Pesticides in Produce," accessed December 19, 2015, http://www.ewg.org/foodnews/summary.php.

24.   Kim Painter, "Loosen Your Belts: U.S. Waist Sizes Keep Expanding," *USA Today*, September 16, 2014; Earl Ford, Leah Maynard, and Chaoyang Li, "Trends in Mean Waist Circumference and Abdominal Obesity Among US Adults, 1999–2012," *Journal of the American Medical Association* 312, no. 11 (2014): 1151–53.

25.   KM Flegal, MD Carroll, BK Kit, and CL Ogden, "Prevalence of Obesity and Trends in the Distribution of Body Mass Index among US Adults, 1999–2010," *Journal of the American Medical Association* 307, no. 5 (2012): 491–97.

26.   Fatima Haggar and Robin Boushey, "Colorectal Cancer Epidemiology: Incidence, Mortality, Survival, and Risk Factors," *Clin Colon Rectal Surg* 22, no. 4 (2009): 191–97, doi: 10.1055/s-0029-1242458.

27.   SS Maruti, JW Lampe, and JD Potter, "A Prospective Study of Bowel Motility and Related Factors on Breast Cancer Risk," *Cancer Epidemiol*

Biomarkers Prev 17 (July 2008): 1746; MS Micozzi et al., "Bowel Function and Breast Cancer in US Women," *Am J Public Health* 79, no. 1 (1989): 73–75.

28.   "The International Shark Attack File 2014 Worldwide Shark Attack Summary," Florida Program for Shark Research, Florida Museum of Natural History, University of Florida, accessed March 31, 2015, http://www.flmnh.ufl.edu/fish/sharks/isaf/2014Summary.html.

29.   David Kennedy and Amanda Just, "The Dentist's Health: Evaluating Occupational Risks from the Use of Amalgam," *The International Academy of Oral Medicine and Toxicology*, accessed April 1, 2015, http://iaomt.org/dentists-health-evaluating-occupational-risks-amalgam/.

30.   "*The State of World Fisheries and Aquaculture 2012*," FAO Fisheries and Aquaculture Department, Food and Agriculture Organization of the United Nations, (Rome, 2012), http://www.fao.org/docrep/016/i2727e/i2727e.pdf.

31.   B Beckermann, M Beneke, and I Seitz, "Comparative Bioavailability of Eicosapentaenoic Acid and Docoshexaenoic Acid from Triglycerides, Free Fatty Acids and Ethyl Esters in Volunteers," *Arzneimittelforschung* 40, no. 6 (1990): 700–704; LD Lawson and BG Hughes, "Human Absorption of Fish Oil Fatty Acids as Triacylglycerols, Free Acids, or Ethyl Esters," *Biochem Biophys Res Commun* 52 (1988): 328–35; S el Boustani et al., "Enteral Absorption in Man of Eicosapentaenoic Acid in Different Chemical Forms," *Lipids* 10 (1987): 711–14.

32.   "What about Krill? FAQs," Ascenta, accessed April 21, 2015, https://www.ascentahealth.com/omega-3-and-you/faqs/misc/.

33.   "Guide to Sourcing Sustainable Omega-3," Ascenta, accessed February 2, 2014, http:// www.ascentahealth.com/omega-3-resources/.

34.   Mandy Oaklander, "Nearly Half of Fast Food Has More Calories Than Ever," *Time*, Jan. 2, 2015, http://time.com/3652114/fast-food-nutrition/.

35. V Bouvard et al., "Carcinogenicity of Consumption of Red and Processed Meat." *Lancet Oncol* 2015 Dec;16(16):1599-600. doi: 10.1016/S1470-2045(15)00444-1.

36. "Full Menu Nutrition: Large Slice Meat Lover's Pizza," Pizza Hut Corporation, accessed November 16, 2015, https://order.pizza-hut.com/nutrition-menu; "Specialty Pizzas Nutrition Information: Large Slice The Meats Pizza," Papa John's Corporation, accessed November 16, 2015, http://www.papajohns.com/company/nutrition/; "Domino's Nutrition Guide: Large Slice MeatZZa Pizza," Domino's Corporation, accessed November 16, 2015, https://cache.dominos.com/olo/3_7_0/assets/build/market/US/_en/pdf/DominosNutritionGuide.pdf.

37. A Reiter, "How Many Slices of Pizza Does the Average American Eat in a Lifetime?" Food Network, Jan 20, 2015, accessed November 1, 2015, http://blog.foodnetwork.com/fn-dish/2015/01/how-many-slices-of-pizza-does-the-average-american-eat-in-a-lifetime/

38. C Robertson et al., "Get Sick, Get Out: The Medical Causes of Home Mortgage Foreclosures," *Health Matrix: Journal of Law-Medicine* 18, no. 65 (2008).

39. "Cancer Prevalence and Cost of Care Projections," National Cancer Institute, accessed November 1, 2015, http://costprojections.cancer.gov/annual.costs.html#f1.

40. S Klein, "Study: Insurance companies hold billions in fast food stock," April 15, 2010, accessed December 19, 2015, http://www.cnn.com/2010/HEALTH/04/15/insurance.fast.food.stock/.

41. T. Collin Campbell and Thomas Campbell, *The China Study: The Most Comprehensive Study of Nutrition Ever Conducted and the Startling Implications for Diet, Weight Loss, and Long-term Health* (Dallas, BenBella Books: 2006).

42. *M Greger. How Not To Die. Discover the Foods Scientifically Proven to Prevent and Reverse Disease.* (New York, Flatiron Books, 2015).

43. "Denny's All American Slam. Nutrition Facts," Denny's Corporation, accessed December 19, 2015, https://www.dennys.com/food/breakfast/all-american-slam/.

44. H Wu and R Sturm, "What's on the Menu? A Review of the Energy and Nutritional Content of US Chain Restaurant Menus," *Public Health Nutrition* 16, no. 1 (January 2013): 87–96.

45. M Oaklander, "Nearly Half of Fast Food Has More Calories Than Ever," Time Magazine, January 2, 2015, accessed January 9th, 2016, http://time.com/3652114/fast-food-nutrition/.

46. M Greger, "Who Says Eggs Aren't Healthy or Safe?" NutritionFacts.org, Accessed February 26, 2016. http://nutritionfacts.org/video/who-says-eggs-arent-healthy-or-safe/.

47. "How to Read Egg Carton Labels: A Brief Guide to Labels and Animal Welfare," The Humane Society of the United States, July 3, 2014, accessed July 6, 2014, http://www.humanesociety.org/issues/confinement_farm/facts/guide_egg_labels.html; "How to Decipher Egg Carton Labels," The Humane Society of the United States, accessed December 19, 2015, http://www.humanesociety.org/issues/confinement_farm/facts/guide_egg_labels.html.

48. Martin Marchello and Judy Driskell, "Nutrient Composition of Grass- and Grain-Finished Bison," *Great Plains Research: A Journal of Natural and Social Sciences* (Spring 2001) 11:65-82.

49. S K Duckett et al., "Effects of Time on Feed on Beef Nutrient Composition," *J Anim Sci* 71, no. 8 (1993): 2079–88.

50. B Prayson, J T McMahon, R A Prayson, "Fast Food Hamburgers: What Are We Really Eating?" *Annals of Diagnostic Pathology* 12, no. 6 (2008): 408–09.

51. Michael Pollan, "How Cooking Can Save Your Life," posted in "The Big Food Discrepancy: Why Are American Foods Routinely More Toxic Than European Versions?" Mercola.com, February 11, 2015, accessed February 16, 2015, http://articles.mercola.com/sites/articles/archive/2015/02/11/mcdonalds-fries-ingredients.aspx.

52. "EWG's 2015 Shopper's Guide to Pesticides in Produce," Environmental Working Group, accessed December 19, 2015, http://www.ewg.org/foodnews/dirty_dozen_list.php.

53. "The Hot-Dog Report," Clear Food, accessed November 16, 2015, http://www.clearfood.com/food_reports/2015/the_hotdog_report

54. Dina Spector, "See What Happens to Millions of Pounds of Las Vegas Buffet Leftovers," *Business Insider*, July 11, 2012, http://www.businessinsider.com/las-vegas-buffet-rc-farms-pigs-bob-combs-2012-7?op=1.

55. "McDonald's Product Nutrition McRib", McDonald's Corporation. Accessed December 19, 2015, http://www.mcdonalds.com/us/en/food/product_nutrition.burgerssandwiches.10.mcrib-.html.

56. A Ossola, "Chinese Factory Will Make Cloned Beef on a Massive Scale," Popular Science, November 30, 2015, accessed December 1, 2015, http://www.popsci.com/chinese-company-will-make-cloned-beef-on-massive-scale?9B9dxX4KzXRkyEhA.03.

57. "Animal Cloning," U.S. Food and Drug Administration, accessed December 19, 2015, http://www.fda.gov/AnimalVeterinary/SafetyHealth/AnimalCloning/.

58. R Weiss, "Studies Fail to Quell Concerns Over Gas Treatment of Meat," *The Washington Post*, July 23, 2006.

59. "Carbon Monoxide: Masking the Truth About Meat?" Food and Water Watch, April 2008. Accessed December 27, 2015, http://abcnews.go.com/GMA/Consumer/story?id=3863064&page=1*https://www.*

foodandwaterwatch.org/sites/default/files/carbon_monoxide_report_apr_2008.pdf.

60.   Ibid; "Proof in the Pink? Meat Treated to Give It Fresh Look," ABCnews.com, accessed December 27, 2015,

61.   "Chickens," United Poultry Concerns, Accessed December 19, 2015, http://www.upc-online.org/chickens/chickensbro.html.

62.   "Chicken, Ground Beef Top List of Riskiest Meats," Center for Science in the Public Interest, April 23, 2013, accessed December 19, 2015, http://cspinet.org/new/201304231.html.

63.   Alexander C. Kaufman, "2 Ways McDonald's 'Quick Fix' Antibiotics Move Falls Short," *Huffington Post*, March 4, 2015. accessed December 19, 2015, http://www.huffingtonpost.com/2015/03/04/mcdonalds-chicken-antibiotics_n_6801642.html.

64.   L DeCuir, "Finally! The FDA Admits That Nearly Over 70% of U.S. Chickens Contain Cancer-Causing Arsenic," MSN.com, January, 15, 2015, accessed December 25, 2015, http://www.msn.com/en-ca/foodanddrink/foodnews/finally-the-fda-admits-that-nearly-over-70percent-of-us-chickens-contain-cancer-causing-arsenic/ar-AA8cWca?ocid=se.

65.   E Group, "The Health Dangers of Arsenic Toxicity," Global Healing Center, December 4, 2015, accessed December 25, 2015, http://www.globalhealingcenter.com/natural-health/health-dangers-arsenic-toxicity/#10.

66.   Nancy Huehnergarth and Bettina Elias Siegel, "Chicken from China? Your Seafood Is Already Being Processed There," *Huffington Post*, May 3, 2014, accessed December 19, 2015, http://www.huffingtonpost.com/nancy-huehnergarth/chicken-seafood-china_b_4871733.html.

67.   Bettina Siegel and Nancy Huehnergarth "Congress: Keep Chinese Chicken Out of Our Schools and Supermarkets!" Change.org,

December 10, 2014, https://www.change.org/p/congress-keep-chinese-chicken-out-of-our-schools-and-supermarkets.

68. Robin McDowell, Margie Mason, and Martha Mendonza, "Slaves Used to Catch Fish That End Up on U.S. Tables," *The World Post*, March 24, 2015, http://www.huffingtonpost.com/2015/03/24/slaves-fish_n_6936070.html.

69. J R Jambeck et al., "Marine Pollution: Plastic Waste Inputs from Land into the Ocean," *Science* 347, no. 6223 (2015): 768–71.

70. Lynne Peeples, "Surprise Finding Heightens Concern over Tiny Bits of Plastic Polluting Our Oceans," *The Huffington Post*, March 23, 2015, http://www.huffingtonpost.com/2015/03/23/plastic-ocean-pollution-fish-health_n_6923872.html.

71. Jamais Cascio, "The Cheeseburger Footprint," Open the Future, accessed December 19, 2015, http://openthefuture.com/cheeseburger_CF.html.

72. Steve Boyan, "How Our Food Choices Can Help Save the Environment," Earth Save, accessed December 19, 2015, http://www.earthsave.org/environment/foodchoices.htm

73. Betty Hallock, "To Make a Burger, You First Need 660 Gallons of Water," *The Los Angeles Times*, Jan. 27, 2014.

74. Infographic, "The Hidden Water We Use: How Much H20 Is Embedded in Everyday Life?" *National Geographic*, accessed March 30, 2015, http://environment.nationalgeographic.com/environment/freshwater/embedded-water/.

75. Shannon Dinny, "Food-Borne Illnesses Cost U.S. $152 Billion Annually: Study," *Huffington Post*, May 5, 2010, http://www.huffingtonpost.com/2010/03/05/food-borne-illnesses-cost_n_487710.html.

76. Lisa Baertlein and P. J. Huffstutter, "McDonald's Is Removing Human Antibiotics from Its U.S. Chicken Supply," *The Huffington Post*, March 4, 2105, http://www.huffingtonpost.com/2015/03/04/mcdonalds antibiotics_n_6800030.html.

77. Centers for Disease Control, *Estimates of Food Borne Illness*, 2011. accessed December 19, 2015, http://www.cdc.gov/foodborneburden/2011-foodborne-estimates.html.

78. Centers for Disease Control, *Antibiotic Resistant Threats in the United States, 2013*, accessed December 19, 2015, http://www.cdc.gov/drugresistance/threat-report-2013/pdf/ar-threats-2013-508.pdf.

79. F Speizer, *The Nurses' Health Study*, Harvard Medical School, accessed December 19, 2015, http://www.channing.harvard.edu/nhs/?page_id=197.

80. Campbell and Campbell, *The China Study*.

81. Ibid.

82. T V Madhavan and C Gopalan, "The Effect of Dietary Protein on Carcinogenesis of Aflatoxin," *Arch Pathol* 85, no. 2 (1968): 133–7.

83. Campbell and Campbell, *The China Study*.

84. P Wells, L Alftergood, and R B Alfin-Slater, "Effect of Varying Levels of Dietary Protein on Tumor Development and Lipid Metabolism in Rats Exposed to Aflatoxin," *J Am Oil Chem Soc* 53 (1964): 559–62.

85. L D Youngman and T C Campbell, "High Protein Intake Promotes the Growth of Hepatic Preneoplastic Foci in Fischer #344 Rats: Evidence That Early Remodeled Foci Retain the Potential for Future Growth," *J Nutr* 121, no. 9 (1991): 1454–61; L D Youngman and T C Campbell, "The Sustained Development of Preneoplastic Lesions Depends on High Protein Intake," *Nutr Cancer* 18, no. 2 (1992): 131–42.

86. "Dietary Reference Intakes: Macronutrients", USDA, accessed December 19, 2015, http://fnic.nal.usda.gov/sites/fnic.nal.usda.gov/files/uploads/macronutrients.pdf.

87. Jessica Jones, "The Protein Myth: Why You Need Less Protein Than You Think," *HuffPost,* Sept. 21, 2012, http://www.huffingtonpost.com/jessica-jones-ms-rd/protein-diet_b_1882372.html.

88. J F Hu et al., "Repression of Hepatitis B Virus (HBV) Transgene and HBV-Induced Liver Injury by Low-Protein Diet," *Oncogene* 15 (1997): 2795–801.

89. Park et al., "A Milk Protein, Casein, as a Proliferation Promoting Factor in Prostate Cancer Cells," *World J Mens Health* 32, no. 2 (2014): 76–82; B C Meinik et al., "The Impact of Cow's Milk-Mediated mTORC1-Signaling in the Initiation and Progression of Prostate Cancer," *Nutr Metab* 9, no. 1 (2012): 74.

90. Campbell and Campbell, *The China Study.*

91. Kathleen Doheny, "Drugs in Our Drinking Water? Experts Put Potential Risks in Perspective after a Report That Drugs Are in the Water Supply," WebMD, March 10, 2008, http://www.webmd.com/a-to-z-guides/features/drugs-in-our-drinking-water; Brian Bienkowski and Environmental Health News, "Only Half of Drugs Removed by Sewage Treatment," *Scientific American,* November 22, 2013, http://www.scientificamerican.com/article/only-half-of-drugs-removed-by-sewage-treatment/.

92. E Del Giudice, "Old and New Views on the Structure of Matter and the Special Case of Living Matter," *Journal of Physics: Conference Series* (2007), http://dx.doi.org/10.1088/1742-6596/67/1/012006; E Del Giudice, A Tedeschi, and G Vitiello, "Coherent Structures in Liquid Water Close to Hydrophilic Surfaces," *Journal of Physics: Conference Series* (2013), doi:10.1088/1742-6596/442/1/012028; E Del Giudice, P Stefanini, and A Tedeschi, "The Interplay of Biomolecules and Water at the Origin of the

Active Behavior of Living Organisms," *Journal of Physics: Conference Series* (2011), doi: 10.1088/1742-6596/329/1/012001; I Bono et al., "Emergence of the Coherent Structure of Liquid Water," *Water* 4, no.3 (2012): 510-532, doi: 10.3390/w4030510; M W Ho, "Quantum Coherent Water, Non-thermal EMF Effects, and Homeopathy," *Science in Society* (2011), http://www.i-sis.org.uk/Quantum_Coherent_Water_Homeopathy.php; M W Ho, "Illuminating Water and Life: Emilio Del Giudice," *Electromagnetic biology and medicine* (2015), doi:10.3109/15368378.2015.1036079; M W Ho, "Life Is Water Electric," *Bioelectromagnetic and Subtle Energy Medicine*, 2nd ed. (Boca Raton, CRC Press, 2014); V L Voeikov and E Del Giudice, "Water Respiration: The Basis of the Living State," *Water Journal* (July 2009), doi: 10.14294/WATER.2009.4; V L Voeikov, "Reactive Oxygen Species-(ROS) Pathogens or Sources of Vital Energy? Part 1. ROS in Normal and Pathologic Physiology of Living Systems," *The Journal of Alternative and Complementary Medicine* 12, no. 2 (March 2006): 111–18, doi:10.1089/acm.2006.12.111; V L Voeikov, "Biological Significance of Active Oxygen-Dependent Processes in Aqueous Systems," *Water and the Cell* (2006): 285–98, doi: 10.1007/1-4020-4927-7_14; V L Voeikov, "Fundamental Role of Water in Bioenergetics," *Biophotonics and Coherent Systems in Biology* (2007): 89–104, doi: 10.1007/978-0-387-28417-0; I V Baskakov and V L Voeikov, "The Role of Electron Excited States in Biochemical Processes," *Biochemistry* 61, no. 7 (1996): 837–44; V L Voeikov, "The Possible Role of Active Oxygen in the Memory of Water," *Homeopathy* 96, no. 3 (July 2007): 196–201; L Montagnier et al., "Electromagnetic Signals Are Produced by Aqueous Nanostructures Derived from Bacterial DNA Sequences," *Interdisciplinary Sciences: Computational Life Sciences* 1, no. 2 (June 2009): 81–90; L Montagnier et al., "DNA Waves and Water," *Journal of Physics: Conference Series* 306, no. 1 (2011), doi: 10.1088/1742-6596/306/1/012007.

93. "Sublingual Immunotherapy Research Bibliography," AllergyChoices Incorporated, accessed December 19, 2015, https://www.allergy-choices.com/research/bibliography/.

94. Robert Odze, "Diagnostic Problems and Advances in Inflammatory Bowel Disease," *Mod Pathol* 16, no. 4 (2003): 347–58.

95. John Cush, Jonathan Kay, and Kathryn Dao, "Does Rheumatoid Arthritis or Biological Therapy Increase Cancer Risk?" *Drug Safety Quarterly* 4, no. 2 (2012).

96. G S Abela, "Cholesterol Crystals Piercing the Arterial Plaque and Intima Trigger Local and Systemic Inflammation," *J Clin Lipidol* 4, no. 3 (2010): 156–64; G S Abela and K Aziz, "Cholesterol Crystals Cause Mechanical Damage to Biological Membranes: A Proposed Mechanism of Plaque Rupture and Erosion Leading to Arterial Thrombosis," *Clin Cardiol* 28, no. 9 (2005): 413–20; G S Abela et al., "Effect of Cholesterol Crystals on Plaques and Intima in Arteries of Patients with Acute Coronary and Cerebrovascular Syndromes," *Am J Cardiol* 103, no. 7 (2009): 959–68.

97. William E. Boden et al., "Optimal Medical Therapy with or without PCI for Stable Coronary Disease," *N Engl J Med* 356 (2007): 1503–16.

98. Jennifer Brown, "Dr. Dean Ornish: Turn Back the Clock on Heart Disease," Everyday Health, February 18, 2014, http://www.everyday-health.com/news/dr-dean-ornish-turn-back-clock-heart-disease/.

99. D Ornish et al., "Effects of Stress Management Training and Dietary Changes in Treating Ischemic Heart Disease, *JAMA* 29, no, 1 (1983): 54–9.

100. D Ornish et al., "Intensive Lifestyle Changes for Reversal of Coronary Heart Disease, *JAMA* 280, no. 23 (1998): 2001–7.

101. D Ornish et al., "Changes in Prostate Gene Expression in Men Undergoing an Intensive Nutrition and Lifestyle Intervention," *Proc Natl Acad Sci USA* 105, no. 24 (2008): 8369–74.

102. D Ornish et al., "Effect of Comprehensive Lifestyle Changes on Telomerase Activity and Telomere Length in Men with Biopsy-Proven Low-Risk Prostate Cancer: 5-year Follow-Up of a Descriptive Pilot Study," *The Lancet Oncology* 14, no. 11 (2013): 1112–20.

103. "Sanjay Gupta Reports: The Last Heart Attack," CNN, August 20, 2011, accessed December 19, 2015, https://www.youtube.com/watch?v=JnDrjY2EgnQ.

104. Robert Odze, "Diagnostic Problems and Advances in Inflammatory Bowel Disease," *Mod Pathol* 16, no. 4 (2003): 347–58.

105. "Why the Use of Glyphosate in Wheat Has Radically Increased Celiac Disease: Interview with Dr. Stephanie Seneff," Mercola.com, Sept 14, 2014, http://articles.mercola.com/sites/articles/archive/2014/09/14/glyphosate-celiac-disease-connection.aspx

106. A Samsel and S Seneff, "Glyphosate's Suppression of Cytochrome P450 Enzymes and Amino Acid Biosynthesis by the Gut Microbiome: Pathways to Modern Diseases," *Entropy* 15 no. 4 (2013): 1416–63; A Samsel and S Seneff, "Glyphosate, Pathways to Modern Diseases II: Celiac Sprue and Gluten Intolerance," *Interdiscip Toxicol* 6, no. 4 (2013): 159–84.

107. Samsel and Seneff, "Glyphosate, Pathways to Modern Diseases II."

108. Ibid.

109. N Swanson et al., "Genetically Engineered Crops, Glyphosate and the Deterioration of Health in the United States of America," *Journal of Organic Systems* 9, no. 2 (2014), http://www.organic-systems.org/journal/92/JOS_Volume-9_Number-2_Nov_2014-Swanson-et-al.pdf.

110. Michael Pollan, *Cooked: A Natural History of Transformation* (New York: Penguin, 2014).

111. William Davis, *Wheat Belly: Lose the Wheat, Lose the Weight, and Find Your Path Back to Health* (New York, Rodale Books, 2014).

112. David Perlmutter, *Grain Brain: The Surprising Truth about Wheat, Carbs and Sugar—Your Brain's Silent Killers* (Boston: Little, Brown: 2013).

113. Dr. Christina Warinner is an archeologist at the University of Oklahoma and the University of Zurich's Centre for Evolutionary Medicine. Web Article: "The 'Paleo Diet': Real or Fad?" accessed December 19, 2015, http://www.meltorganic.com/the-paleo-diet-real-or-fad/.

114. Stephanie Butler, "Going Paleo: What Prehistoric Man Actually Ate," History Channel, Feb. 28, 2014, accessed December 19, 2015, http://www.history.com/news/hungry-history/going-paleo-what-prehistoric-man-actually-ate.

115. David Bassett et al., "Pedometer-Measured Physical Activity and Health Behaviors in United States Adults." *Medicine and science in sports and exercise* 42.10 (2010): 1819–1825.

116. Jo Robinson, *Pasture Perfect: How You Can Benefit from Choosing Meat, Eggs, and Dairy Products from Grass-Fed Animals* (Vashon, Vashon Island Press, 2004).

117. "New Research Discovers That Depression Is an Allergic Reaction," Feelguide, January 6, 2015, http://www.feelguide.com/2015/01/06/new-research-discovers-tha-depression-is-an-allergic-reaction-to-inflammation/.

118. US Surgeon General, *The Health Consequences of Smoking—50 Years of Progress: A Report of the Surgeon General, 2014,* US Department of Health & Human Services, accessed December 19, 2015, http://www.surgeongeneral.gov/library/reports/50-years-of-progress/

119. Denver Nicks, "1 Billion Smokers Light Up Around the Globe: But the Overall Smoking Rate Has Decreased Dramatically since 1980," *Time,* January 8, 2014.

120. Harlan R. Juster et al., "Declines in Hospital Admissions for Acute Myocardial Infarction in New York State after Implementation of a Comprehensive Smoking Ban," *Am J Public Health* 97, no. 11 (2007): 2035–39.

121. Jennifer Hissett et al., "Effects of Changing Guidelines on Prescribing Aspirin for Primary Prevention of Cardiovascular Events," *J Am Board Fam Med* 27, no. 1 (2014): 78–86.

122. Ross Hauser, "Wonder Why? The Acceleration of Articular Cartilage Degeneration in Osteoarthritis by Nonsteroidal Anti-inflammatory Drugs," *Journal of Prolotherapy* 2, no. 1 (2010), 309–22.

123. Ibid.

124. "LiverTox: Clinical and Research Information on Drug Induced Liver Injury," National Library of Medicine, accessed December 19, 2015, http://livertox.nih.gov/NonsteroidalAntiinflammatoryDrugs.htm.

125. "Risks Associated with Non Steroidal Anti-inflammatories (NSAIDs)," American Chiropractor Association, accessed December 19, 2015, http://www.acatoday.org/content_css.cfm?CID=2428.

126. D Adebayo and I Bjarnason, "Is Non-steroidal Anti-inflammatory Drug (NSAID) Enteropathy Clinically More Important Than NSAID Gastropathy? *Postgrad Med J* 82, no. 965 (2006): 186–91.

127. D Mozaffarian et al., "Heart Disease and Stroke Statistics—2015 Update: A Report from the American Heart Association," *Circulation* 131,4 (2015): e29–322.

128. "FDA Drug Safety Communication: FDA Strengthens Warning That Non-aspirin Nonsteroidal Anti-inflammatory Drugs (NSAIDs) Can Cause Heart Attacks or Strokes," FDA, July 9, 2015, http://www.fda.gov/Drugs/DrugSafety/ucm451800.htm.

129. Ibid.

130. T Wiegand et al., "Nonsteroidal Anti-inflammatory Agent Toxicity," *Medscape*, updated March 11, 2015, accessed April 21, 2015, http://emedicine.medscape.com/article/816117-overview.

131. Maggie Fox, "FDA Strengthens Heart Safety Warnings of Painkillers," NBCNews.com, July 9, 2015, http://www.nbcnews.com/health/heart-health/fda-strengthens-heart-safety-warnings-painkillers-n389516.

132. G Singh, "Recent Considerations in Nonsteroidal Anti-inflammatory Drug Gastropathy," *Am J Med* 105, no. 1B (1998): 31S–38S; M Wolfe, D Lichtenstein, and G Singh, "Gastrointestinal Toxicity of Nonsteroidal Antiinflammatory Drugs," *N Engl J Med* 340, no. 24 (1999): 1888–99; G Singh and R Rosen, "NSAID Induced Gastrointestinal Complications: The ARAMIS Perspective," 1997 Arthritis, Rheumatism, and Aging Medical Information System, *J Rheutmatol Suppl* 51 (1998): 8–16; J. Lazarou, B Poemeranz, and P Corey, "Incidence of Adverse Drug Reactions in Hospitalized Patients: A Meta-analysis of Prospective Studies," *JAMA* 279, no. 14 (1998): 1200–5; D Suh et al., "Clinical and Economic Impact of Adverse Drug Reactions in Hospitalized Patients," *Ann Pharmacother* 34, no. 12 (2000): 1373–9; N Moore, C Pollack, P Butkerait, "Adverse Drug Reactions and Drug-Drug Interactions with Over the Counter NSAIDs," *Therapeutics and Clinical Risk Management* 11 (2015): 1061–75; Singh, "Gastrointestinal Complications of Prescription and Over-the-Counter Nonsteroidal Anti-inflammatory Drugs," 115–21.

133. "Risks Associated with Non Steroidal Anti-inflammatories (NSAIDs)," American Chiropractor Association, accessed December 19, 2015, http://www.acatoday.org/content_css.cfm?CID=2428.

134. G Null et al., "Death by Medicine" (2011), accessed December 19, 2015, http://www.webdc.com/pdfs/deathbymedicine.pdf.

135. "Military Deaths in American Wars," Civil War Trust, accessed December 24, 2015, http://www.civilwar.org/education/civil-war-casualties.html?referrer=https://www.google.com/.

136. Ibid; "Casualties in Iraq and Afghanistan," Antiwar.com, accessed December 24, 2015, http://antiwar.com/casualties/; G Null et al.,

"Death by Medicine" (2011), accessed December 19, 2015, http://www.webdc.com/pdfs/deathbymedicine.pdf.

137. G Null et al., "Death by Medicine," *Life Extension Magazine* (March 2004).

138. Infographic, "NSAIDs: The Painful Truth behind Painkillers," Mercola.com, accessed December 27, 2015, http://www.mercola.com/infographics/nsaids.htm.

139. A Kumar et al., "Nuclear factor-kappaB: its role in health and disease, *Journal of Molecular Medicine* 82 (2004): 434–48.

140. S Prasad et al., "Curcumin, a Component of Golden Spice: From Bedside to Bench and Back," *Biotechnol Adv* 32, no. 6 (2014): 1053–64; B Aggarwal et al., "Prevention and Treatment of Colorectal Cancer by Natural Agents From Mother Nature," *Curr Colorectal Cancer Rep* 9, no. 1 (2013): 37–56; R Kannappan et al., "Neuroprotection by Spice-Derived Nutraceuticals: You Are What You Eat!" *Mol Neurobiol* 44, no. 2 (2011): 142–59; A Goel and B Aggarwal, "Curcumin, the Golden Spice from Indian Saffron, Is a Chemosensitizer and Radiosensitizer for Tumors and Chemoprotector and Radioprotector for Normal Organs," *Nutrition and Cancer* 62, no. 7 (201): 919–930; Ajaikumar B. Kunnumakkara et al., "Curcumin Sensitizes Human Colorectal Cancer Xenografts in Nude Mice to Radiation by Targeting Nuclear Factor-KB ^ Regulated Gene Products," *Clin Cancer Res* 14, no. 7 (2008): 2128-36; Amit K. Garg, Thomas A Buchholz, and Bharat B. Aggarwal, *Effects of Natural Polyphenols on Chemoradiotherapy in Cancer* (New Delhi, Jaypee Brothers Medical Publishers, 2009); K Sandur et al., "Curcumin Modulates the Radiosensitivity of Colorectal Cancer Cells by Suppressing Constitutive and Inducible NF-kB Activity," *Int J Radiation Oncology Biol Phys* 75, no. 2 (2009): 534–42; B Aggarwal et al., "Identification of Novel Anti-inflammatory Agents from Ayurvedic Medicine for Prevention of Chronic Diseases: 'Reverse Pharmacology' and 'Bedside to Bench' Approach," *Curr Drug Targets* 12, no. 11 (2011): 1595–1653; A Moussaleff and R Mechoulam, "Boswellia Resin: From

Religious Ceremonies to Medical Uses: A Review of In-vitro, In-vivo and Clinical Trials," *J Pharm Pharmacol* 61, no. 10 (Oct. 2009): 1281–93; R Wang et al., "The Comparative Study of Acetyl-11-keto-beta-boswellic acid (AKBA) and Aspirin in the Prevention of Intestinal Adenomatous Polyposis in APC(Min/+) Mice," *Drug Discov Ther* 8, no. 1 (2014): 25–32; M Takahashi et al., "Boswellic Acid Exerts Antitumor Effects in Colorectal Cancer Cells by Modulating Expression of the let-7 and miR-200 MicroRNA Family," *Carcinogenesis* 33, no. 12 (2012): 2441–9, doi: 10.1093/carcin/bgs286; CY Hsiang et al., "Ginger Extract and Zingerone Ameliorated Trinitrobenzene Sulphonic Acid-Induced Colitis in Mice via Modulation of Nuclear Factor-κB Activity and Interleukin-1β Signaling Pathway," *Food Chem* 136, no. 1 (2013): 170–7; EK Radhakrishnan et al., "[6]-Gingerol Induces Capsase-Dependent Apoptosis and Prevents PMA-Induced Proliferation in Colon Cancer Cells by Inhibiting MAPK/AP-1 Signaling," *PLoS One* 9, no. 8 (2014).

141. A Kumar et al., "Nuclear Factor-kappaB: Its Role in Health and Disease," *J Mol Med (Berl)* 82, no. 7 (2004): 434–48.

142. S C Gupta et al., "Discovery of Curcumin, a Component of Golden Spice, and Its Miraculous Biological Activities," *Clin Exp Pharmacol Physiol* 39, no. 3 (March 2012): 283–99, doi: 10.1111/j.1440-1681.2011.05648.x.

143. A B Kunnumakkara, P Anand, and B B Aggarwal, "Curcumin Inhibits Proliferation, Invasion, Angiogenesis, and Metastasis of Different Cancers Through Interaction with Multiple Cell Signaling Proteins," *Cancer Lett* 269, no. 2 (2008): 199–225, doi: 10.1016/j.canlet.2008.03.009.

144. B Sayantan et al., "Curcumin and Tumor Immune-Editing: Resurrecting the Immune System," *Cell Div* 10 (2015): 6, published online Oct 12, 2015, doi: 10.1186/s13008-015-0012-z.

145. S Prasad et al., "Curcumin," 1053–64.

146. Ibid.

147. Yanyan Li and Tao Zhang, "Targeting Cancer Stem Cells by Curcumin and Clinical Applications," *Cancer Letters* (2014). May 1;346(2):197-205.

148. Sayer Ji, "Are Cancer Stem Cells the Key to Discovering a Cure?", May 10, 2012, accessed December 27, 2015, http://wakeup-world.com/2012/05/10/are-cancer-stem-cells-the-key-to-discovering-a-cure/.

149. Katia Sampieri and Riccardo Fodde, "Cancer Stem Cells and Metastasis," *Seminars in Cancer Biology* 22, no. 3 (2012): 187–93.

150. Goel and Aggarwal, "Curcumin, the Golden Spice," 919–930; K Sandur et al., "Curcumin Modulates the Radiosensitivity," 534–542; Garg, Buchholz, Aggarwal, *Effects of Natural Polyphenols*.

151. Goel and Aggarwal, "Curcumin, the Golden Spice," 919–30.

152. Ibid.

153. B B Aggarwal, S C Gupta, and B Sung, "Curcumin: An Orally Bioavailable Blocker of TNF and Other Pro-inflammatory Biomarkers," *Br J Pharmacol* 169, no. 8 (2013): 1672–92; P Usharani et al., "Effect of NCB-02, Atorvastatin and Placebo on Endothelial Function, Oxidative Stress and Inflammatory Markers in Patients with Type 2 Diabetes Mellitus: A Randomized, Parallel-Group, Placebo-Controlled, 8-Week Study," *Drugs R D* 9, no. 4 (2008): 243–50.

154. P Usharani et al., "Effect of NCB-02," 243–50.

155. Heleen M Wortelboer et al., "Interplay Between MRP Inhibition and Metabolism of MRP Inhibitors: The Case of Curcumin," *J Clin Rheumatol* (2010): Dec; 16(12):1642-51.

156. S Zang et al., "Curcumin: A Promising Agent Targeting Cancer Stem Cells," *Anticancer Agents Med Chem* 14, no. 6 (2014): 787–92.

157.   Goel and Aggarwal, "Curcumin, the Golden Spice," 919–30.

158.   Goel and Aggarwal, "Curcumin, the Golden Spice," 919–930; K Sandur et al., "Curcumin Modulates the Radiosensitivity," 534–542; Garg, Buchholz, Aggarwal, *Effects of Natural Polyphenols*.

159.   USP Pharmacopeial Forum 33, no. 6, (2007). http://www.usp.org/usp-nf/pharmacopeial-forum.

160.   Bosmeric-SR is manufactured in state-of-the-art facilities assessed by NSF International and certified to be in compliance with GMP, as set forth in NSF/ANSI standard 173–2008, Dietary Supplements, Section 8. These requirements are consistent with the published GMP regulations for dietary supplements as defined in 21 CFR ¶ 111.

161.   Sandur et al., "Curcumin, Demethoxycurcumin, Bisdemethoxycurcumin, Tetrahydrocurcumin and Turmerones Differentially Regulate Anti-inflammatory and Anti-proliferative Responses through a ROS-Independent Mechanism," *Carcinogenesis* 28, no. 8 (2007): 1765–73.

162.   R Cooper et al., "Graph on Journal Pharmaceutical Advertisements: Are They Truthful and Are They Adequately Detailed?" *Fourth International Congress on Peer Review in Biomedical Publications*, Sept. 14–16, 2001, http://www.ama-assn.org/public/peer/prc_program2001.htim#truthful; P Norris et al., "Drug Promotion: What We Know, What We Have Yet to Learn," World Health Organization, accessed April 4, 2015, http:www.haiweb.org/18012006/drug-Promodhai12sept.pdf; "Understanding and Responding to Pharmaceutical Promotion: A Practical Guide," World Health Organization/Health Action International Collaborative Project, accessed April 4, 2015, http://www.haiweb.org/10112010/DPM_ENG_Final_SEP10.pdf.

163.   M Kobayashi et al., "Discovery of the Curcumin Metabolic Pathway Involving a Unique Enzyme in an Intestinal Microorganism," *Proc Nat Acad Sci USA* 108 (2011): 6615–20.

164. SK Vareed et al., "Pharmacokinetics of Curcumin Conjugate Metabolites in Healthy Human Subjects," *Cancer Epidemiol Biomarkers Prev* 17, no. 6 (2008): 1411–7; M Shoji et al., "Comparison of the Effects of Curcumin and Curcumin Glucuronide in Human Hepatocellular Carcinoma HepG2 cells," *Food Chem* 151 (2014): 126–32.

165. A Pal et al. "Curcumin Glucuronides: Assessing the Proliferative Activity Against Human Cell Lines," *Bioorg Med Chem* 22, no. 1 (2014): 435–9; JS Dempe et al. "Metabolism of Curcumin and Induction of Mitotic Catastrophe in Human Cancer Cells," *Mol Nutr Food Res* 52 (2008): 1074–81. A *Bioorganic & Medicinal Chemistry* 2013 (DOI 10.1016/j. bmc.2013.11.006).

166. Sandur et al. "Curcumin, demethoxycurcumin," 1765–1773.

167. "Founder's Desk," Sabinsa Corporation, January 1, 2014. http://www. sabinsa.com/founder-letter.html

168. ConsumerLab.com, "In the News, Turmeric and Curcumin Supplements, Press Releases," Feb 5, 2008, Feb 6, 2011, Dec 6, 2013, https://www.consu-merlab.com/reviews/turmeric-curcumin-supplements-spice-review/turmeric/.

169. S Gupta, S Patchva, and B Aggarwal, "Therapeutic Roles of Curcumin: Lessons Learned from Clinical Trials," *AAPS J* 15, no. 1 (2013): 195–218; S Prasad, et al. "Curcumin," 1053–64; S Prasad, B Aggarwal, and A Tyagi, "Recent Developments in Delivery, Bioavailability, Absorption, and Metabolism of Curcumin: The Golden Pigment from Golden Spice, *Cancer Res Treat* 46, no. 1 (2014): 2–18.

170. Goel and Aggarwal, "Curcumin, the Golden Spice," 919–30.

171. Ibid.

172. "Airport Scanners in 2014: Currents of Fear and the End of Privacy," *The Sleuth Journal*, Feb. 13, 2013, accessed April 6, 2015, http://www.

thesleuthjournal.com/airport-scanners-in-2014-currents-of-fear-and-the-end-of-privacy/; Michael Grabell, "TSA Removes X-Ray Body Scanners from Major Airports. Controversial "Backscatter Machines Being Relocated to Smaller Facilities," *Propublica*, NBCNews. com, Oct. 10, 2012, http://www.nbcnews.com/id/49481455/ns/travel-news/t/tsa-removes-x-ray-body-scanners-major-airports/#. VoHgcRorLwc.

173. "RF/MW-Exposed Soldiers Have More Leukemia and Lymphoma," *Microwave News* 15, no. 3 (1995): 1, http://microwavenews.com/news/backissues/m-j95issue.pdf.

174. M Z Siddiqui, "Boswellia Serrata, a Potential Antiinflammatory Agent: An Overview," *Indian J Pharm Sci* 73, no. 3 (2011): 255–61; M Schubert-Zsilavecz, "Boswellia Serrata: An Overall Assessment of In Vitro, Preclinical, Pharmacokinetic and Clinical Data," *Clin Pharmacokinet* 50, no. 6 (2011): 349–69; C Cuaz-Perolin et al., "Antiinflammatory and Antiatherogenic Effects of the NF-kappaB Inhibitor Acetyl-11-keto-beta-boswellic Acid in LPS-Challenged ApoE-/- Mice," *Arterioscler Thromb Vasc Biol* 28, no. 2 (2008): 272–7; A Moussaieff et al., "A Novel Anti-inflammatory Compound Isolated from Boswellia Resin, Inhibits Nuclear Factor-kappa B Activation," *Mol Pharmacol* 72, no. 6 (2007): 1657–64; D Dey et al., "Inhibition of LPS-Induced TNF-α and NO Production in Mouse Macrophage and Inflammatory Response in Rat Animal Models by a Novel Ayurvedic Formulation, BV-9238," *Phytother Res* 28, no. 10 (2014): 1479–85; A Ahangarpour et al., "Effect of Boswellia Serrata Supplementation on Blood Lipid, Hepatic Enzymes and Fructosamine Levels in Type2 Diabetic Patients," *J Diabetes Metab Disord* 13, no. 1 (2014): 29; YS Zang et al., "Acetyl-11-keto-β-boswellic Acid (AKBA) Inhibits Human Gastric Carcinoma Growth Through Modulation of the Wnt/β-catenin Signaling Pathway," *Biochim Biophys Acta* 1830, no. 6 (2013): 3604–15; Y Qurishi et al., "NF-κB Down-Regulation and PARP Cleavage by Novel 3-α-butyryloxy-β-boswellic Acid Results in Cancer Cell Specific Apoptosis and In Vivo Tumor Regression," *Anticancer Agents Med Chem* 13, no. 5 (2013): 777–90; M Takasashi

et al., "Boswellic Acid Exerts Antitumor Effects in Colorectal Cancer Cells by Modulating Expression of the let-7 and miR-200 MicroRNA Family," *Carcinogenesis* 33, no. 12 (2012): 2441–9;

VR Yadav et al., "Boswellic Acid Inhibits Growth and Metastasis of Human Colorectal Cancer in Orthotropic Mouse Model by Downregulating Inflammatory, Proliferative, Invasive and Angiogenic Biomarkers," *Int J Cancer* 130, no. 9 (2012): 2176–84;

B U Mahesh et al., "Antioxidant and Hepatoprotective Effects of Boswellia Ovalifoliolata Bark Extracts," *Chin J Nat Med* 12, no. 9 (2014): 663–71;

R M Hartmann et al., "Boswellia Serrata Has Beneficial Anti-inflammatory and Antioxidant Properties in a Model of Experimental Colitis," *Phytother Res* 28, no. 9 (2014): 1392–8; H P Ammon, "Modulation of the Immune System by Boswellia Serrata Extracts and Boswellic Acids," *Phytomedicine* 17, no. 11 (2010): 862–7.

175. N Kimmatkar et al., "Efficacy and Tolerability of Boswellia Serrata Extract in Treatment of Osteoarthritis of Knee: A Randomized Double Blind Placebo Controlled Trial," *Phytomedicine* 10 (2003): 3–7; S Sontakke et al., "Open, Randomized, Controlled Clinical Trial of Boswellia Serrata Extract as Compared to Valdecoxib in Osteoarthritis of Knee," *Indian J Pharmacol* 39 (2007): 27–9; R R Kulkarni et al., "Treatment of Osteoarthritis with a Herbomineral Formulation: A Double-Blind, Placebo-Controlled, Cross-Over Study," *J Ethnopharmacol* 33 (1991): 91–5; R Etzel, "Special Extract of Boswellia Serrata (H15) in the Treatment of Rheumatoid Arthritis," *Phytomed* 3 (1996): 91–4; G B Singh, S Singh, and S Bani, "New Phytotherapeutic Agent for the Treatment of Arthritis and Allied Disorders with Novel Mode of Action," *4th International Congress on Phytotherapy* (Sept. 10–13, 1992); A Chopra et al., "Randomized Double Blind Trial of an Ayurvedic Plant Derived Formulation for Treatment of Rheumatoid Arthritis," *J Rheumatol* 27 (2000): 1365–72; O Sander, G Herborn, and R Rau, "Is H15 (Resin Extract of Boswellia Serrata, 'Incense') a Useful Supplement to Established Drug Therapy of Chronic Polyarthritis? Results of a Double-Blind Pilot Study," *Z Rheumatol* 57 (1998): 11–6

[in German]; K C Srivastava and T Mustafa, "Ginger (*Zingiber offici-nale*) in Rheumatism and Musculoskeletal Disorders," *Med Hypoth* 39 (1992): 342–8.

176. R M Hartmann, H S Fillmann, and M I Martins, "Boswellia Serrata Has Beneficial Anti-inflammatory and Antioxidant Properties in a Model of Experimental Colitis," *J Complement Integr Med* (July 1, 2013): 1; A Madisch et al., "Boswellia Serrata Extract for the Treatment of Collagenous Colitis. A Double-Blind, Randomized, Placebo-Controlled, Multicenter Trial," *Int J Colorectal Dis* 22, no. 12 (2007): 1445–51;
   I Gupta et al., "Effects of Gum Resin of Boswellia Serrata in Patients with Chronic Colitis," *Planta Med* 67 (2001): 391–95; I Gupta et al., "Effects of Boswellia Serrata Gum Resin in Patients with Ulcerative Colitis," *Eur J Med Res* 2 (1997): 37–43.

177. R Wang et al., "The Comparative Study of Acetyl-11-keto-beta-boswellic Acid (AKBA) and Aspirin in the Prevention of Intestinal Adenomatous Polyposis in APC(Min/+) Mice," *Drug Discov Ther* 8, no. 1 (2014): 25–32; HP Liu, ZH Gao, and SX Cui, "Chemoprevention of Intestinal Adenomatous Polyposis by Acetyl-11-keto-beta-boswellic Acid in APC(Min/+) Mice," *Int J Cancer* 132, no. 11 (June 1, 2013): 2667–81.

178. M E Houssen, A Ragab, and A Mesbah, "Natural Anti-inflammatory Products and Leukotriene Inhibitors as Complementary Therapy for Bronchial Asthma," *Clin Biochem* 43, no. 10–11 (2010): 887–90; I Gupta et al., "Effects of Boswellia Serrata Gum Resin in Patients with Bronchial Asthma: Results of a Double-Blind, Placebo-Controlled, 6-Week Clinical Study," *Eur J Med Res* 3 (1998): 511–4.

179. S Kirste et al., "Boswellia Serrata Acts on Cerebral Edema In-Patient Irradiated for Brain Tumors: A Prospective, Randomized, Placebo-Controlled, Double-Blind Trial," *Cancer* 117, no. 16 (2012): 3788–95; Y Ding et al., "Post Treatment with 11-keo-B-Boswellic Acid Ameliorates Cerebral Ischemia-Refusion Injury. Nrf2/HO-1 Pathway as a Potential Mechanism," *Mol Neurobiol* (Oct. 28, 2014); Y Ding et al., "Neuroprotection by Acety-11-keto-B-Boswellic Acid, in Ischemic Brain Injury Involves

Nrf2/HO-1 Defense Pathway," *Sci Rep* 4 (2014): 7002; A Moussaleff et al., "Protective Effects of Incensole Scetate on Cerebral Ischemic Injury," *Brain Res* 1443 (2012): 89–97; A Moussaleff et al., "Incensole Acetate: A Novel Neuroprotective Agent Isolated from Boswellia Carterii," *J Cereb Blood Flow Metab* 28, no. 7 (2008): 1341–52; D F Flavin, "A Lipoxygenase Inhibitor in Breast Cancer Brain Metastases," *J Neurooncol* 82, no. 1 (2007): 91–3; Y S Park et al., "Cytotoxic Action of Acetyl-11-keto-beta-boswellic Acid (AKBA) on Meningioma Cells," *Planta Med* 68, no. 5 (2002): 397–401; K Hostanska, G Daum, and R Saller, "Cytostatic and Apoptosis-Inducing Activity of Boswellic Acids Toward Malignant Cell Lines in Vitro," *Anticancer Res* 22, no. 5 (2002): 2853–62.

180. A Moussaleff et al., "Incensole acetate, an incense component, elicits psychoactivity by activating TRPV3 channels in the brain," *FASEB J*, 22 (Aug. 2008): 3024–3034.

181. M Z Siddiqui, "Boswellia Serrata, a Potential Antiinflammatory Agent: An Overview," *Indian J Pharm Sci*, 73, no. 3 (2011): 255–61.

182. Ibid.; Schubert-Zsilavecz, "Boswellia Serrata: An Overall Assessment of In Vitro, Preclinical, Pharmacokinetic and Clinical Data," *Clin Pharmacokinet* 50, no. 6 (2011): 349–69; C Cuaz-Perolin et al., "Antiinflammatory and Antiatherogenic Effects of the NF-kappaB Inhibitor Acetyl-11-keto-beta-boswellic Acid in LPS-challenged ApoE-/- Mice," *Arterioscler Thromb Vasc Biol* 28, no. 2 (2008): 272–7; A Moussaieff et al., "A Novel Anti-inflammatory Compound Isolated from Boswellia Resin, Inhibits Nuclear Factor-kappa B Activation," *Mol Pharmacol* 72, no. 6 (2007): 1657–64.

183. "Boswellin PS (Patent Pending): Full Spectrum Anti-Inflammatory Bio-actives from *Boswellia serrata*," Sabinsa Corporation, accessed May 10, 2015, http://boswellin.com/boswellinps.html.

184. Mahima et al., "Immunomodulatory and Therapeutic Potentials of Herbal, Traditional/Indigenous and Ethnoveterinary Medicines," *Pak J Biol Sci* 15, no. 16 (2012): 754–74; D Tejasari, "Evaluation of Ginger

(Zingiber officinale Roscoe) Bioactive Compounds in Increasing the Ratio of T-cell Surface Molecules of CD3+CD4+:CD3+CD8+ In-Vitro," *Malays J Nutr* 13, no. 2 (2007): 161–70; Y Takada, A Murakami, and B B Aggarwal, "Zerumbone Abolishes NF-kappaB and IkappaBalpha Kinase Activation Leading to Suppression of Antiapoptotic and Metastatic Gene Expression, Upregulation of Apoptosis, and Downregulation of Invasion," *Oncogene* 24, no. 46 (2005): 6957–69; B Sung et al., "Zerumbone Abolishes RANKL-Induced NF-kappaB Activation, Inhibits Osteoclastogenesis, and Suppresses Human Breast Cancer-Induced Bone Loss in Athymic Nude Mice," *Cancer Res* 69 no. 4 (2009): 1477–84; S N Omoregie et al., "Antiproliferative Activities of Lesser Galangal (Alpinia officinarum Hance Jam1), Turmeric (Curcuma longa L.), and Ginger (Zingiber officinale Rosc.) against Acute Monocytic Leukemia," *J Med Food* 1, no. 7 (2013): 647–55; K Tsuboi et al., "Zerumbone Inhibits Tumor Angiogenesis via NF-κB in Gastric Cancer," *Oncol Rep* 31, no. 1 (2014): 57–64; Q Liu et al., "6-Shogaol Induces Apoptosis in Human Leukemia Cells through a Process Involving Caspase-mediated Cleavage of eIF2α," *Mol Cancer* 12, no. 1 (2013): 135; M Brahmbhatt et al., "Ginger Phytochemicals Exhibit Synergy to Inhibit Prostate Cancer Cell Proliferation," *Nutr Cancer* 65, no. 2 (2013): 263–72; A Al-Nahain, R Jahan, and M Rahmatullah, "Zingiber Officinale: A Potential Plant against Rheumatoid Arthritis," *Arthritis* (2014): 159089; A Chopra et al., "Ayurvedic Medicine Offers a Good Alternative to Glucosamine and Celecoxib in the Treatment of Symptomatic Knee Osteoarthritis: A Randomized, Double-Blind, Controlled Equivalence Drug Trial," *Rheumatology* 52, no. 8 (2013): 1408–17; T Arablou et al., "The Effect of Ginger Consumption on Glycemic Status, Lipid Profile and Some Inflammatory Markers in Patients with Type 2 Diabetes Mellitus," *Int J Food Sci Nutr* 65, no. 4 (2014): 515–20; R Haniadka et al., "A Review of the Gastroprotective Effects of Ginger (Zingiber officinale Roscoe)," *Food Funct* 4, no. 6 (2013): 845–55; A R Khuda-Bukhsh, S Das, and S K Saha, "Molecular Approaches toward Targeted Cancer Prevention with Some Food Plants and Their Products: Inflammatory and other Signal Pathways," *Nutr Cancer* 66, no. 2 (2014): 194–205; P L Palatty et al., "Ginger in the Prevention of Nausea and Vomiting: A review," *Crit Rev Food Sci Nutr*, 53, no. 7 (2013): 659–69;

J L Ryan et al., "Ginger (Zingiber officinale) Reduces Acute Chemotherapy-Induced Nausea: A URCC CCOP Study of 576 Patients," *Support Care Cancer* 20, no. 7 (July 2012): 1479–89; F Dabaghzadeh, H Khalili, and S Dashti-Khavidaki, "Ginger for Prevention or Treatment of Drug-Induced Nausea and Vomiting," *Curr Clin Pharmacol* (2013); M R Cominetti et al., "[6]-Gingerol as a Cancer Chemopreventive Agent: A Review of Its Activity on Different Steps of the Metastatic Process," *Mini Rev Med Chem* 14, no. 4 (2014): 313–21; F Mohammadi et al., "Protective Effect of Zingiber Officinale Extract on Rat Testis after Cyclophosphamide Treatment," *Andrologia* 46, no. 6 (2014): 680–6; A Angelini et al., "Modulation of Multidrug Resistance P-glycoprotein Activity by Antiemetic Compounds in Human Doxorubicin-Resistant Sarcoma Cells (MES-SA/Dx-5): Implications on Cancer Therapy," *J Biol Regul Homeost Agents* 27, no. 4 (2013): 1029–37; M M Taha et al., "Potential Chemoprevention of Diethylnitrosamine-Initiated and 2-Acetylaminofluorene-Promoted Hepatocarcinogenesis by Zerumbone from the Rhizomes of the Subtropical Ginger (Zingiber zerumbet)," *Chem Biol Interact* 186, no. 3 (Aug. 5, 2010): 295–305; A A Oyagbemi, A B Saba, and O I Azeez, "Molecular Targets of [6]-Gingerol: Its Potential Roles in Cancer Chemoprevention," *Biofactors* 36, no. 3 (2010): 169–78.

185. Mahima et al., "Immunomodulatory and Therapeutic Potentials of Herbal, Traditional/Indigenous and Ethnoveterinary Medicines," *Pak J Biol Sci* 15, no. 16 (2012): 754–74; D Tejasari, "Evaluation of Ginger (Zingiber officinale Roscoe) Bioactive Compounds in Increasing the Ratio of T-cell Surface Molecules of CD3+CD4+:D3+CD8+ In-Vitro," *Malays J Nutr* 13, no. 2 (2007): 161–70;

Y Takada, A Murakami, B B Aggarwal, "Zerumbone Abolishes NF-kappaB and IkappaBalpha Kinase Activation Leading to Suppression of Antiapoptotic and Metastatic Gene Expression, Upregulation of Apoptosis, and Downregulation of Invasion," *Oncogene* 24, no. 46 (2005): 6957–69; B Sung et al., "Zerumbone Abolishes RANKL-Induced NF-kappaB Activation, Inhibits Osteoclastogenesis, and Suppresses Human Breast Cancer-Induced Bone Loss in Athymic Nude Mice," *Cancer Res* 69, no. 4 (2009): 1477–84; S N Omoregie et al., "Antiproliferative Activities of Lesser Galangal (Alpinia officinarum

Hance Jam1), Turmeric (Curcuma longa L.), and Ginger (Zingiber officinale Rosc.) against Acute Monocytic Leukemia," *J Med Food* 16, no. 7 (2013): 647–55; K Tsuboi et al., "Zerumbone Inhibits Tumor Angiogenesis via NF-κB in Gastric Cancer," *Oncol Rep* 31, no. 1 (2014): 57–64; Q Liu et al., "6-Shogaol Induces Apoptosis in Human Leukemia Cells through a Process Involving Caspase-Mediated Cleavage of eIF2α," *Mol Cancer* 12, no. 1 (Nov. 12, 2013): 135; M Brahmbhatt et al., "Ginger Phytochemicals Exhibit Synergy to Inhibit Prostate Cancer Cell Proliferation," *Nutr Cancer* 65, no. 2 (2013): 263–72; A Al-Nahain, R Jahan, and M Rahmatullah, "Zingiber Officinale: A Potential Plant against Rheumatoid Arthritis," *Arthritis* (2014): 159089; A Chopra et al., "Ayurvedic Medicine Offers a Good Alternative to Glucosamine and Celecoxib in the Treatment of Symptomatic Knee Osteoarthritis: A Randomized, Double-Blind, Controlled Equivalence Drug Trial," *Rheumatology* 52, no. 8 (2013): 1408–17; T Arablou et al., "The Effect of Ginger Consumption on Glycemic Status, Lipid Profile and Some Inflammatory Markers in Patients with Type 2 Diabetes Mellitus," *Int J Food Sci Nutr* 65, no. 4 (June 2014): 515–20; R Haniadka et al., "A Review of the Gastroprotective Effects of Ginger (Zingiber officinale Roscoe)," *Food Funct* 4, no. 6 (2013): 845–55; A R Khuda-Bukhsh, S Das, and S K Saha, "Molecular Approaches toward Targeted Cancer Prevention with Some Food Plants and Their Products: Inflammatory and Other Signal Pathways," *Nutr Cancer* 66, no. 2 (2014): 194–205; P L Palatty et al., "Ginger in the Prevention of Nausea and Vomiting: A Review," *Crit Rev Food Sci Nutr* 53, no. 7 (2013): 659–69; J L Ryan et al., "Ginger (Zingiber officinale) Reduces Acute Chemotherapy-Induced Nausea: A URCC CCOP Study of 576 Patients," *Support Care Cancer* 20, no. 7 (July 2012): 1479–89; F Dabaghzadeh, H Khalili, and S Dashti-Khavidaki, "Ginger for Prevention or Treatment of Drug-Induced Nausea and Vomiting," *Curr Clin Pharmacol* (Nov. 11, 2013); M R Cominetti et al., "[6]-Gingerol as a Cancer Chemopreventive Agent: A Review of Its Activity on Different Steps of the Metastatic Process," *Mini Rev Med Chem* 14, no. 4 (2014): 313–21; F Mohammadi et al., "Protective Effect of Zingiber Officinale Extract on Rat Testis after Cyclophosphamide Treatment," *Andrologia* 46, no. 6 (2014): 680–6; A Angelini et al., "Modulation of Multidrug Resistance P-glycoprotein Activity by Antiemetic Compounds in Human

Doxorubicin-Resistant Sarcoma Cells (MES-SA/Dx-5): Implications on Cancer Therapy," *J Biol Regul Homeost Agents* 27, no. 4 (2013): 1029–37; M M Taha et al., "Potential Chemoprevention of Diethylnitrosamine-Initiated and 2-Acetylaminofluorene-Promoted Hepatocarcinogenesis by Zerumbone from the Rhizomes of the Subtropical Ginger (Zingiber zerumbet)," *Chem Biol Interact* 163, no. 3 (2010): 295–305; A A Oyagbemi, AB Saba, and O I Azeez, "Molecular Targets of [6]-gingerol: Its Potential Roles in Cancer Chemoprevention," *Biofactors* 36, no. 3 (2010): 169–78.

186.   Mahima et al., "Immunomodulatory and Therapeutic Potentials of Herbal, Traditional/Indigenous and Ethnoveterinary Medicines," *Pak J Biol Sci* 15, no. 16 (2012): 754–74; D Tejasari, "Evaluation of Ginger (Zingiber officinale Roscoe) Bioactive Compounds in Increasing the Ratio of T-cell Surface Molecules of CD3+CD4+:CD3+CD8+ In-Vitro," *Malays J Nutr* 13, no. 2 (2007): 161–70; Y Takada, A Murakami, and B B Aggarwal, "Zerumbone Abolishes NF-kappaB and IkappaBalpha Kinase Activation Leading to Suppression of Antiapoptotic and Metastatic Gene Expression, Upregulation of Apoptosis, and Downregulation of Invasion," *Oncogene* 24, no. 46 (2005): 6957–69; B Sung et al., "Zerumbone Abolishes RANKL-Induced NF-kappaB Activation, Inhibits Osteoclastogenesis, and Suppresses Human Breast Cancer-Induced Bone Loss in Athymic Nude Mice," *Cancer Res* 69, no. 4 (2009): 1477–84; S N Omoregie et al., "Antiproliferative Activities of Lesser Galangal (Alpinia officinarum Hance Jam1), Turmeric (Curcuma longa L.), and Ginger (Zingiber officinale Rosc.) against Acute Monocytic Leukemia," *J Med Food* 16, no. 7 (2013): 647–55; K Tsuboi et al., "Zerumbone Inhibits Tumor Angiogenesis via NF-κB in Gastric Cancer," *Oncol Rep* 31, no. 1 (2014): 57–64; Q Liu et al., "6-Shogaol Induces Apoptosis in Human Leukemia Cells through a Process Involving Caspase-Mediated Cleavage of eIF2α," *Mol Cancer* 12, no. 1 (2013): 135; M Brahmbhatt et al., "Ginger Phytochemicals Exhibit Synergy to Inhibit Prostate Cancer Cell Proliferation," *Nutr Cancer* 65, no. 2 (2013): 263–72; A Al-Nahain, R Jahan, and M Rahmatullah, "Zingiber officinale: A Potential Plant against Rheumatoid Arthritis," *Arthritis* (2014): 159089; A Chopra et al., "Ayurvedic Medicine Offers a Good Alternative to Glucosamine and Celecoxib in the Treatment of Symptomatic Knee Osteoarthritis:

A Randomized, Double-Blind, Controlled Equivalence Drug Trial," *Rheumatology* 52, no. 8 (2013): 1408–17; T Arablou et al., "The Effect of Ginger Consumption on Glycemic Status, Lipid Profile and Some Inflammatory Markers in Patients with Type 2 Diabetes Mellitus," *Int J Food Sci Nutr* 65, no. 4 (2014): 515–20; R Haniadka et al., "A Review of the Gastroprotective Effects of Ginger (Zingiber officinale Roscoe)," *Food Funct* 4, no. 6 (2013): 845–55; A R Khuda-Bukhsh, S Das, and S K Saha, "Molecular Approaches toward Targeted Cancer Prevention with Some Food Plants and Their Products: Inflammatory and other Signal Pathways," *Nutr Cancer* 66, no. 2 (2014): 194–205; P L Palatty et al., "Ginger in the Prevention of Nausea and Vomiting: A Review," *Crit Rev Food Sci Nutr* 53, no. 7 (2013): 659–69; J L Ryan et al., "Ginger (Zingiber officinale) Reduces Acute Chemotherapy-Induced Nausea: A URCC CCOP Study of 576 Patients," *Support Care Cancer* 20, no. 7 (2012): 1479–89; F Dabaghzadeh, H Khalili, and S Dashti-Khavidaki, "Ginger for Prevention or Treatment of Drug-Induced Nausea and Vomiting," *Curr Clin Pharmacol* (Nov. 11, 2013); M R Cominetti et al., "[6]-gingerol as a Cancer Chemopreventive Agent: A Review of Its Activity on Different Steps of the Metastatic Process," *Mini Rev Med Chem* 14, no. 4 (2014): 313–21; F Mohammadi et al., "Protective Effect of Zingiber officinale Extract on Rat Testis after Cyclophosphamide Treatment," *Andrologia* 46, no. 6 (2014): 680–6; A Angelini et al., "Modulation of Multidrug Resistance P-glycoprotein Activity by Antiemetic Compounds in Human Doxorubicin-Resistant Sarcoma Cells (MES-SA/Dx-5): Implications on Cancer Therapy," *J Biol Regul Homeost Agents* 27, no. 4 (2013): 1029–37; M M Taha et al., "Potential Chemoprevention of Diethylnitrosamine-Initiated and 2-Acetylaminofluorene-Promoted Hepatocarcinogenesis by Zerumbone from the Rhizomes of the Subtropical Ginger (Zingiber zerumbet)," *Chem Biol Interact* 163, no. 3 (2010): 295–305; A A Oyagbemi, A B Saba, and O I Azeez, "Molecular Targets of [6]-gingerol: Its Potential Roles in Cancer Chemoprevention," *Biofactors* 36, no. 3 (2010): 169–78.

187. J Rhode, S Fogoros, and S Zick, "Ginger Inhibits Cell Growth and Modulates Angiogenic Factors in Ovarian Cancer Cells," *BMC Complement Altern Med* 7 (2007): 44.

188. B Sung et al., "Cancer Cell Signaling Pathways Targeted by Spice-Derived Nutraceuticals," *Nutr Cancer* 64, no. 2 (2012): 173–97; S C Gupta et al., "Regulation of Survival, Proliferation, Invasion, Angiogenesis, and Metastasis of Tumor Cells through Modulation of Inflammatory Pathways by Nutraceuticals," *Cancer Metastasis Rev* 29, no. 3 (2010): 405–34; B B Aggarwal et al., "Molecular Targets of Nutraceuticals Derived from Dietary Spices: Potential Role in Suppression of Inflammation and Tumorigenesis," *Exp Biol Med (Maywood)* 234, no. 8 (2009): 825–49.

189. S Prasad, A K Tyagi, and B B Aggarwal, "Recent Developments in Delivery, Bioavailability, Absorption and Metabolism of Curcumin: The Golden Pigment from Golden Spice," *Cancer Res Treat* 46, no. 1 (2014): 2–18.

190. Y Liu et al., "Inhibitory Effects of Black Pepper (Piper nigrum) Extracts and Compounds on Human Tumor Cell Proliferation, Cyclooxygenase Enzymes, Lipid Peroxidation and Nuclear Transcription Factor-kappa-B," *Nat Prod Commun* 5, no. 8 (2010): 1253–7; Y Panahi et al., "Effects of Curcuminoids-Piperine Combination on Systemic Oxidative Stress, Clinical Symptoms, and Quality of Life in Subjects with Chronic Pulmonary Complications Due to Sulfur Mustard: A Randomized Controlled Trial," *J Diet Suppl* (2016): 13(1):93-105; G Shoba et al., "Influence of Piperine on the Pharmacokinetics of Curcumin in Animals and Human Volunteers," *Planta Med* 64, no. 4 (1998): 353–56; Vladimir Badmaev, Muhammed Majeed, and Edward P. Norkus, "Piperine, an Alkaloid Derived from Black Pepper, Increases Serum Response of Beta-Carotene During 14-Days of Oral Beta-Carotene Supplementation," *Nutrition Research* 19, no. 3 (1999): 381–388; Vladimir Badmaev, Muhammed Majeed, and Lakshmi Prakash, "Piperine Derived from Black Pepper Increases the Plasma Levels of Coenzyme Q10 Following Oral Supplementation," *J Nutr Biochem* 11 (2000): 109–113; M T Do et al., "Antitumor Efficacy of Piperine in the Treatment of Human HER2-Overexpressing Breast Cancer Cells," *Food Chem* 141, no. 3 (2013): 2591–9; A Samykutty et al., "Piperine, a Bioactive Component of Pepper Spice Exerts Therapeutic Effects on

Androgen Dependent and Androgen Independent Prostate Cancer Cells," *PLoS One* 8, no. 6 (2013): e65889; P B Yaffe et al., "Piperine Impairs Cell Cycle Progression and Causes Reactive Oxygen Species-Dependent Apoptosis in Rectal Cancer Cells," *Exp Mol Pathol* 94, no. 1 (2013): 109–14; C D Doucette et al., "Piperine, a Dietary Phytochemical, Inhibits Angiogenesis," *J Nutr Biochem* 24, no. 1 (2013): 231–9; Y P Hwang et al., "Suppression of Phorbol-12-myristate-13-acetate-induced Tumor Cell Invasion by Piperine via the Inhibition of PKCα/ERK1/2-Dependent Matrix Metalloproteinase-9 Expression," *Toxicol Lett* 203, no. 1 (May 30, 2011): 9–19; M S Butt et al., "Black Pepper and Health Claims: A Comprehensive Treatise," *Crit Rev Food Sci Nutr* 53, no. 9 (2013): 875–86; P Rinwa and A Kumar, "Piperine Potentiates the Protective Effects of Curcumin against Chronic Unpredictable Stress-Induced Cognitive Impairment and Oxidative Damage in Mice," *Brain Res*, 1488 (Dec. 7, 2012): 38–50; P Rinwa, A Kumar, and S Garg, "Suppression of Neuroinflammatory and Apoptotic Signaling Cascade by Curcumin Alone and in Combination with Piperine in Rat Model of Olfactory Bulbectomy Induced Depression," *PLoS One* 8, no. 4 (2013): e61052.

191. Michael F. Holick, "Vitamin D Deficiency," *N Engl J Med* 357 (2007): 266–28.

192. E Hyppönen, E Läärä, and A Reunanen, "Intake of Vitamin D and Risk of Type 1 Diabetes: A Birth-Cohort Study," *Lancet* 358, no. 9292 (2001): 1500–3.

193. J M Lappe et al., "Vitamin D and Calcium Supplementation Reduces Cancer Risk: Results of a Randomized Trial," *Am J Clin Nutr* 85, no. 6 (2007): 1586–91.

194. V Vetivicka, *Beta Glucan: Nature's Secret*, 2nd ed. (Louisville, Vaclav Vetvicka, 2011).

195. V Vetvicka and J Vetvickova, "1,3-Glucan: Silver Bullet or Hot Air?" *Open Glycoscience* 3 (2010): 1–6; V Vetvicka and J Vetvickova, "Comparison

of Immunological Effects of Commercially Available Beta-glucans," *Applied Scientific Reports* 1 (2014): 2, 1–7.

196. W Bohn, "The Technology Development History and Current Significance of the 'Physical BEMER Vascular Therapy' in Medicine," *Compliment Integr Med* 10, Supplement (2013): S1–S3.

197. Rainer Klopp, "Clinical Studies on the Physical Stimulation of Flexible Arteriolar Wall Movement with Disturbed Autorhythmic and Centrally Controlled in Patients with Deficiencies in the Regulation of Blood Circulation of Organs," BEMER International Conference, Budapest, Hungary, April 17–28, 2013; Balogh Imre, "Dentofit 2000: Using BEMER Therapy in Endocrine and Metabolic Syndromes," BEMER International Conference, Budapest, Hungary, April 17–28, 2013;

C Klopp, W Niemer, and J Schulz, "Complementary-Therapeutic Stimulation of Deficient Autorhythmic Arteriolar Vasomotion by Means of Biorhythmically Physical Stimulus on the Microcirculation and Immune System in 50-Year-Old Rehabilitation Patients," *Compliment Integr Med* 10, Supplement (2013): S29–S37; Rozsos István, "Lower Limb Circulatory Disorders and Efficient Supplementary Therapy BEMER Therapy—Experiences of 5 years," BEMER International Conference, Budapest, Hungary, April 17–28, 2013; Miléder Margit, "Possible Application of the BEMER Therapy in Late Diabetes Complications," BEMER International Conference, Budapest, Hungary, April 17–28, 2013; Liezl Naudé, "Independent Evaluation of BEMER Physical Vascular Regulation Therapy: The Specialist Forum," *WoundCare* (June 2013): 9–13; Kovács Matild, "BEMER Therapy in Rehabilitation," BEMER International Conference, Budapest, Hungary, April 17–28, 2013; Bernát Sándor Iván, "Efficacy of the BEMER Therapy and Pentoxyphyllin Infusion Therapy in Lower Limb Obliterative Arterial Disease," BEMER International Conference, Budapest, Hungary, April 17–28, 2013.

198. RB Pelka, C Jaenicke, and J Gruewald, "Impulse Magnetic-Field Therapy for Erectile Dysfunction: A Double-Blind, Placebo-Controlled Study," *Adv Ther* 19, no. 1 (2002): 53–60.

199. W Bohn, L Hess, R Burger, "The Effects of the 'Physical BEMER Vascular Therapy' a Method for the Physical Stimulation of the Vasomotion of Precapillary Microvessels in Case of Impaired Microcirculation on Sleep, Pain and Quality of Life with Different Clinical Pictures on the Basis of Three Scientifically Validated Scales," *Compliment Integr Med* 10, Supplement (2013): S5–S12; J Piatkowski, S Kern, and T Ziemssen, "Effect of BEMER Magnetic Field Therapy on the Level of Fatigue in Patients with Multiple Sclerosis: A Randomized, Double-Blind Controlled Trial," *J Altern Complement Med* 15, no. 5 (2009): 507–11, doi: 10.1089/acm.2008.0501; R Haase, J Piatkowski, and T Ziemssen, "Long-Term Effects of Bio-Electromagnetic-Energy Regulation Therapy on Fatigue in Patients with Multiple Sclerosis," *Altern Ther Health Med* 17, no. 6 (2011): 22–28.

200. David Rakel, *Integrative Medicine* 3rd ed. Chapter 11,(Philadelphia, Saunders/Elseiver, 2012); David Rakel, *Integrative Medicine* 4th ed. Chapter 13,(Philadelphia, Saunders/Elseiver, 2016 - pending publication.)

201. A M Mulligan et al., "Insulin Receptor Is an Independent Predictor of a Favorable Outcome in Early Stage Breast Cancer," *Breast Cancer Res Treat* 106, no. 1 (2007): 39–47; J A Emond et al., "Risk of Breast Cancer Recurrence Associated with Carbohydrate Intake and Tissue Expression of IGF-1 Receptor," *Cancer Epidemiol Biomarkers Prev* 23, no. 7 (2014): 1273–9; D B Boyd, "Insulin and Cancer," *Integr Cancer Ther* 2, no. 4 (2003): 315–29; S Sieri et al., "Dietary Glycemic Index, Glycemic Load, and the Risk of Breast Cancer in an Italian Prospective Cohort Study," *Am J Clin Nutr* 86, no. 4 (2007): 1160–6; M Lajous et al., "Carbohydrate Intake, Glycemic Index, Glycemic Load, and Risk of Postmenopausal Breast Cancer in a Prospective Study of French Women," *Am J Clin Nutr* 87, no. 5 (May 2008): 1384–91; S H Yun et al., "The Association of Carbohydrate Intake, Glycemic Load, Glycemic Index, and Selected Rice Foods with Breast Cancer Risk: A Case-Control Study in South Korea," *Asia Pac J Clin Nutr* 19, no. 3 (2010): 383–92; R A Krajcik et al., "Insulin-like Growth Factor I (IGF-I), IGF-Binding

Proteins, and Breast Cancer," *Cancer Epidemiol Biomarkers Prev* 11, no. 12 (2002): 1566–73.

202. Link to Pubmed with citations provided by sugarscience.org, accessed May 10, 2015, http://goo.gl/XnNV6U.

203. S W Ng, M M Slining, and B M Popkin, "Use of Caloric and Noncaloric Sweeteners in US Consumer Packaged Foods, 2005-2009," *Journal of the Academy of Nutrition and Dietetics* 112, no. 11 (2012): 1828–34.

204. "Sugar Consumption at a Crossroads," Credit Suisse Research Institute: Thought Leadership from Credit Suisse Research and the World's Foremost Experts, September 2013, accessed January 14, 2014, https://doc.research-and-analytics.csfb.com/docView?language=ENG&source=ulg&format=PDF&document_id=1022457401&serialid=atRE31ByPkIjEXa/p3AyptOvIGdxTK833tLZ1E7AwlQ=.

205. Ibid.

206. "Is Sugar Toxic?" CBS News, accessed April 2, 2012, http://www.cbsnews.com/8301-18560_162-57407294/is-sugar-toxic/?pageNum=2&tag=contentMain;contentBody.

207. Quanhe Yang, Zefeng Zhang, Edward W. Gregg, "Added Sugar Intake and Cardiovascular Diseases Mortality Among US Adults," *JAMA Internal Medicine* (2014).

208. Meredith Melnick, "American Soda Consumption: Half of Us Drink It Everyday, Study Says," *The Huffington Post*, July 25, 2012, http://www.huffingtonpost.com/2012/07/25/half-of-americans-drink-soda-everyday-consumption_n_1699540.html#slide=1074464.

209. Alice Walton, "How Much Sugar Are Americans Eating?" *Forbes*, accessed January 29, 2014, http://www.forbes.com/sites/alicegwalton/2012/08/30/how-much-sugar-are-americans-eating-infographic/.

210. G Null, "Sugar: Killing Us Sweetly. Staggering Health Consequences of Sugar on Health of Americans," Global Research, February 3, 2014, accessed December 27, 2014, http://www.globalresearch.ca/sugar-killing-us-sweetly/5367250.

211. "Nutrition Catalog," Baskin Robbins, accessed April 11, 2015, https://www.baskinrobbins.com/content/baskinrobbins/en/nutritioncatalog.html.

212. Shakira F Suglia, Sara Solnick, and David Hemenway, "Soft Drinks Consumption Is Associated with Behavior Problems in 5-Year-Olds," The Journal of Pediatrics, 163, no. 5 (2013):1323-8, doi: 10.1016/j.jpeds.2013.06.023.

213. S Solnick and D Hemanway, "The 'Twinkie Defense': The Relationship Between Carbonated Non-diet Soft Drinks and Violence Perpetration among Boston High School Students," Inj Prev 18, no.4 (2011):259-63, doi:10.1136/injuryprev-2011-040117.

214. S Solnick and D Hemanway, "Soft Drinks, Aggression, and Suicidal Behavior in US High School Students," Int J Inj Contr Saf Promot 21, no. 3 (2014): 266–73.

215. Shakira F Suglia, Sara Solnick, and David Hemenway, "Soft Drinks Consumption Is Associated with Behavior Problems in 5-Year-Olds," The Journal of Pediatrics, 163, no. 5 (2013):1323-8, doi: 10.1016/j.jpeds.2013.06.023.

216. C Colantuoni et al., "Evidence That Intermittent, Excessive Sugar Intake Causes Endogenous Opioid Dependence," Obes Res 10, no. 6 (2002): 478–88.

217. P Frisina and A. Sclafani, "Naltrexone Suppresses the Late but Not Early Licking Response to a Palatable Sweet Solution: Opioid Hedonic Hypothesis Reconsidered," Pharmacol Biochem Behav 74, no. 1 (2002): 163l; A S Levine et al., "Naltrexone Infusion Inhibits the Development of Preference for a High-Sucrose Diet." Am J PhysiolRegulIntegr Comp

Physiol 283, no. 5 (2002): R1149–54; N Pecoraro et al., "Brief Access to Sucrose Engages Food-Entrainable Rhythms in Food-Deprived Rats," *Behav Neurosci* 116, no. 5 (2002): 757–76; G Bartley, "Neural Systems for Reinforcement and Inhibition of Behavior: Relevance to Eating, Addiction, and Depression," *Well-being: Foundations of Hedonic Psychology* (New York, Russell Sage Foundation, 1999): 558–572; D B Matthews et al., "Effects of Sweetened Ethanol Solutions on Ethanol Self-Administration and Blood Ethanol Levels," *Pharmacol Biochem Behav* 68, no. 1 (2001): 13–21; A Rogowski et al., "Sucrose Self-Administration Predicts Only Initial Phase of Ethanol-Reinforced Behaviour in Wistar Rats," *Alcohol* 37, no. 5 (2002): 436–40; G A Olson et al., "Naloxone and Fluid Consumption in Rats: Dose-Response Relationships for 15 Days," *Pharmacol Biochem Behav* 23, no. 6 (1985): 1065–8; M Cichelli and M Lewis, "Naloxone Nonselective Suppression of Drinking of Ethanol, Sucrose, Saccharin, and Water by Rats," *Pharmacol Biochem Behav* 72, no. 3 (2002): 699; F J Files et al., "Sucrose, Ethanol, and Sucrose/Ethanol Reinforced Responding under Variable-Interval Schedules of Reinforcement," *Alcohol Clin Exp Res* 19, no. 5 (1995): 1271–8; C L Czachowski, "Independent Ethanol- and Sucrose-Maintained Responding on a Multiple Schedule of Reinforcement," *Alcohol ClinExp Res* 23, no. 3 (March 1999): 398–403.

218. J W Grimm et al., "Effect of Cocaine and Sucrose Withdrawal Period on Extinction Behavior, Cue-Induced Reinstatement, and Protein Levels of the Dopamine Transporter and Tyrosine Hydroxylase in Limbic and Cortical Areas in Rats," *BehavPharmacol* 13, no. 5–6 (2002): 379–88.

219. A Cerami, H Vlassara, and M Brownlee, "Glucose and Aging," *Scientific American*, May 1987, 90.

220. L Melton, "AGE Breakers, Rupturing the Body's Sugar-Protein Bonds Might Turn Back the Clock," *Sci Am* 283, no. 1 (2000): 16.

221. GH Anderson et al., "Inverse Association Between the Effect of Carbohydrates on Blood Glucose and Subsequent Short-Term Food Intake in Young Men," *Am J ClinNutr* 76, no. 5 (2002): 1023–30.

222. Ibid.

223. S Rostler, "Excess Blood Sugar May Boost Free Radical Production," Atkins Diet & Low Carbohydrate website, 2000. http://www.lowcarb. ca/articles/article001.html; P Mohanty et al., "Glucose challenge stimulates reactive oxygen species (ROS) generation by leucocytes," *J Clin Endocrinol Metab*, 85, no. 8 (2000): 2970-3.

224. B J Hoogwerf et al., "Blood Glucose Concentrations < or = 125 mg/ dl and Coronary Heart Disease Risk," *Am J Cardiol* 89, no. 5 (2002): 596–9; A Norhammar et al., "Glucose Metabolism in Patients with Acute Myocardial Infarction and No Previous Diagnosis of Diabetes Mellitus: A Prospective Study," *Lancet* 359, no. 9324 (2002): 2140–4; H C McGill Jr. et al., "Obesity Accelerates the Progression of Coronary Atherosclerosis in Young Men," *Circulation* 105, no. 23 (2002): 2712–8; P Ziccardi et al., "Reduction of Inflammatory Cytokine Concentrations and Improvement of Endothelial Functions in Obese Women after Weight Loss over One Year," *Circulation* 105, no. 7 (2002): 804–9.

225. V S Malik et al., "Sugar-Sweetened Beverages and Risk of Metabolic Syndrome and Type 2 Diabetes: A Meta-Analysis," *Diabetes Care* 33, no. 11 (2010): 2477–83.

226. T T Fung et al., "Sweetened Beverage Consumption and Risk of Coronary Heart Disease in Women," *Am J Clin Nutr* 89, no. 4 (2009): 1037–42.

227. KL Stanhope et al., "Consumption of Fructose and High Fructose Corn Syrup Increase Postprandial Triglycerides, LDL-Cholesterol, and Apolipoprotein-B in Young Men and Women," *J Clin Endocrinol Metab* 96, no. 10 (2011): E1596–1605.

228. M Maersk et al., "Sucrose-Sweetened Beverages Increase Fat Storage in the Liver, Muscle, and Visceral Fat Depot: A 6-Mo Randomized Intervention Study," *Am J Clin Nutr* 95, no. 2 (2012): 283–89.

229. Quanhe Yang, Zefeng Zhang, and Edward W. Gregg, "Added Sugar Intake and Cardiovascular Diseases Mortality among US Adults," *JAMA Intern Med* 174, no. 4 (2014): 516–24.

230. S Schoenthaler et al., "The Impact of Low Food Additive and Sucrose Diet on Academic Performance in 803 New York City Public Schools," *Int J Biosocial Res* 8, no. 2 (1986).

231. "Program for the International Student Assessment (PISA) Results from 2012, United States, Key Findings," The Organization for Economic Co-operation and Development (OECD), accessed May 10, 2015, http://www.oecd.org/unitedstates/PISA-2012-results-US.pdf

232. S Schoenthaler, "Detention Home Double-Blind Study: Sugar Goes on Trial," *Int J Biosocial Res* 3, no. 1 (1982): 1–9; S Schoenthaler, "Northern California Diet-Behavior Program: An Empirical Examination of 3,000 Incarcerated Juveniles in Stanislaus County Juvenile Hall," *Int J Biosocial Res* 5, no. 2 (1983): 99–108.

233. Ibid.; S Schoenthaler, "The Los Angeles Probation Department Diet-Behavior Program: An Empirical Analysis of Six Institutional Settings," *Int J Biosocial Res* 5, no. 2 (1983): 88–89.

234. S Schoenthaler, "Alabama Diet-Behavior Program: An Empirical Evaluation at Coosa Valley Regional Detention Center," *Int J Biosocial Res* 5, no 2 (1983): 78–87; S Schoenthaler, "The Los Angeles Probation Department Diet-Behavior Program: An Empirical Analysis of Six Institutional Settings," *Int J Biosocial Res* 5, no. 2 (1983): 88–89.

235. D S Ludwig, K E Peterson, and S L Gortmaker, "Relation Between Consumption of Sugar-Sweetened Drinks and Childhood Obesity: A Prospective, Observational Analysis," *Lancet* 357, no. 9255 (2001): 505–8.

236. Ibid.; F Bellisle, et al., "How Sugar-Containing Drinks Might Increase Adiposity in Children," *Lancet* 357, no. 9255 (2001): 490–1

237. Sara N. Bleich et al., "Reducing Sugar-Sweetened Beverage Consumption by Providing Caloric Information: How Black Adolescents Alter Their Purchases and Whether the Effects Persist," *American Journal of Public Health,* 104, no. 12 (2014):2417-24.

238. Petter Lundborg, Paul Nystedt, and Dan-Olof Rooth, "Body Size, Skills, and Income: Evidence From 150,000 Teenage Siblings," *Demography* 51, no. 5 (2014): 1573–96.

239. A Sheiham, "Dietary Effects on Dental Diseases," *Public Health Nutr* 4, no. 2B (2001): 569–91; C Jones et al., "Sugar, Drinks, Deprivation and Dental Caries in 14-Year-Old Children in the Northwest of England in 1995," *Community Dent Health* 16, no. 2 (1999): 68–71; I L Parajas, "Sugar Content of Commonly Eaten Snack Foods of School Children in Relation to Their Dental Health Status," *J Philipp Dent Assoc* 51, no. 1 (1999): 4–21; C S Rodrigues and A Sheiham, "The Relationships Between Dietary Guidelines, Sugar Intake and Caries in Primary Teeth in Low Income Brazilian 3-Year-Olds: A Longitudinal Study," *Int J Paediatr Dent* 10, no. 1 (2000): 47–55; S L Huumonen et al., "High-Sucrose Diet Reduces Defensive Reactions of the Pulpo-Dentinal Complex to Dentinal Caries in Young Rats," *Acta Odontol Scand* 59, no. 2 (2001): 83–7; W T Spruill, "PDA Establishes Position Statement on Cola Contracts in Schools," *Pa Dent J* 67, no. 5 (2000): 29–32; R K Johnson and C Frary, "Choose Beverages and Foods to Moderate Your Intake of Sugars: The 2000 Dietary Guidelines for Americans—What's All the Fuss About?" *J Nutr* 131, no. 10 (2001): 2766S–2771S; R S Levine, "Caries Experience and Bedtime Consumption of Sugar-Sweetened Food and Drinks—A Survey of 600 Children," *Community Dent Health* 18, no. 4 (2001): 228–31; W Van Wyk, I Stander, and I Van Wyk, "The Dental Health of 12-Year-Old Children Whose Diets Include Canned Fruit from Local Factories: An Added Risk for Caries?" *SADJ* 56, no. 11 (2001): 533–7; M A Falco, "The Lifetime Impact of Sugar Excess and Nutrient Depletion on Oral Health," *Gen Dent* 49, no. 6 (2001): 591–5; A Sayegh et al., "Food and Drink Consumption, Sociodemographic Factors and Dental Caries in 4–5-Year-Old Children in Amman, Jordan," *Br Dent J* 193, no. 1 (2002): 37–42; M Nobre Dos Santos et al., "Relationship among Dental Plaque Composition, Daily Sugar Exposure, and Caries in the Primary Dentition," *Caries Res* 36, no. 5 (2002): 347–52.

240. A Sanchez et al., "Role of Sugars in Human Neutrophilic Phagocytosis," *Am J Clin Nutr* 26, no. 11 (1973): 1180–4.

241. Ibid.

242. N Yabunaka et al., "Elevated Serum Content of Macrophage Migration Inhibitory Factor in Patients with Type 2 Diabetes," *Diabetes Care* 23, no. 2 (2000): 256–8.

243. G G Donders, "Lower Genital Tract Infections in Diabetic Women," *Curr Infect Dis Rep* 4, no. 6 (2002): 536–39.

244. Norman Kretchmer and Claire B. Hollenbeck, *Sugars and Sweeteners* (Boca Raton, CRC Press: 1991): v; H Beckles, *A History of Barbados from Amerindian Settlement to Nation State* (Cambridge: Cambridge Univ. Press, 1990); R E Chardon, "Sugar Plantations in the Dominican Republic, 1770–1844," *Geographical Review* 74, no. 4 (1984); P D Curtin, *The Rise and Fall of the Plantation Complex: Essays in Atlantic History* (Cambridge: Cambridge Univ. Press, 1990); R Dunn, *Sugar and Slaves: The Rise of the Planter Class in the English West Indies, 1624–1713* (Chapel Hill, The University of North Carolina Press, 1972).

245. E Han and L M Powell, "Consumption Patterns of Sugar-Sweetened Beverages in the United States," *J Acad Nutr Diet* 113, no. 1 (2013): 43–53.

246. California Center for Public Health Advocacy, PolicyLink, UCLA Center for Health Policy Research, *Designed for Disease: The Link Between Local Food Environments and Obesity and Diabetes*, , April 2008, http://www.policylink.org/sites/default/files/DESIGNEDFORDISEASE_FINAL.PDF;

247. K Morland, A V Diez Roux, and S Wing, "Supermarkets, Other Food Stores, and Obesity: The Atherosclerosis Risk in Communities Study," *Am J Prev Med* 30, no. 4 (2006): 333–39; Lori Dorfman and Hilary Abramson, "Sugar Water Gets a Facelift: What Marketing Does for Soda," Berkeley Media Studies Group, September 2009, http://www.preventioninstitute.org/component/jlibrary/article/id-171/127.html.

248. J Leibowitz et al., "A Review of Food Marketing to Children and Adolescents," Federal Trade Commission, December 2012, https://www.ftc.gov/sites/default/files/documents/reports/review-food-marketing-children-and-adolescents-follow-report/121221foodmarketingreport.pdf.

249. Ibid.

250. SN Zenk et al., "Relative and Absolute Availability of Healthier Food and Beverage Alternatives across Communities in the United States," *Am J Public Health* 104, no. 11 (2014): 2170–8.

251. Ibid.

252. O Warburg, "On the Origin of Cancer Cells," *Science* 123 (Feb. 1956): 309–14.

253. Ibid.

254. A Belfiore and R Malaguarnera, "Insulin Receptor and Cancer," *Endocr Relat Cancer* 18, no. 4 (2011): R125–47.

255. PL Pedersen, "3-Bromopyruvate (3BP) a Fast Acting, Promising, Powerful, Specific, and Effective 'Small Molecule' Anti-cancer Agent Taken from Labside to Bedside: Introduction to a Special Issue," *J Bioenerg Biomembr* 44, no. 1 (2012): 1–6; S Ganapathy-Kanniappan et al., "3-bromopyruvate: A New Targeted Antiglycolytic Agent and a Promise for Cancer Therapy," *Curr Pharm Biotechnol* 11, no. 5 (2010): 510–7; Y Ko et al., "A Translational Study 'Case Report' on the Small Molecule 'Energy Blocker' 3-bromopyruvate (3BP) as a Potent Anticancer Agent: From Bench Side to Bedside," *J Bioenerg Biomembr* 44 (2012): 163–70; Y Ko et al., "Advanced Cancers: Eradication in All Cases Using 3-bromopyruvate Therapy to Deplete ATP," *Biochemical and Biophysical Research Communications* 324 (2004): 269–75; S P Mathupala, Y H Ko, and P L Pedersen, "Hexokinase II: Cancer's Double-Edged Sword Acting as Both Facilitator and Gatekeeper of

Malignancy When Bound to Mitochondria," *Oncogene* 25 (2006): 4777–86; P Pedersen, "Warburg, Me and Hexokinase 2: Multiple Discoveries of Key Molecular Events Underlying One of Cancers' Most Common Phenotypes, the 'Warburg Effect,' i.e., Elevated Glycolysis in the Presence of Oxygen," *J Bioenerg Biomembr* 39 (2007): 211–22; S P Mathupala, Y H Ko, and P L Pedersen, "The Pivotal Roles of Mitochondria in Cancer: Warburg and Beyond and Encouraging Prospects for Effective Therapies," *Biochimica et Biophysica Acta* 1797 (2010): 1225–30.

256. Amit K. Garg, Thomas A. Buchholz, and Bharat B. Aggarwal, *Effects of Natural Polyphenols on Chemoradiotherapy in Cancer* (New Delhi, Jaypee Brothers Medical Publishers: 2009); K Sandur et al., "Curcumin Modulates the Radiosensitivity of Colorectal Cancer Cells by Suppressing Constitutive and Inducibe NF-kB Activity," *Int J Radiation Oncology Biol Phys* 75, no. 2 (2009): 534–542; Goel and Aggarwal, "Curcumin, the Golden Spice," 919–930; Ajaikumar B. Kunnumakkara et al., "Curcumin Sensitizes Human Colorectal Cancer Xenografts in Nude Mice to Radiation by Targeting Nuclear Factor-KB ^ Regulated Gene Products," *Clin Cancer Res* 14, no. 7 (2008).

257. Y Sun et al., "Treatment-Induced Damage to the Tumor Microenvironment Promotes Prostate Cancer Therapy Resistance through WNT16B," *Nat Med* 18, no. 9 (2012): 1359–68; L M Johnson, D K Price, and W D Figg, "Treatment-Induced Secretion of WNT16B Promotes Tumor Growth and Acquired Resistance to Chemotherapy: Implications for Potential Use of Inhibitors in Cancer Treatment," *Cancer Biol Ther* 14, no. 2 (2013): 90–91; S Acharyya et al., "A CXCL1 Paracrine Network Links Cancer Chemoresistance and Metastasis," *Cell* 150, no. 1 (2012): 165–78; J Chen et al., "A Restricted Cell Population Propagates Glioblastoma Growth after Chemotherapy," *Nature* 488, no. 7412 (2012): 522–6.

258. Sara N. Bleich et al., "Diet-Beverage Consumption and Caloric Intake Among US Adults, Overall and by Body Weight," *American Journal of Public Health* 104, no. 3 (2014): e72–e78.

259. S Fowler, K Williams, and H Hazuda. "Diet Soda Intake Is Associated with Long-Term Increases in Waist Circumference in a Biethnic Cohort of Older Adults: The San Antonio Longitudinal Study of Aging," *Journal of the American Geriatrics Society* 63, no. 4 (2015): 708–15; Bleich et al. "Diet-Beverage Consumption," 104; K Doyle, "Drinking Diet Soda Linked to a Widening Waistline with Age," *Scientific American*, March 18, 2015;

260. David Zinkzenco, "The 10 Saltiest Meals in America," *The Huffington Post*, Oct. 24, 2014, http://www.huffingtonpost.com/david-zinczenko/the-10-saltiest-foods-in-_b_5948684.html.

261. "The 13 Amazing Health Benefits of Himalayan Crystal Salt, the Purest Salt on Earth (and Why You Want to Avoid Conventional Salt)," Mercola, accessed October 30, 2014, http://products.mercola.com/himalayan-salt/.

262. Ibid.

263. Ibid.; B Hendel and P Ferreira, "*Water & Salt: The Essence Of Life: The Healing Power of Nature*," (Munich, Natural Resources, 2003).

264. Ibid.

265. "Swami Vivekananda Yoga Anusandhana Samsthana," S-VASYA Deemed University, http://svyasa.edu.in/research/research-publications/; K E Riley and C L Park, "How Does Yoga Reduce Stress? A Systematic Review of Mechanisms of Change and Guide to Future Inquiry," *Health Psychol Rev* (April 15, 2015): 1–18; G A Kelly and K S Kelley, "Meditative Movement Therapies and Health-Related Quality-of-Life in Adults: A Systematic Review of Meta-Analyses," *PLoS One* 10, no. 6 (2015); J E Bower and M R Irwin, "Mind-Body Therapies and Control of Inflammatory Biology: A Descriptive Review," *Brain Behav Immun* 51, (2016); V Kayuri et al., "Irritable Bowel Syndrome: Yoga as Remedial Therapy," *Evid Based Complement Alternat Med* (2015); L Desveaux et al., "Yoga in the Management of Chronic Disease: A

Systematic Review and Meta-analysis," *Med Care* 53, no. 7 (2015): 653–61; R Desai, A Tailor, and T Bhatt, "Effects of Yoga on Brain Waves and Structural Activation: A Review," *Complement Ther Clin Pract* 21, no. 2 (2015): 112–18; Y Klainin et al., "Effects of Relaxation Interventions on Depression and Anxiety among Older Adults: A Systematic Review," *Aging Ment Health* (Jan. 9, 2015): 1–13; P Chu et al., "The Effectiveness of Yoga in Modifying Risk Factors for Cardiovascular Disease and Metabolic Syndrome: A Systematic Review and Meta-Analysis of Randomized Controlled Trials," *Eur J Prev Cardiol* (Dec. 15, 2014); M Sharma and P Branscum, "Yoga Interventions in Pregnancy: A Qualitative Review," *J Altern Complement Med* 21, no. 4 (2015): 208–16.

266. B Kligler et al., "Cost Savings in Inpatient Oncology Through an Integrative Medicine Approach," *The American Journal of Managed Care* 17, no. 2 (2011): 779–84; J Friedman et al., "Decreased Medication Use and Cost Savings in Inpatient Oncology through a Yoga-Based Integrative Medicine Approach," *BMC Complement Altern Med* 12, Supplement 1 (2012): P59.

267. J E Bower et al., "Yoga Reduces Inflammatory Signaling in Fatigued Breast Cancer Survivors: A Randomized Controlled Trial," *Psychoneuroendocrinology* 43 (2014): 20–9; M Dharmawardene et al., "A Systematic Review and Meta-Analysis of Meditative Interventions for Informal Caregivers and Health Professionals," *BMJ Support Palliat Care* (March 26, 2015); B Holzel et al., "Mindfulness Practice Leads to Increases in Regional Brain Gray Matter Density," *Psychiatry Res* 191, no. 1 (2011): 36–43; T De Meyer et al., "Studying Telomeres in a Longitudinal Population Based Study," *Frontiers in Bioscience* 13 (2008): 2960–70; Robert E. Herron, "Changes in Physician Costs among High-Cost Transcendental Meditation Practitioners Compared with High-Cost Nonpractitioners over 5 Years," *American Journal of Health Promotion* 26, no. 1 (2011): 56–60; Z Bai et al., "Investigating the Effect of Transcendental Meditation on Blood Pressure: A Systematic Review and Meta-Analysis," *J Hum Hypertens* (Feb. 12, 2015); I B Ray et al., "Meditation and Coronary Heart Disease: A Review of the Current Clinical Evidence," *Ochsner J* 14, no. 4 (2014): 696–703; F A Jain et al.,

"Critical Analysis of the Efficacy of Meditation Therapies for Acute and Subacute Phase Treatment of Depressive Disorders: A Systematic Review," *Psychosomatics* 56, no. 2 (2015): 140–52.

268. E Santarnecchi et al., "Interaction between Neuroanatomical and Psychological Changes after Mindfulness-Based Training," *PLOS One,* October 20, 2014.

269. Alena Hall, "Meditation Is Even More Powerful Than We Originally Thought," *Huffington Post,* Nov. 11, 2014, http://www.huffingtonpost.com/2014/11/11/meditation-reduces-stress-harvard-study_n_6109404.html.

270. Ibid.

271. American Academy of Pain Management, *The Pain Practitioner: Integrative Pain Management for Optimal Patient Care* 2, no. 3 (2012).

272. Ibid.

273. "What Is Functional Medicine?" The Institute of Functional Medicine, accessed December 31, 2015, https://www.functionalmedicine.org/What_is_Functional_Medicine.

274. L M Moberg, P M Nilsson, and G Samsioe, "Use of Proton Pump Inhibitors (PPI) and History of Earlier Fracture Are Independent Risk Factors for Fracture in Postmenopausal Women: The WHILA Study," *Maturitas* 78, no. 4 (2014): 310–5; J R Lewis et al., "Long-Term Proton Pump Inhibitor Therapy and Falls and Fractures in Elderly Women: A Prospective Cohort Study," *J Bone Miner Res* 29, no. 11 (2014): 2489–97; Tetsuhide Ito and Robert T. Jensen, "Association of Long-term Proton Pump Inhibitor Therapy with Bone Fractures and Effects on Absorption of Calcium, Vitamin B12, Iron, and Magnesium," *Curr Gastroenterol Rep* 12, no. 6 (2010): 448–57; J B Richards and D Goltzman, "Proton Pump Inhibitors: Balancing the Benefits and Potential Fracture Risks," *CMAJ* 179 (Aug. 12, 2008): 306–7; S E Gulmez et al., "Use of Proton

Pump Inhibitors and the Risk of Community-Acquired Pneumonia: A Population-Based Case Control Study," *Arc Intern Med* 167, no. 9 (2007): 950–5; C Bavishi and H L Dupont, "Systematic Review: The Use of Proton Pump Inhibitors and Increased Susceptibility to Enteric Infection," *Aliment Pharmacol Ther* 34, no. 11–12 (2011): 1269–81; R Fossmark et al., "Rebound Acid Hypersecretion after Long-Term Inhibition of Gastric Acid Secretion," *Aliment Pharmacol Ther* 21, no. 2 (2005): 149–54; S L Gray et al., "Proton Pump Inhibitors Use, Hip Fracture, and Change in Bone Mineral Density in Post-menopausal Women: Results from the Women's Health Initiative," *Arc Intern Med* 170, no. 9 (2010): 765–71; D T Eurich et al., "Recurrent Community-Acquired Pneumonia in Patients Starting Acid-Suppressing Drugs," *Am J Med* 123, no. 1 (2010): 47–53; B S Skikne, S R Lynch, and S D Cook, "Role of Gastric Acid in Food Iron Absorption," *Gastroenterology* 81, no. 6 (1981): 1068–71; K E McColl, "Effect of Proton Pump Inhibitors on Vitamins and Iron," *Am J Gastroenterol* 104, Supplement 2 (March 2009): S5–9; T Ito and R T Jensen, "Association of Long-Term Proton Pump Inhibitor Therapy with Bone Fractures and Effects on Absorption of Calcium, Vitamin B12, Iron, and Magnesium," *Curr Gastroenterol Rep* 12, no. 6 (2010): 448–57; S Oh, "Proton Pump Inhibitors—Uncommon Adverse Effects," *Aust Fam Physician* 40, no. 9 (2011): 705–8; J R Saltzman et al., "Effect of Hypochlorhydria Due to Omeprazole Treatment or Atrophic Gastritis on Protein-Bound Vitamin B12 Absorption," *J Am Coll Nutr* 13 (1994): 584–91; M Alleyne, M K Horne, and J L Miller, "Individualized Treatment for Iron-Deficiency Anemia in Adults," *Am J Med* 121 (2008): 943–8; F Bronner and D Pansu, "Nutritional Aspects of Calcium Absorption," *J Nutr* 129, no. 1 (1999): 9–12; M W Hess et al., "Systematic Review: Hypomagnesaemia Induced by Proton Pump Inhibition," *Aliment Pharmacol Ther* 36 (2012): 405–13; R M Russel et al., "Effect of Antacid and H2 Receptor Antagonists on the Intestinal Absorption of Folic Acid," *J Lab Clinc Med* 112 (1988): 458–63; B J Iskandar et al., "Folic Acid Supplementation Enhances Repair of the Adult Central Nervous System," *Ann Neurol* 56, no. 2 (2004): 221–7; G C Sturniolo et al., "Inhibition of Gastric Acid Secretion Reduces Zinc Absorption in Man," *J Am Coll Nutr* 10, no. 4 (1991): 372–5; C S Eom et al., "Use of Acid-Suppressive Drugs and Risk of Fracture: A Meta-Analysis of Observational Studies," *Ann Fam Med* 9 (2011): 257–67; S Kopic and J P Geibel, "Gastric Acid, Calcium Absorption, and Their Impact on Bone Health," *Physiol Rev* 93, no. 1 (2013): 189–268; Y X Yang, "Chronic Proton Pump Inhibitor Therapy and Calcium Metabolism," *Curr Gastroenterol Rep* 14, no. 6 (2012): 473–9; C Bolton-Smith et al., "Two-Year Randomized Controlled Trial of Vitamin K1 (Phylloquinone) and Vitamin D3 Plus Calcium on the Bone Health of Older Women," *J Bone Miner Res* 22, no. 4 (2007): 509–19; M Aseeri et al., "Gastric Acid Suppression by Proton Pump Inhibitors as a Risk Factor for *Clostridium difficile*-Associated Diarrhea in Hospitalized Patients," *Am J Gastroenterol* 103, no. 9 (2008): 2308–13; J F Pohl, "*Clostridium difficile* Infection and Proton Pump Inhibitors," *Curr Opin Pediatr* 24, no. 5 (2012): 627–31; J Theisen et al., "Suppression of Gastric Acid Secretion in Patients with Gastroesophageal Reflux Disease Results in Gastric Bacterial Overgrowth and Deconjugation of Bile Acids," *J Gastrointes Surg* 4, no. 1 (2000): 50–4; S Dial et al., "Use of Gastric Acid-Suppressive Agents and the Risk of Community-Acquired *Clostridium difficile*-Associated Disease," *JAMA* 294, no. 23 (2005): 2989–95; R J Laheij et al., "Risk of Community-Acquired Pneumonia and Use of Gastric Acid-Suppressives Drugs," *JAMA* 292, no. 16 (2004): 1955–60;

S J Herzig et al., "Acid Suppressive Medication Use and the Risk for Hospital-Acquired Pneumonia," *JAMA* 301, no. 20 (2009): 2120–8; C Reimer et al., "Proton Pump Inhibitors Therapy Induces Acid-Related Symptoms in Healthy Volunteers after Withdrawal of Therapy," *Gastroenterology* 137, no. 1 (2009): 80–7.

275. B Goldman, "Some heartburn drugs may boost risk of heart attack, study finds," Stanford Medicine News Center, accessed December 31, 2015, https://med.stanford.edu/news/all-news/2015/06/some-heartburn-drugs-may-boost-risk-of-heart-attack-study-finds.html.

276. M Bouvier et al., "Effects of Consumption of a Milk Fermented by the Probiotic *Bifidobacterium animalis* DN-173 010 on Colonic Transit Time in Healthy Humans," *Bioscience and Microflora* 20, no. 2 (2001): 43–48; P Marteau et al., "*Bifidobacterium animalis*, Strain DN-173 010

Shortens the Colonic Transit Time in Healthy Women. A Double-Blind Randomized Controlled Study," *Aliment Pharmacol Ther* 16 (2002): 587–59.

277. "Nutrition Facts Labels," Activia, accessed December 31, 2015, http://activia.us.com/probiotic-yogurt.

278. V Vetvicka, *Beta Glucan: Nature's Secret* 2nd ed. (Louisville, Vaclav Vetvicka, 2011).

279. V Vetvicka and J Vetvickova. "1,3-Glucan: Silver Bullet or Hot Air?" *Open Glycoscience* 3 (2010): 1–6, http://benthamopen.com/contents/pdf/TOGLYJ/TOGLYJ-3-1.pdf; V Vetvicka and J Vetvickova. "Comparison of Immunological Effects of Commercially Available Beta-Glucans," *Applied Scientific Reports* 1, no. 2(2014): 1–7, http://www.hoajonline.com/journals/pdf/2054-9903-1-2.pdf.

280. M Fredrikson et al., "Production Process for High-Quality Pea-Protein Isolate with Low Content of Oligosaccharides and Phytate," *J Agric Food Chem* 49, no. 3 (2001): 1208–12; N Gausserès et al., "[15N]-Labeled Pea Flour Protein Nitrogen Exhibits Good Ileal Digestibility and Postprandial Retention in Humans," *J Nutr* 127, no. 6 (1997): 1160–65.

281. Y Zhang et al., "A Major Inducer of Anticarcinogenic Protective Enzymes from Broccoli: Isolation and Elucidation of Structure," *Proc Natl Acad Sci USA* 89, no. 6 (1992): 2399–403; K L Cheung and A N Kong, "Molecular Targets of Dietary Phenethyl Isothiocyanate and Sulforaphane for Cancer Chemoprevention," *AAPS J* 12, no. 1 (2010): 87–97; "Sulforophane Glucosinolate: Monograph," *Altern Med Rev* 15, no. 4 (2010): 352–60.

282. A Boots, G Haenen, A Bast. "Health Effects of Quercetin: From Antioxidant to Nutraceutical," *Eur J Pharmacol* 582, no. 2–3 (2008): 325–37; A Boots, et al., "The Quercetin Paradox," *Toxicol Appl Pharmacol* 222, no. 1 (2007): 89–96; M Chan, et al., "Synergy between Ethanol and

Grape Polyphenols, Quercetin, and Resveratrol, in the Inhibition of the Inducible Nitric Oxide Synthase Pathway," *Bio Pharm* 60, no. 10 (2000): 1539–48; C Chuang, et al., "Quercetin Is Equally or More Effective Than Resveratrol in Attenuating Tumor Necrosis Factor-{Alpha}-Mediated Inflammation and Insulin Resistance in Primary Human Adipocytes," *Am J Clin Nutr* 92, no. 6 (2010): 1511–21; F Dajas. "Life or Death: Neuroprotective and Anticancer Effects of Quercetin," *J Ethnopharmacol* 143, no. 2 (2012): 383–96; R Edwards et al., "Quercetin Reduces Blood Pressure in Hypertensive Subjects," *J Nutr* 137, no. 11 (2007): 2405–11; S Egert et al., "Quercetin Reduces Systolic Blood Pressure and Plasma Oxidized Low-Density Lipoprotein Concentrations in Overweight Subjects with a High-Cardiovascular Disease Risk Phenotype: A Double-Blinded, Placebo-Controlled Cross-Over Study," *Br J Nutr* 102, no. 7 (2009): 1065–74; M Gates et al., "A Prospective Study of Dietary Flavonoid Intake and Incidence of Epithelial Ovarian Cancer," *Int J Cancer* (Apr 30, 2007); T Guardia et al., "Anti-Inflammatory Properties of Plant Flavonoids: Effects of Rutin, Quercetin, and Hesperidin on Adjuvant Arthritis in Rat," *Farmaco* 56, no. 9 (2001): 683–87; R Kleemann et al., "Anti-inflammatory, Anti-proliferative and Anti-atherosclerotic Effects of Quercetin in Human In Vitro and In Vivo Models," *Atherosclerosis* 218, 1 (2011): 44–52; P Knekt et al., "Quercetin Intake and the Incidence of Cerebrovascular Disease," *Eur J Clin Nut* 54, no. 5 (2000): 415–17; T Lam et al., "Dietary Quercetin, Quercetin-Gene Interaction, Metabolic Gene Expression in Lung Tissue and Lung Cancer Risk," *Carcinogenesis* 31, no. 4 (2010): 634–42; D Lamson, M Brignall, "Antioxidants and Cancer III: Quercetin," *Alt Med Rev* 5, no. 3 (2000): 196–208; I Mackraj, T Govender, S Ramesar, "The Antihypertensive Effects of Quercetin in a Salt-Sensitive Model of Hypertension," *J Cardiovasc Pharmacol* 51, no. 3 (2008): 239–45; R Owen, et al., "The Antioxidant/Anticancer Potential of Phenolic Compounds Isolated from Olive Oil," *Eur J Cancer* 36, no. 10 (2000): 1235–47; S Ramos. "Effects of Dietary Flavonoids on Apoptotic Pathways Related to Cancer Chemoprevention," *J Nutr Biochem* 18, no. 7 (2007): 427–42; P Ruiz et al., "Quercetin Inhibits TNF-Induced NF-kappaB Transcription Factor Recruitment to Proinflammatory Gene Promoters in Murine Intestinal Epithelial Cells," *J Nutr* 137, no. 5 (2007): 1208–15; D Staedler et al., "Drug Combinations with Quercetin:

Doxorubicin Plus Quercetin in Human Breast Cancer Cells," *Cancer Chemother Pharmacol* 68, no. 5 (2011): 1161–72;

S Thornhill and A Kelly, "Natural Treatment of Perennial Allergic Rhinitis," *Alt Med Rev* 5, no. 5 (2000): 448–54; P Wang et al., "Effects of Quercetin on the Apoptosis of the Human Gastric Carcinoma Cells," *Toxicol in Vitro* 26, no. 2 (2012): 221–8; N Xing, Y Chen, S Mitchell, C Young, "Quercetin Inhibits the Expression and Function of the Androgen Receptor in LNCaP Prostate Cancer Cells," *Carcinogenesis* 22, no. 3 (2001): 409–14.

283. S Pai, "Cannabinoid Medicine from Industrial Hemp Oil: Another Practical and Legal Cannabidiol (CBD) Alternative," *Cancer Strategies Journal* 2, no. 3 (2014): 1–7.

284. Bharat B. Aggarwal et al., "Identification of Novel Anti-inflammatory Agents from Ayurvedic Medicine for Prevention of Chronic Diseases 'Reverse Pharmacology' and 'Bedside to Bench' Approach," *Curr Drug Targets* 12, no. 11 (2011): 1595–1653.

285. J D Feusner et al., "Effects of Cranial Electrotherapy Stimulation on Resting State Brain Activity," *Brain and Behavior* (2012): 1–10; A G Taylor et al., "A Randomized, Controlled Double-Blind Pilot Study of the Effects of Cranial Electrotherapy Stimulation on Activity in Brain Pain-Processing Regions in Individuals with Fibromyalgia," *Explore* 9, no. 1 (2013): 32–40; R Kennerly, "Changes in Quantitative EEG and Low Resolution Tomography following Cranial Electrotherapy Stimulation" (PhD dissertation, University of North Texas, 2006); Y Chen et al., "Results of Cranial Electrotherapy Stimulation to Children with Mixed Anxiety and Depressive Disorder," *Shanghai Archives of Psychiatry* 19, no. 4 (2007): 203–05; R G Lande and C Gragnani, "Efficacy of Cranial Electrotherapy Stimulation for the Treatment of Insomnia: A Randomized Pilot Study," *Complementary Therapies in Medicine* 21, no. 1 (2013): 8–13; R C Cork et al., "The Effect of Cranial Electrotherapy Stimulation (CES) on Pain Associated with Fibromyalgia," *The Internet Journal of Anesthesiology*, 8, no. 2 (2004); D H Rintala et al., "Feasibility of Using Cranial Electrotherapy Stimulation for Pain in Persons with Parkinson's Disease," *Parkinson's*

Disease May 5, (2010); T H Barclay and R D Barclay, "A Clinical Trial of Cranial Electrotherapy Stimulation for Anxiety and Comorbid Depression," *Journal of Affective Disorders* 164 (2014): 171–77; R R Mellen and W Mackey, "Reducing Sheriff's Officer's Symptoms of Depression Using Cranial Electrotherapy Stimulation (CES): A Control Experimental Study," *The Correctional Psychologist* 41, no. 1 (2009): 9–15; R L Winick, "Cranial Electrotherapy Stimulation (CES): A Safe and Effective Low Cost Means of Anxiety Control in a Dental Practice," *General Dentistry* 47, no. 1 (1999): 50–55; Kolesos On, Osionwo Ho, Akkhigbe, "The Role of Relaxation Therapy and Cranial Electrotherapy Stimulation in the Management of Dental Anxiety in Nigeria," *ISOR Journal of Dental and Medical Sciences* 10, no. 4 (2013): 51–57; R Kennerly, "Changes in Quantitative EEG and Low Resolution Tomography following Cranial Electrotherapy Stimulation" (PhD dissertation, University of North Texas, 2006).

286. J Funk et al., "Efficacy and Mechanism of Action of Turmeric Supplements in the Treatment of Experimental Arthritis," *Arthritis Rheum* 54, no. 11 (2006): 3452–64.

287. S Vemur and CT Rhode, "Preparation and Characterization of Liposomes as Therapeutic Delivery Systems: A Review," *Pharm Acta Helv* 70, no. 2 (1995): 95–111.

288. G Began, et al., "Interaction of Curcumin with Phosphatidylcholine: A Spectrofluorometric Study," *J Agric Food Chem* 47, no. 12 (1999): 4992–97.

289. A Liua et al., "Validated LC/MS/MS Assay for Curcumin and Tetrahydrocurcumin in Rat Plasma and Application to Pharmacokinetic Study of Phospholipid Complex of Curcumin," *J Pharm Biomed Anal* 40, no. 3 (2006): 720–27.

290. J Cuomo et al., "Comparative Absorption of a Standardized Curcuminoid Mixture and Its Lecithin Formulation," *J Nat Prod* 74, no. 4 (2011): 664–69.

291. J S Dempe et al., "Metabolism of Curcumin and Induction of Mitotic Catastrophe in Human Cancer Cells," *Mol Nutr Food Res* 52, no. 9 (2008): 1074–81.

292 J Cuomo et al., "Comparative Absorption of a Standardized Curcuminoid Mixture and Its Lecithin Formulation," *J Nat Prod* 74, no. 4 (2011): 664–69.

293 . V S Gota et al., "Safety and Pharmacokinetics of a Solid Lipid Curcumin Particle Formulation in Osteosarcoma Patients and Healthy Volunteers," *J Agric Food Chem* 58, no. 4 (2010): 2095–99.

294. Ibid.

295. C Schiborr et al., "The Oral Bioavailability of Curcumin from Micronized Powder and Liquid Micelles Is Significantly Increased in Healthy Humans and Differs between Sexes," *Mol Nutr Food Res* 58, no. 3 (2014): 516–27.

296. S D Kirlian and V Kirlian, "Photography and Visual Observations by Means of High-Frequency Currents," *Journal of Scientific and Applied Photography* 6 (1961): 397–403; L Schroeder and S Ostrander, *Psychic Discoveries Behind the Iron Curtain* (London, Abacus, 1977), 124–9; T Moss and K Johnson, "Bioplasma of Corona Discharge," in *Galaxies of Life: The Human Aura in Acupuncture and Kirlian Photography*, ed. S Krippner and D Rubin (New York: Gordon and Breach Science Publishers, Inc., 1973), 8–192; L W Konikiewicz, *Introduction to Electrography* (Harrisburg, PA: Leonard's Associates Press, 1979), 22–89.

297. L W Konikiewicz and L C Grif, *Bioelectrography: A New Method for Detecting Cancer and Monitoring Body Physiology* (Harrisburg, PA: Leonard's Associates Press, 1984), 35–188.

298. E Jakovleva and K Korotkov, *Electrophotonic Analysis in Medicine. GDV Bioelectrography Research* (Seattle, Amazon Digital Services Inc, 2012), 1–160.

299. C Augner et al., "Gas Discharge Visualization (GDV): Eine auf physikalischen Methoden und Meridiananalysen basierende Technik zur Untersuchung von Stressreaktionen und energetischen Schwachstellen—Zwischenbericht laufender Forschung (GDV: A Technique Based on Physical Methods and Meridian Analyses to Detect Stress Reactions and Energetic Weaknesses. Report of Ongoing Research)," *German Journal of Acupuncture & Related Techniques* 53 (2010): 14–20; P V Bundzen et al., "Psychophysiological Correlates of Athletic Success in Athletes Training for the Olympics," *Human Physiology* 31 (2005): 316–23; I L Ciesielska, "The Precursory Analysis of the Influence of Garments on Corona Discharge Created around a Human Fingertip," *Textile Research Journal* 80 (2010): 216–25; M Cowan and B Nunley, "The Effects of Crystal Bowl Toning on the Chakras as Measured by the Gas Discharge Visualization Technique (GDV) and Scores on the Profile of Mood States Scale," *Subtle Energies and Energy Medicine* 16 (2005): 37–40; S Gibson and B Williams, "The Effect of Music and Focused Meditation on the Human Energy Field as Measured by the Gas Discharge Visualization (GDV) Technique and Profile of Mood States," *Subtle Energies and Energy Medicine* 16 (2005): 57–60; B Haydon and B Nunley, "A GDV Comparison of Human Energy Fields before and after Stimulation of Shealy's Rings of Fire, Earth, Water, Air, Crystal," *Subtle Energies and Energy Medicine* 16 (2005): 69–72; G W Hacker et al., "Biomedical Evidence of Influence of Geopathic Zones on the Human Body: Scientifically Traceable Effects and Ways of Harmonization," *Forsch Komplementärmed Klass Naturheilkd* 12 (2005): 315–27;

J Polushin et al., "Monitoring Energy Levels during Treatment with GDV Technique," *J of Science of Healing Outcome* 2 (2009): 5–15; G V Rgeusskaja and U I Listopadov, "Medical Technology of Electrophotonics—Gas Discharge Visualization—in Evaluation of Cognitive Functions," *J of Science of Healing Outcome* 2 (2009): 15–17; B Rubik and A Brooks, "Digital High-Voltage Electrophotographic Measures of the Fingertips of Subjects Pre and Post-Qigong," *Evidence Based Integrative Medicine* 2 (2005): 245–48; K Korotkov et al., "Bioelectrographic Correlates of the Direct Vision Phenomenon," *J of Alternative and Complementary Medicine* 11 (2005): 885–93.

About the Author

Sunil Pai, MD is Board Certified in Holistic Integrative Medicine. After his residency in Family Medicine at the University of New Mexico and becoming Board Certified in Family Medicine, he became a Fellow of the Program in Integrative Medicine at University of Arizona (Class 2002) directed by Dr. Andrew Weil. He was the first in New Mexico to undergo this specialty training as well as the youngest in the country. He is certified by Dr. Deepak Chopra as a Primordial Sound Meditation Instructor and a Creating Health (Ayurveda Lifestyle) Instructor. He is also certified in Functional Medicine, Physiological Regulating Medicine, Medical Acupuncture and Neuro-Acupuncture through Stanford University School of Medicine and Dr. Jason Hao. Dr. Pai is the Vice President of the Neuro-Acupuncture Institute, a non-profit organization focusing on teaching physicians neuro-acupuncture which is focused for pain conditions and neurological dysfunction such as stroke, multiple sclerosis, Parkinson's and traumatic brain injury. Dr. Pai also specializes in Auriculotherapy focusing on treatment of both food and inhalant allergies using sublingual immunotherapy or SAAT. Dr. Pai is also certified in Plant-Based Nutrition from Cornell University and the T. Colin Campbell Foundation and teaches each patient about the health benefits of eating whole food plant based diets. Dr. Pai has undergone specialized training in Ayurvedic Medicine at the Sri Dharmasthala Manjunatheshwara College of Ayurveda, and Intensive Yoga Therapies at the Vivekananda Yoga Anusandhana Samsthana in India.

Sunil Pai, MD is an deacon of the House of Sanjevani Integrative Medicine Health & Lifestyle Center located in Albuquerque, New Mexico, an Integrated Auxiliary of the Priory of Santa Fe. As a 508 (c)(1)(a) church organization, they provide full service health and lifestyle education and Integrative Medicine services with emphasis in indigenous and natural medicines. Sanjevani is also certified by the Physicians Committee for Responsible Medicine (PCRM) as an Educational Alliance Partner for delivering evidence based, clinical plant based nutritional programs.

Dr. Pai specializes in custom formulation of dietary supplements including vitamins, minerals, Ayurvedic herbs, medical foods, and homeopathics using safe, clinically effective ingredients. He has been a consultant to various nutraceutical companies as well as functional medicine testing companies. Over the past 16 years, Dr. Pai has studied the processing of raw materials from farm to manufacturing and from the bench top research to clinical studies. His interest in the benefits of natural therapies led to the development of an entire line of dietary supplements which are safe, natural and clinically effective. His flagship product, Bosmeric-SR', is considered the strongest natural supplement for pain and inflammation support available worldwide. The all-natural, patented ingredients in a bi-layered tablet provides an immediate action within 20 minutes and sustained release over an 8 hour period.

Dr. Pai is also a Clinical Assistant Professor at the Department of Family and Community Medicine at the University of New Mexico School of Medicine and conducts seminars and workshops on a variety of health conditions. Dr. Pai is a highly requested speaker at national medical and health conferences and is actively publishing in in the field of Integrative Medicine. Dr. Pai is one of a select group of Integrative Medicine physicians in the U.S. and only MD in New Mexico to be published in all 4 editions of David Rakel's Integrative Medicine [Chapter: "Peripheral Neuropathy"] published by Saunders, and in Benjamin Klinger and Roberta Anne Lee's Integrative Medicine: Principles in Practice [Chapter: "Ayurvedic Medicine"] published by McGraw- Hill. In addition some of his key publications "Plant Based Diet and Natural Anti-Inflammatories Help, Prevent and Treat Cancer" and "Cannabinoid Medicine From Industrial Hemp Oil: Another Practical and Legal Cannabidiol (CBD) Alternative" has led him to be recognized leader in developing integrative cancer protocols using natural compounds. Dr. Pai was recently was featured in the internet documentary series "The Truth About Cancer: The Quest for the Cures Continues" (2014) and "The Truth About Cancer: The Global Quest." (2015). Dr. Pai's current projects include coordinating clinical trials internationally using 3-BP, a novel anti-cancer agent. In addition he is providing dietary protocols and formulating supportive supplemental products in a variety of holistic and integrative cancer clinics to help improve health outcomes.

Dr. Pai lives in Albuquerque, New Mexico and his hobbies include cooking, hiking, yoga, music trivia and playing both guitar and drums.

33577434R00250

Made in the USA
San Bernardino, CA
06 May 2016